Nutrition and Arthritis

Margaret Rayman
BSc, DPhil (Oxon), RPHNutr
Division of Nutrition, Dietetics and Food Science
School of Biomedical and Molecular Sciences
University of Surrey, Guildford, UK

Alison Callaghan
BSc, SRD
Senior Dietitian
Queen Elizabeth The Queen Mother Hospital, Kent, UK

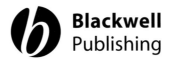

Blackwell Publishing

Blackwell Publishing Ltd
Editorial Offices:
Blackwell Publishing Ltd, 9600 Garsington Road, Oxford OX4 2DQ, UK
   Tel: +44 (0)1865 776868
Blackwell Publishing Professional, 2121 State Avenue, Ames, Iowa 50014-8300, USA
   Tel: +1 515 292 0140
Blackwell Publishing Asia Pty Ltd, 550 Swanston Street, Carlton, Victoria 3053, Australia
   Tel: +61 (0)3 8359 1011

First published 2006 by Blackwell Publishing Ltd
2   2007

ISBN: 978-1-4051-2418-8

Library of Congress Cataloging-in-Publication Data
Rayman, Margaret.
Nutrition and arthritis / Margaret Rayman, Alison Callaghan.
    p. ; cm.
Includes bibliographical references and index.
ISBN-13: 978-1-4051-2418-8 (pbk. : alk. paper)
ISBN-10: 1-4051-2418-0 (pbk. : alk. paper)
1. Arthritis—Nutritional aspects.   2. Arthritis—Diet therapy.
[DNLM: 1. Arthritis—diet therapy.   2. Nutrition Therapy.   WE 344 R267n 2006]
I. Callaghan, Alison.   II. Title.

RC933.R332 2006
616.7'220654—dc22
2005035552

A catalogue record for this title is available from the British Library

Set in 10/12.5pt Sabon by Graphicraft Limited, Hong Kong
Printed and bound in India by Replika Press Pvt. Ltd

The publisher's policy is to use permanent paper from mills that operate a sustainable forestry policy,
and which has been manufactured from pulp processed using acid-free and elementary chlorine-free
practices. Furthermore, the publisher ensures that the text paper and cover board used have met
acceptable environmental accreditation standards.

For further information on Blackwell Publishing, visit our website:
www.blackwellpublishing.com

'Leave your drugs in the chemist's pot if you can heal the patient with food.'
Hippocrates, the Father of Medicine

Contents

Appendices

Acknowledgements

We want to express our thanks to Dr Gail Darlington, one of the earliest researchers in the field of nutrition and arthritis, for encouraging us to write this book and for allowing us to use her dietary programme for the detection of food intolerance. Dr Dorothy Pattison has very kindly provided this dietary programme for us in the user-friendly format she used with arthritic patients when working as a senior dietician.

Our thanks are also due to Alexander Thompson who largely put together the section on how to interpret the statistical data on studies quoted in this book and provided the statistical terms for the glossary, to John Rayman who took on the exacting job of compiling the index and to Miriam Rayman for the cover photograph of the fish.

We are grateful to the Arthritis Research Campaign for allowing us to use some of their excellent figures to illustrate the text and to the many other researchers and publications who gave permission for their figures and tables to be used.

We want to acknowledge the co-operation we have had from our employers, the University of Surrey, East Kent Hospitals NHS Trust and Canterbury and Coastal PCT.

Last but by no means least, we thank our families and friends for their support and willingness to put up with our apparently reclusive behaviour over the period of writing this book.

Margaret Rayman
Alison Callaghan

Abbreviations

AA	Arachidonic acid
ACR	American College of Rheumatology
ADAM-TS4, ADAM-TS5	Cartilage aggrecanases
ADAPT	Arthritis, diet and activity promotion trial
AGEs	Advanced glycation end-products
ALA	α-linolenic acid
ARA	American Rheumatism Association
ARC	Arthritis Research Campaign
BCSO	Blackcurrant seed oil
BMI	Body mass index
CI	Confidence interval
COT UK	Committee on toxicity of chemicals in food, consumer products and the environment
COX	Cyclo-oxygenase
CRP	C-Reactive protein
CSFII	Continuing food survey of intakes by individuals
CVD	Cerebrovascular disease
DGLA	Dihomo-γ-linolenic acid
DHA	Docosahexaenoic acid
DMARD	Disease modifying antirheumatic drug
DNA	Deoxyribonucleic acid
DPA	Docosapentaenoic acid
DRIA test	Dynamometric challenge test
ECG	Epicatechin gallate
EGCG	Epigallocatechin gallate
EPA	Eicosapentaenoic acid
EPIC	European Prospective Investigation of Cancer
EPO	Evening primrose oil
ERT	Oestrogen replacement therapy
ESR	Erythrocyte sedimentation rate
FAO	Food and Agriculture Organization
FDA	Food and Drug Administration
FFQ	Food frequency questionnairre
FSA	Food Standards Agency
GAG	Glycosaminoglycan
GAIT	Glucosamine/chondroitin Arthritis Intervention Trial

GALT	Gut-associated lymphoid tissue
GI	Gastrointestinal
GLA	Gamma-linolenic acid (γ-linolenic acid)
GP	General practitioner
GPx	Glutathione peroxidase
GSH	Glutathione
HAQ	Health assessment questionnaire
HBA$_1$c	Haemoglobin A$_1$c
HDL	High density lipoprotein
HLA	Human leucocyte antigen
HRT	Hormone replacement therapy
IBS	Irritable bowel syndrome
Ig	Immunoglobulin
IL	Interleukin
IU	International units
JECFA	Joint Expert Committee on Food Additives
JSN	Joint space narrowing
LA	Linoleic acid
LDL	Low density lipoprotein
LGG	*Lactobacillus rhamnosus GG*
LT	Leukotriene
MBP	Mannose-binding protein
MCP	Metacarpophalangeal
MDA	Malondialdehyde
MHC	Major histocompatability complex
MMP	Metalloproteinase
MSM	Methylsulfonylmethane
MTP	Metatarsophalangeal
MUFA	Monounsaturated fatty acid
MUST	Malnutrition Universal Screening Tool
n-3	Series of fatty acids in which the last double bond in the chain is 3 carbon atoms from the methyl end of the molecule (e.g. α-linolenic acid)
n-6	Series of fatty acids in which the last double bond in the chain is 6 carbon atoms from the methyl end of the molecule (e.g. linoleic acid)
n-9	Series of fatty acids in which the only double bond in the chain is 9 carbon atoms from the methyl end of the molecule (e.g. oleic acid)
NADPH	Nicotinamide adenine dinucleotide phosphate (reduced form)
NCCAM	National Centre for Complementary and Alternative Medicine
NF	Nuclear factor
NHANES	National Health and Nutrition Examination Survey
NIAMS	National Institute of Arthritis and Musculoskeletal and Skin Diseases

NICE	National Institute for Health and Clinical Excellence
NIH	National Institutes of Health
NO·	Nitric oxide
NOAR	Norfolk Arthritis Register
NSAID	Non-steroidal anti-inflammatory drug
NZGLM	New Zealand green-lipped mussel
O_2^-	Superoxide
OA	Osteoarthritis
OH·	Hydroxyl radical
ONOO$^-$	Peroxynitrite
PCB	Polychlorinated biphenyl
PGE	Prostaglandin
PHA	Phytohaemagglutanin
PIP	Proximal interphalangeal
PUFA	Polyunsaturated fatty acid
QOL	Quality of life
RA	Rheumatoid arthritis
RCT	Randomised controlled trial
RDA	Recommended dietary allowance
RE	Reticuloendothelial
RE	Retinol equivalents
RF	Rheumatoid factor
RNA	Ribonucleic acid
RNI	Reference nutrient intake
RNS	Reactive nitrogen species
ROS	Reactive oxygen species
RR	Relative risk
SACN	Scientific Advisory Committee on Nutrition
SBA	Soya bean agglutinin
SFA	Saturated fatty acid
SMR	Standardised mortality rate
SOD	Superoxide dismutase
TDI	Total daily intake
TEQ	Toxic equivalent
Th	T helper cell
TIMP	Tissue inhibitor of metalloproteinases
TNF	Tumour necrosis factor
TRAP	Ability of the fresh serum to resist attack from peroxyl radicals
UVB	Ultraviolet B rays
VAS	Visual analogue scale
VEGF	Vascular endothelial growth factor
WHO	World Health Organization
WOMAC	Western Ontario and McMaster Universities index for assessment of OA

1 Introduction

'Musculoskeletal conditions are prevalent and their impact is pervasive. They are the most common cause of severe long-term pain and physical disability, affecting hundreds of millions of people around the world. They significantly affect the psychosocial status of affected people as well as their families and carers. They are a major cause of years lived with disability in all continents and economies' (Woolf & Pfleger, Bulletin of the World Health Organization, 2003).

1.1 The range of rheumatic diseases

There are over 200 forms of rheumatic disease (ARC 2002), a term used to encompass both arthritis and rheumatism. Arthritis is defined in the Oxford English Dictionary as 'inflammation of joints'. The American Rheumatism Association (Hill 1998) has listed the common rheumatic diseases as shown in Table 1.1.

Table 1.1 Common rheumatic diseases (adapted from Hill 1998).

Inflammatory joint disease	• Rheumatoid arthritis (RA) • Felty's syndrome • Juvenile chronic arthritis
Spondyloarthropathies	• Psoriatic arthropathy • Ankylosing spondylitis • Reiter's syndrome • Behcet's syndrome
Crystal deposition diseases	• Gout • Pyrophosphate arthropathy
Joint failure	• Osteoarthritis (OA)
Metabolic bone disease	• Osteoporosis
Connective tissue diseases	• Systemic lupus erythematosus • Scleroderma • Polymyositis • Dermatomyositis
Non-articular conditions	• Polymyalgia rheumatica • Giant cell arteritis • Raynaud's phenomenon • Sjögren's syndrome
Soft tissue rheumatism	• Fibromyalgia • Carpal tunnel syndrome • Tennis and golfer's elbow

Arthritic conditions vary in prevalence from common to rare. They are part of the spectrum of musculoskeletal complaints that are the second most frequent reason for consulting a doctor and in most countries constitute between 10% and 20% of primary care consultations (Woolf & Pfleger 2003). They place a tremendous burden on individuals, health systems, and social care systems. In this book, we shall deal primarily with osteoarthritis (OA) and rheumatoid arthritis (RA), the most common arthritic diseases amenable to dietary analysis.

1.2 Rheumatoid arthritis (RA): description

RA is a chronic, systemic, inflammatory autoimmune disorder that mainly affects synovium of the diarthrodial joints (Lee & Weinblatt 2001; West 2002). Its pathogenesis is not fully understood. Symmons and colleagues (2003a) give the following description:

> 'Symmetrical inflammatory polyarthritis is the primary clinical manifestation. The arthritis usually begins in the small joints of the hands and the feet, spreading later to the larger joints. The inflamed joint lining or synovium extends and then erodes the articular cartilage and bone, causing joint deformity and progressive physical disability. Extra-articular features include nodules, pericarditis, pulmonary fibrosis, peripheral neuropathy and amyloidosis.'

To be diagnosed with RA the individual must meet four or more of the American Rheumatism Association criteria listed below, which, in the case of the first four, must have been present for at least six weeks (Arnett et al. 1988; David & Lloyd 1999; West 2002) (see Chapter 2 for full classification criteria):

(1) Morning stiffness in and around joints of at least one hour duration before maximal improvement
(2) Arthritis of three or more joint areas indicated by swelling and tenderness or deformity
(3) Arthritis (swelling) of the hand joints – wrist, metacarpophalangeal (MCP) or proximal interphalangeal (PIP)
(4) Symmetrical arthritis in at least one area
(5) Rheumatoid nodules
(6) Serum rheumatoid factor positive
(7) Radiographic erosions or periarticular osteopenia in hand or wrist joints.

1.3 Osteoarthritis (OA): description

OA is the most common articular disorder and accounts for more disability among the elderly than any other disease (West 2002). It is also referred to as osteoarthrosis, degenerative joint disease, hypertrophic arthritis, degenerative disc disease and generalised osteoarthritis (West 2002).

There is no single definition of OA as it is not a simple disease entity, but it can be described as a slowly progressive chronic disease affecting the hands and diarthrodial, weightbearing joints such as the knees, hips and spine. It is characterised by loss of articular cartilage within synovial joints and is associated with hypertrophy of bone (osteophytes and subchondral bone sclerosis) and thickening of the joint capsule (Woolf & Pfleger 2003). Clinical characteristics are joint pain, tenderness, limitation of movement, crepitus, occasional effusion and variable degrees of local inflammation, which is generally mild (West 2002; Woolf & Pfleger 2003). There are no systemic symptoms (West 2002). The pathological changes associated with OA are now thought to be due to an active reparative process rather than a destructive process as previously believed.

1.4 Incidence and prevalence

As there is a general lack of routinely collected data, the true incidence or indeed prevalence of musculoskeletal conditions such as OA and RA is difficult to ascertain. The overall estimate of the incidence and prevalence of RA and OA varies according to the source quoted. It is difficult to gather incidence values for OA owing to problems in defining the disease and its onset (Woolf & Pfleger 2003). However, though there is variation in data, as OA is a much more common disease than RA, the numbers of patients involved is huge and the disease therefore has a wide-ranging impact on society.

In the US population, 30% have symptoms of arthritis, 20% have symptoms of arthritis that require medication, 5–10% have disability from arthritis, 0.5% are totally disabled by arthritis and 0.02% die from a rheumatic disease (West 2002). RA cases are estimated at 20 million worldwide, around 12 000 new cases being diagnosed each year in the UK alone (ARC 2002; Goff & Barasi 1999). RA affects 0.3–1% of the general population in the USA and Europe (Woolf & Pfleger 2003). Data collected mainly from populations of Anglo-Saxon origin show an incidence range of RA from around 20–300 per 100 000 adults per year (Symmons et al. 2003a; Woolf & Pfleger 2003). Symmons and colleagues (2003b) estimate that 10% of the world's population who are 60 years or older have symptomatic problems that can be attributed to OA. In the population of the UK, cases of OA are estimated as between 7.1 million and 13 million, i.e. up to 29% of the total population (ARC 2002).

RA is more prevalent in women than in men (Symmons et al. 2003a). Estimates from Australian data show 295/100 000 women affected vs. 171/100 000 men (Woolf & Pfleger 2003). All new cases of inflammatory polyarthritis in the Norwich Health Authority of the UK are notified to the Norfolk Arthritis Register from which the annual incidence rate in the early 1990s was estimated to be 36/100 000 for women and 14/100 000 for men (Symmons et al. 1994). The overall minimum prevalence of RA in the UK was determined in 2001 as 1.16% in women and 0.44% in men, suggesting a slight fall in prevalence in women since 1961 (Symmons et al. 2002). OA is also more prevalent in women than in men: worldwide, approximately 9.6% of men and 18.0% of women aged 60 or over have symptomatic OA (Woolf & Pfleger 2003). Radiographic studies of US and European populations aged 45 or over show knee OA in 14.1% of men and 22.8% of women (Woolf & Pfleger 2003).

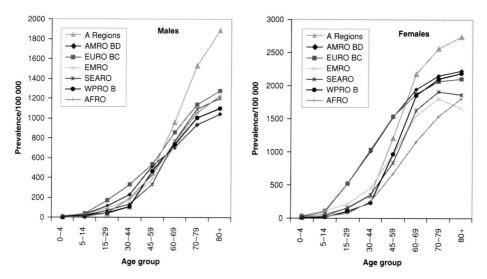

Figure 1.1 RA prevalence rates, age group and sex, broad regions, 2000 (reproduced with permission from Symmons et al. 2003b). A regions: developed countries in north America, western Europe, Japan, Australia, New Zealand; AMRO BD: developing countries in the Americas; Euro BC: developing countries in Europe; EMRO: eastern Mediterranean and north Africa; SEARO: south-east Asia; WPRO B: western Pacific; AFRO: sub-Saharan Africa.

While the prevalence of RA varies from 0.3–1% in industrialised countries, it lies at the lower end of this range in developing countries (Figure 1.1, Symmons et al. 2003a). The disease is apparently absent in areas of rural Nigeria while a prevalence as high as 5% has been reported in American Indians (Toivanen 2003). As with RA, OA is more prevalent in Europe and the US than in other parts of the world (Woolf & Pfleger 2003): Figure 1.2 shows estimates of prevalence of OA of the knee for seven regions of the world (Symmons et al. 2003b).

OA, and to a lesser extent RA, occur in the later years of life. The incidence and prevalence of RA generally rise with increasing age until around age 70, then decline (Symmons et al. 2000a). Data from the UK Norfolk Arthritis Register showed that the incidence of RA in men rose steeply with age whereas in women it rose up to age 45, plateaued until age 75, and fell in the very elderly (Symmons et al. 1994). The prevalence of OA increases indefinitely with age because the condition is not reversible (Woolf & Pfleger 2003). According to West (2002), between 50% and 80% of those aged over 65 years have radiographic evidence of OA, while 78% of cases of OA and 61% of cases of RA occur in those 55 years and over (ARC 2002).

Although arthritis is largely a disease of older people, cases do occur earlier in life, notably idiopathic juvenile arthritis. Arthritis in the younger age groups is less prevalent – 12 000 cases of juvenile idiopathic arthritis diagnosed in the UK up to 2002 (ARC 2002).

A number of authors have reported a decline in both the incidence and severity of RA since the middle of the last century (Toivanen 2003) suggesting that an

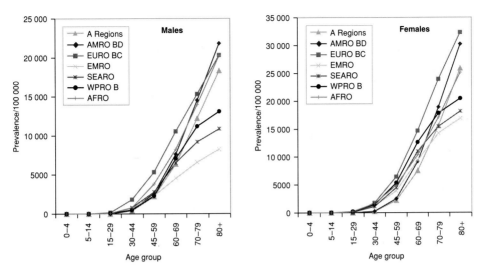

Figure 1.2   Knee OA prevalence rates, age group and sex, broad regions, 2000 (reproduced with permission from Symmons et al. 2003b). A regions: developed countries in north America, western Europe, Japan, Australia, New Zealand; AMRO BD: developing countries in the Americas; Euro BC: developing countries in Europe; EMRO: eastern Mediterranean and N Africa; SEARO: south-East Asia; WPRO B: western Pacific; AFRO: sub-Saharan Africa.

environmental factor may play a role in the aetiology of the condition. For instance, the incidence rate fell progressively over four decades of study in Rochester, Minnesota: from 61.2/100 000 in 1955–64 to 32.7/100 000 in 1985–94 (Doran et al. 2002). The fall in incidence that has been seen particularly in women since the 1960s has been attributed to a protective effect of the oral contraceptive pill (Symmons et al. 2002). There is also a suggestion that these changes may be related to the introduction of antibiotics, implying an involvement of bacterial infection in the onset or severity of the disease (Toivanen 2003).

1.5   Mortality

Mortality data is easily available as a death certificate is a legally required, routinely collected document. However, the use of this type of data is of limited value when investigating RA and OA. The death certificate records the disease or condition directly leading to death and indicates other significant conditions contributing to death, but not actually related to cause of death. RA and OA, being long-term illnesses, are often not included on the death certificate as an underlying cause of death. This limits analysis of the data owing to the under-reporting of the true prevalence of the two conditions. The longer the natural history of the disease, the less information can be provided by mortality statistics on causative factors in disease.

In 1999, UK mortality data recorded 3554 deaths – 935 male and 2619 female – where the underlying cause of death was identified as disease/s of the musculoskeletal and connective tissue (Office for National Statistics, 1999). Of these 925 male deaths, RA was identified as the underlying cause in 129, while OA was the underlying cause in 50. Of the 2619 female deaths, RA was identified as the underlying cause in 551 while OA was the underlying cause in 264.

OA, by itself, is not a life threatening disease, although drugs used in treatment, such as NSAIDs, can lead to excess mortality (Symmons et al. 2003b). There is little doubt that people with RA have a lower life expectancy than others in the same population of comparable age and sex (Gabriel et al. 2003). Excess mortality of 29% was first reported in 1953 and more recent studies have found similar figures: compared to others in the population, a standardised mortality rate (SMR) of 1.27 (95% CI 1.13, 1.41) was found in a cohort of Minnesota residents diagnosed with RA (American College of Rheumatology/American Rheumatism Association 1987 criteria, Arnett et al. 1988) between 1955 and 1994 (Gabriel et al. 2003). However, one study in the Netherlands showed no increased mortality over a follow-up period of up to 10 years from disease onset, leading the authors to conclude either that the study required longer follow-up time to show excess mortality or that recent more aggressive therapeutic strategies and treatment of co-morbidities had improved disease outcome (Kroot et al. 2000).

Excess mortality is more pronounced in women than in men, with SMRs of 1.41 and 1.08 respectively (Gabriel et al. 2003). RA has been shown to shorten life expectancy by 6–10 years (ARC 2002). Wolfe and colleagues (1994) found mortality rates to be at least twofold greater in 3501 RA patients from four different centres in the US, being linked to clinical severity. The global average case fatality rate for RA is around 1 per 1000 prevalent cases for both males and females, though these case fatality rates do not include the cardiovascular deaths and other deaths for which RA is an underlying cause (Symmons et al. 2003a). The main causes of excess deaths are infection, renal, cerebrovascular and cardiovascular disease, the last probably attributable to the cumulative inflammatory burden of RA (Symmons et al. 2003a; Wolfe et al. 1994).

In the Minnesota study referred to above, the presence of one or more extra-articular manifestations of RA increased the risk of death by a factor of 4.4 compared to others of the same age and sex, while co-morbidities (e.g. cardiovascular disease) were also statistically significant predictors of mortality (Gabriel et al. 2003). Surprisingly perhaps, studies appear to show little or no indication of improvement in survival of RA patients over the last decades (Gabriel et al. 2003).

1.6 Morbidity

Although limited mortality is attributed directly to RA and OA, the morbidity (ill effects of the disease process) associated with these diseases is very great though it can vary considerably in intensity between individuals. While at present there is no system available in the UK to monitor the musculoskeletal health of the population, various sources exist to assess morbidity. These include: hospital discharge data, health interview surveys, hospital statistics, morbidity statistics from general practice and sickness absence information. Notable co-morbidities associated with

RA are cardiovascular disease, infection, osteoporosis and peptic ulcer disease: these can be aggravated by treatment with immunosuppressive therapy, glucocorticoid or NSAID use (Mikuls 2003).

Joint stiffness and pain are the most prominent symptoms of musculoskeletal conditions. In RA, joints such as fingers, wrists and knees are affected (Martin 1998), whereas in OA, joints that are weightbearing, such as the hips and knees, are most affected (Thomas 2001). Joints may ache, or be stiff, swollen or painful, impeding movement and preventing sleep. Though pain can be controlled or reduced, usually via analgesics (discussed in Chapter 4), the implications of painful, stiff and swollen joints are far-reaching, affecting many aspects of an individual's life. Thus simple daily tasks such as eating, drinking, preparing food, dressing and washing become very difficult. It is this disability and pain that undoubtedly has the greatest impact on quality of life, many sufferers becoming more dependent on others as the severity of their condition increases and their mobility becomes further impaired.

Arthritis often causes reduced mobility and a lower level of physical activity, resulting in some degree of defined physical disability (Martin 1998). In Canada, the USA and Western Europe, the prevalence of physical disabilities caused by a musculoskeletal condition is estimated to be 4–5% in the adult population (Woolf & Pfleger 2003). In 1990, OA was the eighth leading non-fatal burden of disease in the world, accounting for 2.8% of total years of living with disability and by the year 2020, increases in life expectancy and ageing populations are expected to make osteoarthritis the fourth leading cause of disability (Woolf & Pfleger 2003).

Reduced mobility contributes to the loss of bone mineral density that is associated with the condition of RA. Steroid use, particularly at higher doses, exacerbates bone loss (Kay et al. 2004). Postmenopausal women, the group most affected by RA, already have an increased risk of osteoporosis (Mikuls 2003). Stress fractures are a significant cause of morbidity in RA, particularly in those that have been exposed to high steroid doses in the past (Kay et al. 2004).

1.7   Economic cost of arthritis

Morbidity related to arthritis has an economic cost both to the individual and to society. Arthritis and related conditions were the most common reason for working days lost for both males and females (behind mental disorders for both genders) (ARC 2002). Within 10 years of disease onset, at least 50% of RA patients in developed countries are unable to hold down a full time job (Woolf & Pfleger 2003). Of individuals with arthritis aged 18–64 years, 30% are unable to work or cannot work because of their disease (West 2002). Figures provided by the UK Department of Work and Pensions show that of 206 million working days that were lost in 1999–2000, 36 million were lost due to OA and 9.4 million due to RA, equivalent to a production loss greater than £18 billion (ARC 2002), thus amounting to a huge deficit in economic terms. Costs are also incurred in the form of incapacity benefit and severe disability allowance paid to those with arthritis and related conditions. Arthritis cost the NHS an estimated £1.1 billion in 1998–99 from prescription costs, consultations and knee/hip/limb replacements (ARC 2002). The cost to the US health economy of all musculoskeletal conditions is estimated at more than $254 billion a year (United States Bone and Joint Decade web site 2005). Thus, arthritis and related conditions have a significant economic impact on society as a whole.

1.8 The aim of this book

The institution of the Bone and Joint Decade (2000–2010), a multidisciplinary global initiative proposed at a conference in Lund, Sweden in 1998, and co-sponsored by the World Health Organization (WHO), is indicative of the inadequately recognised significance of this area of health. The goal of the Decade is to improve the health-related quality of life for people with musculoskeletal disorders throughout the world by raising awareness of the growing burden of musculoskeletal disorders on society, by empowering patients, promoting cost effective prevention and treatment and advancing understanding through research (Woolf 2000). With a considerable proportion of the population affected by arthritis, and that proportion likely to grow as our population ages, any means of reducing the development or progression of arthritis or of safely relieving its debilitating symptoms is worth exploring. This book should be seen in this context.

Although perceptions are changing, rheumatologists have traditionally been sceptical about dietary approaches to OA and RA (Martin 1998). However, we aim to show here that dietary advice and intervention do clearly have a place in rheumatology. To this end, we will describe dietary interventions that have had beneficial effects on musculoskeletal health. In the context of adverse side effects of NSAIDs, and more recently, of Cox-2 inhibitors, the alternative approach of successful dietary manipulation could be a safer and more appropriate option for a substantial number of people.

In this book, we will restrict ourselves to a consideration of OA and RA. The reasons for this are firstly, that these are the most common rheumatic diseases, and secondly, that there is little or no dietary information or studies on diets or nutrients relating to other forms of arthritis. For similar reasons, we will not address the issue of juvenile arthritis, which is further complicated by the necessity of considering the provision of nutrients for growth.

In Chapter 2, we outline the classification, describe the clinical features and briefly explain the pathology of OA and RA so that disease processes that may be affected by diet can be understood. We also describe methods of disease assessment that have been used in the studies that will be described in subsequent chapters. We have included a chapter on aetiology and risk factors (Chapter 3) because it is relevant to an understanding of the disease mechanisms. For the sake of completeness, we will briefly outline current methods of disease management and treatment (Chapter 4).

The remaining chapters will discuss nutritional aspects of OA and RA in some detail. We will look at whether current diets in OA and RA patients are adequate (Chapter 5); we will examine some popular nutritional approaches (Chapter 6);

we will then assess the evidence for the use of: exclusion, elemental, vegetarian and vegan diets in RA (Chapter 7); micronutrients in OA and RA (Chapter 8); fish oils in RA (Chapter 9); glucosamine and chondroitin in OA (Chapter 10); and other dietary supplements on the market that are claimed to be of benefit in arthritis (Chapter 11). Chapter 12 summarises our nutritional recommendations and the level of evidence supporting them.

By providing this information for rheumatologists, GPs, dietitians and nutritionists, we aim to ensure that patients are provided with evidence based recommendations on diet and supplements that may help to reduce the risk of disease progression and relieve symptoms in a risk-free manner. At the moment, there is little informed advice available for sufferers to help them decide which of the plethora of so-called remedies are worthwhile and so they are at the mercy of marketing ploys that exploit their vulnerability.

References

Arnett FC, Edworthy SM, Bloch DA, McShane DJ, Fries JF, Cooper NS et al. (1988) The American Rheumatism Association 1987 revised criteria for the classification of rheumatoid arthritis. *Arthritis and Rheumatism* **31**(3), 315–324.

Arthritis Research Council (ARC) (2002) Arthritis: The Big Picture. www.arc.org.uk/about_arth/bigpic.htm

David C, Lloyd J (1999) *Rheumatological Physiotherapy*, 1st edition. London, Mosby, pp. 3–9, 55–61, 65–81 and 83–96.

Doran MF, Pond GR, Crowson CS, O'Fallon WM, Gabriel SE (2002) Trends in incidence and mortality in rheumatoid arthritis in Rochester, Minnesota, over a forty-year period. *Arthritis and Rheumatism* **46**(3), 625–31.

Gabriel SE, Crowson CS, Kremers HM, Doran MF, Turesson C, O'Fallon WM, Matteson EL (2003) Survival in rheumatoid arthritis. *Arthritis and Rheumatism* **48**, 54–8.

Goff LM, Barasi M (1999) An assessment of the diets of people with rheumatoid arthritis. *Journal of Human Nutrition and Dietetics* **12**, 93–101.

Hill J (1998) *Rheumatology, a creative approach*, 1st edition. Edinburgh, Churchill Livingstone.

Kay LJ, Holland TM, Platt PN (2004) Stress fractures in rheumatoid arthritis: a case series and case-control study. *Annals of the Rheumatic Diseases* **63**(12), 1690–92.

Kroot EJA, Van Leeuwen MA, Van Rijswijik MH, Prevoo MLL, Van't Hof MA, Van de Putte LBA, Van Riel PLCM (2000) No increased mortality in patients with rheumatoid arthritis: up to 10 years of follow up from disease onset. *Annals of the Rheumatic Diseases* **59**, 954–58.

Lee DM, Weinblatt ME (2001) Rheumatoid arthritis. *The Lancet* **358**, 903–11.

Martin RH (1998) The role of nutrition and diet in rheumatoid arthritis. *Proceedings of the Nutrition Society* **57**(2), 231–4.

Mikuls TR (2003) Co-morbidity in rheumatoid arthritis. Best Practice Research. *Clinical Rheumatology* **17**, 729–52.

Office for National Statistics (1999) *Mortality statistics – cause*. England and Wales DH 2 Number 26. London, The Stationery Office.

Symmons D, Barrett E, Bankhead C, Scott D, Silman A (1994) The incidence of rheumatoid arthritis in the United Kingdom: results from the Norfolk Arthritis register. *British Journal of Rheumatology* **33**, 735–9.

Symmons D, Turner G, Webb R, Asten P, Barrett E, Lunt M, Scott D, Silman A (2002) The prevalence of rheumatoid arthritis in the United Kingdom: new estimates for a new century. *Rheumatology* **41**, 793–800.

Symmons D, Mathers C, Pfleger B (2003a) *The Global Burden of Rheumatoid Arthritis in the Year 2000*. Geneva, World Health Organization. www3.who.int/whosis/menu.cfm?path=

evidence,burden,burden_gbd2000docs,burden_gbd2000docs_diseasedoc,burden_gbd2000docs_diseasedoc_ra&language=English

Symmons D, Mathers C, Pfleger B (2003b) *Global Burden of Osteoarthritis in the Year 2000*. Geneva, World Health Organization. www3.who.int/whosis/menu.cfm?path=evidence,burden, burden_gbd2000docs,burden_gbd2000docs_diseasedoc,burden_gbd2000docs_diseasedoc_oa&language= english

Thomas B (2001) The manual of dietetic practice, 3rd edition. Oxford, Blackwell Science, Chapter 4.32: 588–92.

Toivanen P (2003) Normal intestinal microbiota in the aetiopathogenesis of rheumatoid arthritis. *Annals of the Rheumatic Diseases* **62**, 807–11.

United States Bone and Joint Decade web site (2005) www.usbjd.org/patients_public/index.cfm?pg=faq.cfm

West SG (2002) Rheumatology Secrets, 2nd edition. Philadelphia, Hanley and Belfus.

Wolfe F, Mitchell DM, Sibley JT, Fries JF, Bloch DA, Williams CA, Sspitz PW, Haga M, Kleinheksel SM, Cathey MA (1994) The mortality of rheumatoid arthritis. *Arthritis and Rheumatism* **37**(4), 481–94.

Woolf AD (2000) The bone and joint decade 2000–2010. *Annals of the Rheumatic Diseases* **59**, 81–2.

Woolf AD and Pfleger B (2003) Burden of major musculoskeletal conditions. *Bulletin of the World Health Organization* **81**, 646–656.

2 Classification, pathology and measures of disease assessment

2.1 Classification of OA

According to Symmons et al. (2003a), the Subcommittee on Osteoarthritis of the American College of Rheumatology (ACR) Diagnostic and Therapeutic Criteria Committee defined osteoarthritis (OA) as:

'*A heterogeneous group of conditions that lead to joint symptoms and signs which are associated with defective integrity of articular cartilage, in addition to related changes in the underlying bone at the joint margins.*'

Criteria for the classification of OA of the knee and hip are shown in Tables 2.1 and 2.2 (Symmons et al. 2003a).

2.2 Classification of RA

The criteria for the classification of rheumatoid arthritis (RA) have been difficult to establish owing to the lack of a distinct clinical, laboratory or radiological marker (Symmons et al. 2003b). The American Rheumatism Association (ARA)

Table 2.1 ACR classification of OA of the knee* (Symmons et al. 2003a).

Clinical	
1	Knee pain for most days of prior month
2	Crepitus on active joint motion
3	Morning stiffness < 30 min in duration
4	Age > 38 years (> 50 from current ACR site)
5	Bony enlargement of the knee on examination
	OA present if items 1, 2, 3, 4, or 1, 2, 5 or 1, 4, 5 are present
Clinical and radiological	
1	Knee pain for most days of prior month
2	Osteophytes at joint margins (X-ray)
3	Synovial fluid typical of osteoarthritis (laboratory)
4	Age > 40 years (> 50 from current ACR site)
5	Morning stiffness < 30 min
6	Crepitus on active joint motion
	OA present if items 1, 2 or 1, 3, 5, 6 or 1, 4, 5, 6 are present

* Modified from Altman et al. (1986), Altman et al. (1991)

Table 2.2   ACR classification of OA of the hip* (Symmons et al. 2003a).

Clinical and radiological	
1	Hip pain for most days of the prior month
2	Erythrocyte sedimentation rate < 20 mm/h (laboratory)
3	Radiographic femoral and/or acetabular osteophytes
4	Radiographic hip joint space narrowing
	OA present if items 1, 2, 3, or 1, 2, 4 or 1, 3, 4 are present

* Modified from Altman et al. (1986), Altman et al. (1991)

Table 2.3   The 1987 revised ARA/ACR criteria for the classification of rheumatoid arthritis (Symmons et al. 2003b)*.

Criterion	Short title	Definition
1	Morning stiffness	Morning stiffness in and around the joints, lasting at least 1 hour before maximal improvement. At least 3 joints
2	Arthritis of 3 or more joint areas	Areas simultaneously have had soft tissue swelling or fluid (not bony overgrowth alone) observed by a physician. The 14 possible areas are right or left PIP, MCP, wrist, elbow, knee, ankle, and MTP joints
3	Arthritis of hand joints	At least 1 area swollen (as defined above) in a wrist, MCP or PIP joint
4	Symmetric arthritis	Simultaneous involvement of the same joint areas [as defined in (2)] on both sides of the body (bilateral involvement of PIPs, MCPs, or MTPs is acceptable without absolute symmetry)
5	Rheumatoid nodules	Subcutaneous nodules, over bony prominences, or extensor in juxta-articular regions, observed by a physician
6	Serum rheumatoid factor	Demonstration of abnormal amounts of serum rheumatoid factor or any method for which the result has been positive in < 5% of normal control subjects
7	Radiographic changes	Radiographic changes typical of rheumatoid arthritis on posteroanterior hand and wrist radiographs, which must include erosions or unequivocal bony decalcification localised in or most marked adjacent to the involved joints (osteoarthritis changes alone do not qualify)

* For classification purposes, a patient shall be said to have rheumatoid arthritis if he/she has satisfied at least four of these seven criteria. Criteria 1 through 4 must have been present for at least 6 weeks. Patients with two clinical diagnoses are not excluded. PIP, proximal interphalangeal joints; MCP, metacarpophalangeal joints, wrist, elbow, knee, ankle; MTP, metatarsophalangeal joints

first proposed criteria in 1958 which were modified by the American College of Rheumatology (ACR) in 1987 (Symmons et al. 2003b). The revised criteria are listed in Table 2.3: to be diagnosed with RA, an individual must meet four or more criteria.

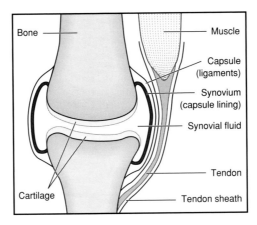

Figure 2.1   A normal joint (illustration reproduced by kind permission of the Arthritis Research Campaign, www.arc.org.uk).

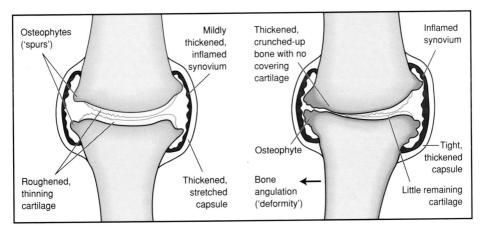

Figure 2.2   Joints affected by mild and severe OA (illustration reproduced by kind permission of the Arthritis Research Campaign, www.arc.org.uk).

2.3   Pathology of OA

2.3.1   General features of OA

OA is a degenerative joint disease that involves not only articular cartilage but also synovium, joint capsule, bone, periarticular muscles and ligaments (Nuki 2002). The pathological process in OA is a dynamic one with increased turnover of cartilage matrix components involving erosion by matrix metalloproteinases, reforming by chondrocyte activity, joint remodelling, incomplete repair and formation of new bone as well as degeneration of articular tissues (Nuki 2002). OA most commonly affects the joints of the hand, spine, knee, foot and hip. Figure 2.1 depicts a normal joint while Figure 2.2 depicts joints affected by mild and severe OA.

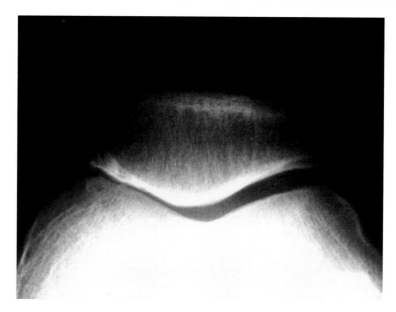

Figure 2.3 Skyline X-ray image of a bent osteoarthritic left knee taken along the leg from the direction of the foot: note the complete absence of joint space on the medial side denoting asymmetric loss of cartilage consequent on pronation of the foot (courtesy of Corrin Buland and Neil Chapman, Radiography Department, Royal Surrey County Hospital).

Clinically, OA is characterised by joint pain, tenderness, limitation of movement, crepitus, occasional effusion, and variable degrees of local inflammation (Symmons et al. 2003a). There is irregularly distributed loss of cartilage, particularly in areas of increased load, resulting in loss of joint space, sclerosis of subchondral bone, subchondral cysts, marginal osteophytes (bony outgrowths), increased blood flow and synovial inflammation (Symmons et al. 2003a). Figure 2.3 shows complete loss of patello-femoral joint space in an osteoarthritic knee joint on X-ray.

Early in the course of the disease, fragmentation of the cartilage surface occurs with the appearance of vertical clefts. There is cloning of chondrocytes, variable crystal deposition, remodelling, and eventual violation of the tidemark (the line between the articular and calcified cartilage zones) by blood vessels (Symmons et al. 2003a).

2.3.2   Structure of cartilage

Prior to discussing the pathogenesis of OA, it is necessary to have some understanding of the structure of cartilage. The functional properties of cartilage result from its unique structure of chondrocytes embedded in a matrix of collagen and proteoglycan (Creamer & Hochberg 1997). The collagen-proteoglycan matrix provides a structural framework for the tissue and gives it its important compressive and tensile properties. Cartilage is composed of a highly charged solid phase known as the extracellular matrix, an electrolyte fluid, and relatively few cells. Major extracellular matrix constituents include large proteoglycans, noncollagenous proteins, small proteoglycans, and collagen. The most abundant proteoglycan in cartilage is

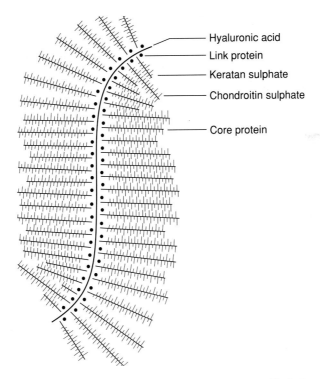

— Hyaluronic acid
— Link protein
— Keratan sulphate
— Chondroitin sulphate

— Core protein

Figure 2.4 Proteoglycan structure showing aggrecan monomers with their glycosaminoglycan (GAG) sidechains (reproduced with permission from Stryer 1988).

aggrecan, representing up to 10% of its dry weight (articular cartilage is up to 75% water). The aggrecan monomer has glycosaminoglycan (GAG) sidechains made up most commonly of chondroitin sulphate and keratan sulphate attached to a poly-peptide backbone called the core protein (Das & Hammad 2000). Aggrecan is highly hydrophilic but also of low viscosity, ideally suited to its function of load dispersal (Creamer & Hochberg 1997). Around 140 aggrecan monomers are bound through their core proteins to a very long filament of hyaluronate giving a proteoglycan aggregate that has the appearance of a 'bottle brush' (Figure 2.4). Collagen fibrils, mainly type II collagen which binds other macromolecules such as types IX and XI collagen, form the tissue network and make up two-thirds of the dry weight of articular cartilage (Creamer & Hochberg 1997; Eyre 2004). Though these latter two forms of collagen are only present in small amounts, they are critical for cartilage stability. The relationship between the components of cartilage can be seen in Figure 2.5.

2.3.3 Pathogenesis of OA

2.3.3.1 Cartilage degradation

Though OA has multiple causes and risk factors, it is clear that when the articular cartilage is lost, the joint fails (Eyre 2004). In OA, there is reduced synthesis and

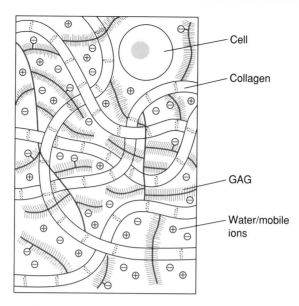

Cell

Collagen

GAG

Water/mobile
ions

Figure 2.5 Glycosaminoglycans (GAG) cartilage structure (reproduced with permission from Beth Israel Deaconess Medical Center, Boston website (2005)).

increased catabolism of cartilage matrix compared to that in normal individuals. Loss of cartilage results in joint space narrowing (JSN) which has been shown in a number of studies to range from 0.06–0.6 mm per year in patients with knee OA, though a large, long-term study indicates a rate of narrowing nearer 0.1 mm per year (Reginster et al. 2001). However, it is worth bearing in mind that when joint space loss is mild to moderate, it reflects meniscal extrusion rather than hyaline cartilage erosion (McAlindon 2001). Nuki (2002) gives the following description of OA pathogenesis.

'In OA, there is an early increase in cartilage matrix hydration reflecting disruption of the collagen fibre network.'

When cartilage becomes too hydrated it swells, its mechanical properties are altered and it loses its resilience to injury.

'Disruption of the collagen fibre network is accompanied by loss of tensile strength in the superficial zone of the cartilage. Chondrocyte activation with the release of the pro-inflammatory cytokines IL-1β, TNF-α and the metalloproteinase, stromelysin (MMP-3), can follow mechanical stimulation of cartilage and there is evidence for elevation of collagenase-1 (MMP-1), collagenase-2 (MMP-8) and collagenase-3 (MMP-13) in OA cartilage.'

Wear particles of cartilage matrix such as fragments of the glycoprotein, fibronectin, which in OA is increased in quantity and ease of degradation, have been shown to be active in stimulating the release of stromelysin and the catabolic cytokines IL-1α (interleukin) and β, TNF-α (tumour necrosis factor) and IL-6 from articular cartilage explants *in vitro* with resultant depletion of cartilage proteoglycan (Chevalier 1993; Nuki 2002). Thus:

'Matrix components released in the process of matrix degradation may them-selves augment cartilage metabolism. The cartilage aggrecanases ADAM-TS4 and ADAM-TS5 which are present in osteoarthritic cartilage are capable of degrading cartilage aggrecan without involvement of matrix metalloproteinases.'
(Nuki 2002).

2.3.3.2 Nitric oxide synthesis damages chondrocytes

Cytokines such as IL-1 cause the release of inflammatory mediators including nitric oxide from human articular chondrocytes: nitric oxide synthase has been found in chondrocytes from cartilage affected by OA (Creamer & Hochberg 1997) while stronger nitrotyrosine staining was observed in degenerating regions compared with intact regions from the same OA cartilage explants (Yudoh et al. 2005).

Nitric oxide may be directly toxic to articular cartilage; it interferes with growth factor stimulation and causes downregulation of IL-1 receptor antagonist synthesis, induction of caspase-3 and apoptosis of chondrocytes (Creamer & Hochberg 1997; Nuki 2002). In this context, a key role for leptin, which functions both as a hormone and a cytokine, has recently been demonstrated in OA (Otero et al. 2005). Leptin is upregulated in OA tissue where, in concert with other pro-inflammatory cytokines, it exhibits a detrimental effect on articular cartilage by promoting nitric oxide synthesis in chondrocytes (Otero et al. 2005). Several studies have also implicated leptin in the pathogenesis of RA (Otero et al. 2005).

2.3.3.3 Sulphation pattern of GAGs in articular cartilage

It has been suggested that sulphate deficiency is involved in the development of OA. Rizzo and colleagues (1995) found sulphur concentration in arthritic cartilage to be about one-third of the level in normal tissue. Reduction in sulphate concentration in the medium from 0.3 mM (physiological) to 0.2 mM resulted in 33% reduction of GAG synthesis in human articular cartilage (van der Kraan et al. 1990). Altered sulphation patterns in GAGs such as chondroitin sulphate and keratan sulphate from OA cartilage have been described by some workers but not by others (Sauerland et al. 2003). It seems that while the internal sulphation patterns of chondroitin sulphate are unchanged in OA, the number of 4,6-disulphated N-acetyl-galactosamine residues at the ends of chondroitin sulphate chains is significantly diminished, which may alter aggrecan fine structure affecting articular cartilage function (Sauerland et al. 2003).

2.3.3.4 Bone changes

There is some discussion as to whether the subchondral bone changes seen in OA are involved in its pathogenesis. Subchondral bone is sclerotic ('stiffened' bone) yet undermineralised in OA, indicating abnormal bone cell metabolism and this could precede cartilage degradation and loss (Lajeunesse 2004). Indirect evidence for this comes from a guinea pig model of OA, where changes in subchondral bone occur before cartilage changes are apparent (Creamer & Hochberg 1997). The alternative view is that although osteoarthritic bone tissue shows subchondral stiffening, containing increased denatured collagen and having reduced matrix mechanical properties, this is compatible with the process of normal bone adaptation (Day et al. 2004). The involvement of bone is also apparent from the inverse association between OA and diseases of low bone mineral density such as osteoporosis (Creamer & Hochberg 1997).

2.3.3.5 Inflammation

Inflammation is increasingly recognised as contributing to the symptoms and progression of OA (Bonnet & Walsh 2005). Expression of nuclear factor NF-κB, a transcription factor required for the expression of various pro-inflammatory genes, has been found in OA synovium (Creamer & Hochberg 1997). Chronic, acute or subclinical inflammation of the synovium resulting from infiltration of inflammatory cells such as macrophages and T-cells, upregulates the production of inflammatory cytokines such as IL-1 and IL-6. These in turn result in release of matrix metalloproteinases, such as collagenases and stromelysin, as well as prostaglandins and plasminogen activators (Creamer & Hochberg 1997). IL-6 produced by synovial cells, osteoblasts and chondrocytes can augment inflammatory angiogenesis and stimulate the production of CRP, a marker of inflammation, on entering the circulation (Bonnet & Walsh 2005). Both CRP and IL-6 have been identified in the circulation and synovial fluid respectively of OA patients (Bonnet & Walsh 2005). Inflammation exacerbates cartilage degradation in OA as evidenced by the fact that patients in whom radiological scores progress rapidly tend to have higher serum CRP concentrations at baseline than those in whom the disease progresses more slowly (Bonnet & Walsh 2005).

2.3.3.6 Angiogenesis

Inflammation is known to stimulate angiogenesis resulting in vascularisation of articular cartilage and osteophytes, which are avascular in normal adults (Bonnet & Walsh 2005). Growth of sensory nerves follows angiogenesis in many tissues and may contribute to the pain experienced in OA (Bonnet & Walsh 2005). Inflammation may also sensitise nerves present in the joint.

2.3.3.7 Oxidative stress

Oxidative stress is associated with inflammation for which there is evidence in OA (see above). Immunostaining for nitrotyrosine, a product of the interaction of peroxynitrite with protein tyrosine residues, correlated with the severity of histological changes to OA cartilage, suggesting a correlation between oxidative damage and articular cartilage degeneration (Yudoh et al. 2005). Increased oxidative stress associated with ageing makes chondrocytes more susceptible to erosion of chondrocyte telomere length and mitochondrial degeneration, leading to loss of function and oxidant-mediated chondrocyte death (Martin et al. 2004). This may help explain the increased risk of osteoarthritis with age (see section 3.3) and after joint trauma and inflammation (Martin et al. 2004).

2.4 Pathology of RA

2.4.1 General features of RA

Though rheumatoid arthritis is a chronic multisystem disorder, it shares many pathogenetic features with osteoarthritis, including synovial activation with release of pro-inflammatory cytokines into the synovial fluid (Reines 2004). Symmons and colleagues (2003b) describe rheumatoid arthritis as a systemic autoimmune disease where the primary manifestation is symmetrical inflammatory polyarthritis. It usually begins in the small joints of the hands and feet and spreads later to the larger joints. The inflamed joint lining, or synovium, proliferates as 'pannus', extending across the joint and becoming heavily infiltrated with inflammatory cells, including T- and B-lymphocytes, macrophages and mast-cells. Joint effusion may occur. Soft tissue too becomes inflamed resulting in laxity of ligaments and tendons. New blood vessel growth occurs accompanied by invasion of articular cartilage and bone by pannus, causing joint deformity and progressive physical disability (Symmons et al. 2003b). Figure 2.6 shows a representation of a rheumatoid joint.

As in OA, cartilage integrity is damaged by proteolytic enzymes such as collagenases, stromelysin and gelatinases. Bone, composed primarily of type I collagen, is eroded by invading synovium through the action of proteases and prostaglandin (PGE_2 (see Chapter 9) produced from synovial fibroblasts (Bathon 1998–2005). Radiographically, bone erosion can be seen while the cartilage thickness is progressively reduced.

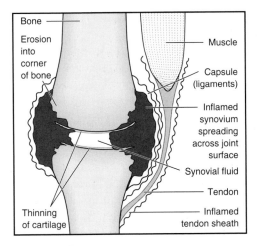

Figure 2.6 A rheumatoid joint (illustration reproduced by kind permission of the Arthritis Research Campaign, www.arc.org.uk).

As a systemic disease, RA is often accompanied by fatigue, weight loss, muscle pain, low grade fever and excessive sweating. Severe cases have extra-articular features that include rheumatoid nodules, pericarditis, pulmonary fibrosis, peripheral neuropathy, Sjögren's syndrome and amyloidosis (Symmons et al. 2003b). Rheumatoid subcutaneous nodules are the most characteristic extra-articular lesion of the disease, occurring in 20 to 30% of cases, almost exclusively in seropositive patients (Bathon 1998–2005).

2.4.2 Immunopathogenesis and production of inflammatory mediators

There are various theories as to the pathways involved in the initiation and propagation of RA but it is certain that immune system activation is involved. The account that follows is taken largely from the Johns Hopkins Arthritis web site (Bathon 1998–2005).

As an autoimmune disease, RA incidence is linked to genes on the major histocompatibility complex (MHC), a large complex of genes that encodes the major histocompatibility glycoproteins (Devereux 2002). The MHC is the molecular basis by which T-cells recognise intracellular pathogens in order to effect an immune response (Devereux 2002). Human MHC, known as the human leucocyte antigen (HLA) system has two structural variants, MHC class I and MHC class II. Susceptibility to RA is associated with having a particular conserved amino acid sequence at positions 70–74, known as the shared epitope – in the MHC class II HLA alleles, DR4 or DR1 (Howell et al. 2002). The shared epitope consists of glutamine (Q), lysine or arginine (K or R), arginine (R), alanine (A), and alanine (A).

The major function of the MHC class II molecules such as DR4 is to present antigen to CD4[+] T-helper (Th) cells (Bathon 1998–2005). Antigen is first taken up and processed by an antigen-presenting cell such as a macrophage, B cell or dendritic cell. Then, complexed to an MHC class II molecule on the surface of an antigen-presenting cell, it is presented to the CD4[+] Th cell. Recognition by the T-cell receptor initiates the host response.

While CD4[+] cells are known to be the predominant T-cell subtype found in the rheumatoid synovium, the identity of the arthritogenic antigen presented by DR4/DR1 in RA is still a matter of speculation. The conserved Q(K/R)RAA sequence could convey disease susceptibility by serving as a binding epitope for a specific arthritogenic peptide, either endogenous or exogenous, or providing a specific epitope for T-cell receptor interaction, or by itself acting as an immunogen. Several lines of evidence have suggested participation of viral or bacterial antigens such as peptides from Epstein–Barr virus, *E. coli*, *Proteus mirabilis*, *Lactobacillus lactis*, *Brucella ovis* that contain the 'shared epitope' amino acid motif and can therefore be described as 'molecular mimics' (Cordain et al. 2000). Alternatively, foreign antigens might mimic host antigens. An immune response to the foreign antigen would break tolerance to the self-antigen that it mimics, leading to autoreactivity against self. Furthermore, antibodies, such as rheumatoid factor (RF) directed against immunoglobulins, and against type II collagen, support the concept of autoreactivity against self, although these phenomena may be a result of disease rather than a cause of it (Bathon 1998–2005).

While T-cells may be important in initiating the disease, chronic inflammation appears to be self-perpetuated by the interaction of synovial macrophages and fibroblasts in a T-cell independent manner (Bathon 1998–2005). Cytokines produced by macrophages and fibroblasts (connective tissue cells) are expressed in abundance in RA synovium and synovial fluid (Bathon 1998–2005). Activated macrophages continuously secrete IL-1 and tumour necrosis factor (TNF), which activate the fibroblasts to secrete large amounts of cytokines IL-6, IL-8 and GM-CSF (granulocyte-macrophage colony stimulating factor), prostaglandins and proteases (Bathon 1998–2005). IL-1 and TNF also have systemic effects, some of which are mediated by IL-6, causing fever, muscle wasting and decreased appetite (Bathon 1998–2005).

IL-6 stimulates the maturation of B-cells to immunoglobulin-secreting plasma cells that secrete rheumatoid factor (RF). It also suppresses albumin synthesis by the liver and stimulates the synthesis of acute phase proteins, raising the erythrocyte sedimentation rate (ESR) (Bathon 1998–2005).

IL-8 acts as a chemotactic stimulus for neutrophils that are recruited to the synovial cavity. In their activated state, they release reactive oxygen species (ROS) that depolymerise hyaluronic acid, a component of synovial fluid, and inactivate endogenous inhibitors of proteases, promoting joint damage (Bathon 1998–2005).

As the pannus invades contiguous bone and cartilage, prostaglandins, notably PGE_2, and proteases (collagenases, stromelysin and gelatinase) are secreted from fibroblasts, causing degradation of proteoglycan and collagen of cartilage and bone (Bathon 1998–2005). This destructive effect is increased by IL-1 and TNF which suppress the synthesis of these matrix molecules and activate chondrocytes to secrete proteolytic enzymes, thus compounding the damage (Bathon 1998–2005). The importance of TNF in the pathology of RA is demonstrated by the dramatic improvement seen on treatment with monoclonal antibody to TNF-α (Caughey et al. 1996).

There may also be a role for leptin – a hormone and a cytokine – in the pathophysiology of RA. Leptin has been reported to modulate the immune response, inflammation, and Th-cell activity in the cellular immune response (Otero et al. 2005).

Th1 and Th2 helper cells are thought to direct different immune response pathways, the cellular-immunity and humoral-immunity pathways respectively, that are differentiated by the cytokines they secrete. While RA is generally considered to be a Th1 (T helper 1) dominant disease, this clear cut distinction has been questioned (Gerli et al. 2002; Kidd 2003).

2.4.3   Autoantibodies: rheumatoid factor

Rheumatoid factors (RF) are autoantibodies (principally IgM-RF, but also IgA-RF and IgG-RF) directed against the Fc portion of IgG. However, it is thought that RF may have another entirely different specificity separate to that of self-IgG-Fc and that the reactivity with IgG-Fc probably occurs because of similarities with an unidentified antigen – a foreign protein or a self-protein (Sutton et al. 1998; Cordain et al. 2000). According to Williams (1992), antibodies to *viral* Fc receptors (surface molecules expressed on different cell types that bind with the Fc region of an immunoglobulin) may provide the initial stimulus for RF production in RA. There is also a suggestion that RF production may occur in response to gastrointestinally related antigens such as milk or wheat (Cordain et al. 2000). An alternative view is that IgG itself has acquired some antigenicity owing to free radical damage (see 2.4.7; Kus et al. 1995).

When RF contributes to the generation of the inflammatory aspects of RA, it probably does so by forming immune complexes that are themselves able to bring about the inflammatory response (Williams 1992). Furthermore, RF-producing B cells could bring immunogenic foreign antigens to inflammatory sites owing to their propensity to bind and ingest antigens trapped in immune complexes (Albani & Carson 1996). They are potent antigen-presenting cells and their presence within the joint would determine amplification of immune and inflammatory responses (Albani & Carson 1996).

Only around 70 to 90% of RA patients have RF (Matsumoto 2005) and it may also be present in individuals with other chronic diseases or following immunisation. Though the RF titre does not correlate with disease activity, a high titre is an indication of a striking involvement of B-cell activation and such patients tend to have more aggressive disease, with more severe joint inflammation, extra-articular manifestations, and greater functional disability (Dorner et al. 2004). RF-negative patients, on the other hand, generally exhibit a milder disease course (Bathon 1998–2005; West 2002).

In individuals who went on to develop RA, autoantibodies both to IgM-RF and also to cyclic citrullinated peptide (CCP) were found in serum samples taken a median of 4.5 years before RA disease onset (Hal Scofield 2004). The negative predictive value of these tests was 75% and the positive predictive value 100%. Thus these autoantibodies that bind self-protein could be used for the prediction of RA in healthy individuals.

2.4.4 Glycosylation patterns of immunoglobulins and complement activation

The carbohydrate part of serum glycoproteins is altered in RA (Matei & Matei 2000–2001). The immunoglobulin A (IgA) isolated from young women with RA showed an altered arrangement of the oligosaccharide chains at the surface of the glycoprotein and its serum level was six times greater than the level in control women (Matei & Matei 2000–2001).

Immunoglobulin G (IgG) consists of four polypeptide chains linked by disulphide bridges (Axford et al. 2003). The different sugars associated with IgG can be grouped into three sets depending on whether they contain 0, 1, or 2 galactose residues on their outer arms. In RA, there is an increase in the number of IgG-G0 structures that lack the terminal galactose residue, causing the N-acetyl glucosamine residues to be revealed at the ends of the arms. It appears that galactosylation is reduced in RA patients because of a significant defect in the galactosyltransferase enzyme that results in reduced activity (Alavi et al. 2004). RFs have been found to bind hypogalactosylated IgG selectively, explaining why immune complexes are abundant in RA (Axford et al. 2003).

A further consequence of loss of bound galactose is that the terminal N-acetyl glucosamine residues on aggregated IgG-G0 isoforms become available for specific recognition by the mannose-binding protein (MBP), a soluble lectin of the collectin family (Rudd et al. 2001). MBP is a plasma protein secreted by the liver as an acute phase protein. It is a central part of the innate immune system, being able to recognise intact antigens and subsequently activate the complement system by the lectin pathway. When it binds to the terminal N-acetyl glucosamine of IgG-G0 residues, the complement system is inappropriately activated with consequent pro-inflammatory effects (Malhotra et al. 1995; Siassi et al. 2005). Increased levels of hypogalactosylated IgG in early synovitis have been linked to the development of RA (Axford 1999).

2.4.5   Dietary lectins, gut translocation and the shared epitope

Intestinal inflammation frequently accompanies RA. In this context, a number of authors have suggested a pathological role for dietary lectins that can exhibit toxic and inflammatory effects on the gut (Freed 1999; Cordain et al. 2000). Lectins are glycoproteins obtained particularly from the seeds of leguminous plants, but also from many other plant and animal sources. They are found in common dietary staples such as cereal grains and legumes (Cordain et al. 2000). Lectins such as concanavalin A and phytohaemagglutinin are familiar laboratory reagents. Dietary lectins are resistant to cooking and digestive enzymes resulting in residual lectin activity and luminal concentrations, which are quite high (Freed 1999). Furthermore, they can get past the gut wall and can be presented by macrophages to competent lymphocytes of the immune system (Freed 1999; Cordain et al. 2000). There is also evidence that lectins stimulate class II HLA antigens on cells that do not normally display them and stimulate T-cell proliferation (Freed 1999; Cordain et al. 2000).

The interaction of lectins with enterocytes and lymphocytes facilitates the translocation of dietary and gut-derived pathogenic antigens to peripheral tissues causing persistent immunological stimulation (Cordain et al. 2000). Legume and cereal lectins alter the gut microflora causing both inflammation and increased intestinal permeability. They facilitate the preferential growth of bacteria such as *Escherichia (E.) coli* and *Lactobacillus lactis* which contain the Q(K/R)RAA shared epitope. Thus, in susceptible individuals, cross-reactivity between bacterial or other exogenous peptides with amino acid motifs similar to those of the HLA-DR4 and HLA-DR1 shared epitope may be able to break immunological tolerance resulting in the expression of RA (Cordain et al. 2000).

Given that we all eat lectins, Freed (1999) himself has raised the question of why we do not all suffer from RA. He suggests that biological variation in the glycoconjugates that coat our cells together with the fact that these are normally protected behind a fine screen of sialic acid molecules attached to the glycoprotein tips should make us safe. While there are apparently numerous case reports of alleviation of RA symptoms with grain-free diets (Cordain et al. 2000), this does not prove that the effect is lectin-related: suitable human studies are needed to prove the hypothesis. We shall return to the subject of dietary lectins in Chapter 7.

2.4.6   Abnormal gut microflora

Intestinal flora differ between RA patients and normal controls (for references, see Peltonen et al. 1997; Toivanen 2001, 2003). Moreover, individuals with RA apparently maintain a high frequency of small intestinal bacterial overgrowth, particularly with anaerobic bacterial species (Cordain et al. 2000).

Patients with newly developed RA were found to have significantly different flora in the faeces than non-rheumatoid controls, those with erosive RA showing the most difference (Toivanen 2001). Gram-positive anaerobic bacteria that have a thick peptidoglycan layer surrounding the cell were primarily responsible for the differences. These differences may be regulated to some extent by the host genome, suggesting that patients with RA might favour intestinal bacteria that are capable of inducing RA (Toivanen 2001, 2003). Some bacterial cell wall peptidoglycans can induce arthritis and can also stimulate production of RF (Toivanen 2003). Bacterial adhesion to the intestinal epithelial surface may be linked to the recognition of specific proteins or glycoproteins on the epithelial cells while bacteria that cannot bind are shed (Toivanen 2003).

The majority of RA patients were found to have abnormally abundant faecal flora of atypical *Clostridium perfringens* compared to controls (Darlington & Ramsey 1993; Kjeldsen-Kragh 1999) while antibodies to *Proteus mirabilis*, a normal commensal component of the human bowel flora and a common cause of urinary tract infection, were described in patients with active RA by Ebringer and colleagues (1985). They suggested that RA was a consequence of cross-reactivity between a sequence of amino acids in *Proteus mirabilis* and HLA-DR antigens associated with RA that contained a similar sequence of amino acids – the 'shared epitope' theory (see section 2.4.2 and 2.4.5).

There is only a single layer of gut epithelial cells separating the individual from enormous amounts of bacterial antigens (Kjeldsen-Kragh 1999). Continuous seeding of bacterial products from the gut may be the source of the bacterial degradation products present in the synovium of RA patients that could contribute to synovial inflammation, erosion, exposition of cartilage antigens and autoimmunity in susceptible individuals (Toivanen 2001).

2.4.7   Reactive oxygen and nitrogen species involved in damage to the rheumatoid joint

The arthritic joint is undoubtedly a site of oxidative stress (Halliwell & Gutteridge 1999) resulting in the alteration of biomolecules, some of which contribute to disease perpetuation (Kus et al. 1995). Oxidative stress is inextricably linked with inflammatory processes: the ability of fresh sera to resist attack by peroxyl radicals (TRAP) was found to be significantly lower in patients with RA than in healthy controls. TRAP values varied inversely with a combination of visual analogue scale, duration of early morning stiffness, grip strength and articular index, reflecting inflammatory activity (Situnayake et al. 1991). Mechanisms that generate reactive oxygen and nitrogen species (ROS, RNS) in the rheumatoid joint are described by Kus and colleagues (1995) and Halliwell and Gutteridge (1999) and are summarised below.

2.4.7.1   Phagocytosis

In the inflamed arthritic joint, there is a significant increase in phagocytic cell populations such as polymorphonuclear neutrophils (PMNs) and macrophages. These activated phagocytes produce ROS and RNS in the respiratory burst with a view to destroying harmful pathogens and antigens.

2.4.7.2   Hypoxia reperfusion injury and joint pH

Walking on an inflamed rheumatoid joint such as the knee, generates intra-articular pressure in excess of capillary perfusion pressure, resulting in a sharp drop in oxygen concentration within the joint (Blake et al. 1989). With rest, oxygen is reintroduced to the tissue resulting in episodes of hypoxia reperfusion that occur with each step.

The ischaemia that occurs within the inflamed joint causes the conversion of xanthine dehydrogenase to xanthine oxidase (Roy & McCord 1983), which on subsequent oxygen exposure (reperfusion), produces the reductant, superoxide ($O_2^{\cdot-}$). Superoxide is capable of slowly releasing iron from ferritin (or from transferrin) (Aust et al. 1985), which is available in the synovium in active RA as a consequence of recurrent traumatic microbleeding (Blake et al. 1990). The amount of ferritin within synovial macrophages was shown to be significantly associated with the activity of early rheumatoid disease at the time of biopsy (Morris et al. 1995). Furthermore, ischaemia is characterised by an acidotic state induced by the conversion of glucose to lactate. Indeed, there is an inverse relationship between joint pH and degree of arthritic inflammation in RA patients (Bobkov et al. 1999). Protein-bound iron, including that bound to transferrin, can be released more readily at this lowered pH (Aust et al. 1985).

'Catalytic' iron can be measured in about 40% of synovial fluid samples aspirated from inflamed RA knee joints and in 25% of synovial lining cells from RA patients (Morris et al. 1995; Halliwell & Gutteridge 1999). Iron has the capacity to form the highly toxic and destructive hydroxyl radical ($OH^{\cdot}$) from $O_2^{\cdot-}$ and hydrogen peroxide by the Fenton reaction, causing tissue damage within the joint (Blake et al. 1990).

2.4.7.3   Involvement of nitric oxide and peroxynitrite

Nitric oxide ($NO^{\cdot}$), an inflammatory mediator produced in inflammatory joints through the action of cytokines, spontaneously oxidises to form nitrite under aqueous aerobic conditions (Farrell et al. 1992). Synovial fluid nitrite was significantly higher than serum nitrite, implying nitric oxide synthesis by the synovium. Reaction of O_2^- with nitric oxide results in the formation of the highly destructive peroxynitrite ($ONOO^-$), and contributes to the pathological process (Sakurai et al. 1995). Evidence of the involvement of peroxynitrite has been seen in elevated nitrotyrosine (a product of the interaction of peroxynitrite and protein tyrosine residues) levels in rheumatoid synovium (Halliwell & Gutteridge 1999) and in the increased concentrations of nitrite in synovial fluid and serum.

2.4.7.4 Consequences of the production of reactive oxygen and nitrogen species in the RA joint

There are a number of undesirable consequences of the presence of ROS and RNS in the rheumatoid joint, some of which are listed below (Kus et al. 1995).

(1) Interaction with lipids leads to the formation of lipid hydroperoxides and oxidatively modified LDL. The degradation of the unstable lipid hydroperoxides in the presence of transition metal ions such as iron results in the production of cytotoxic aldehydes: such products have been detected in rheumatoid serum and synovial fluid.
(2) There is a suggestion that IgG is oxidatively modified causing it to become antigenic to a point where it may trigger the production of RF. The resulting antigen antibody complex can stimulate O_2^- release from PMNs.
(3) Oxidatively modified α_1-antitrypsin is inactivated and therefore unable to inhibit the activity of elastase that is then free to digest tissue components such as collagen, fibronectin and proteoglycans.
(4) $OH^\cdot$ can react with deoxyguanosine in DNA to produce 8-hydroxydeoxyguanosine which is capable of initiating autoimmunity. There is evidence for significantly higher levels of 8-hydroxydeoxyguanosine in lymphocyte DNA from RA patients than from healthy subjects.
(5) The decreased viscosity of hyaluronic acid in the synovial fluid from RA patients is attributed to interaction with $OH^\cdot$ (Corsaro et al. 2004).
(6) NF-κB, a transcription factor that can turn on several genes involved in the inflammatory process, can be activated by ROS.

2.4.8   Lipid abnormalities and cardiovascular risk in RA

As explained in Chapter 1, the risk of cardiovascular death in RA patients compared with an age-matched population is doubled (Gonzalez-Gay et al. 2004). Cerebrovascular risk is the second leading cause of death (Sattar et al. 2003). Though there are many similarities between RA and atherosclerosis, the accelerated atherogenesis associated with RA is not fully explained by the classical risk factors for atherosclerosis (Pasceri & Yeh 1999; Sattar et al. 2003). The following features of RA are associated with cardiovascular and cerebrovascular risk and are mostly linked to the systemic inflammatory response (Sattar et al. 2003).

2.4.8.1   C-Reactive Protein (CRP)

This acute phase reactant is indicative of inflammation and is raised in RA. It is an independent predictor of the risk of myocardial infarction and stroke (Manzi & Wasco 2000).

2.4.8.2   Dyslipidaemia

The lipid pattern in RA is highly atherogenic despite low total cholesterol. Triglycerides are high, high density lipoprotein (HDL) cholesterol is low and there is a mass of small dense low density lipoprotein (LDL) particles that correlate positively with the degree of inflammation, giving an overall pattern that is highly atherogenic (Sattar et al. 2003). Significantly increased plasma concentrations of lipoprotein(a), an independent atherogenic factor that binds macrophages and promotes their transformation into foam cells, have also been reported in RA (Kus et al. 1995). Mechanisms underlying the dyslipidaemia are likely to relate to pro-inflammatory cytokine effects.

2.4.8.3   Endothelial dysfunction

There is evidence for endothelial dysfunction in RA patients, probably provoked by inflammation (Gonzalez-Gay et al. 2004). As vascular endothelial injury is synonymous with atherosclerosis, this may lead to subsequent cardiovascular events. The extent of endothelial dysfunction is dependent on HLA-DR genotype, with the HLA-DRB1 shared epitope alleles (see 2.3.2), particularly HLA-DRB1*0404, conferring particular susceptibility (Gonzalez-Gay et al. 2004).

2.4.8.4   Oxidised LDL in the joint and the formation of fatty streaks

Cytokines can directly promote oxidative modification of LDL (Sattar et al. 2003). Oxidised lipoproteins are cytotoxic to endothelial cells (Kus et al. 1995). Macrophages take up oxidised LDL via the scavenger receptor to form foam cells which, when they accumulate in the artery wall, lead to the formation of fatty streaks. Such fatty streaks were identified around blood vessels within the subintimal lining of rheumatoid synovial tissue (Kus et al. 1995).

2.4.8.5   Adhesion molecules

Oxidatively modified LDL, TNF-α, IL-1 and IL-6 upregulate adhesion molecules that are important in the migration of inflammatory cells to rheumatoid synovium (Kus et al. 1995; Manzi & Wasco 2000). These adhesion molecules have a role in recruiting T-cells, monocytes and macrophages to the site of vascular injury, a key step in the formation of atherosclerotic plaque (Manzi & Wasco 2000).

2.4.8.6   Haemostatic changes

The potential for blood clotting is raised in RA patients (Sattar et al. 2003). A prolonged low level acute phase response causes a decrease in plasma albumin and an increase in globulin and haemostatic proteins, including fibrinogen (Manzi & Wasco 2000). TNF-α causes the expression of tissue factor on monocytes and possibly endothelium, thereby initiating the coagulation cascade, whereas IL-6 can increase the levels of fibrinogen (Sattar et al. 2003). Fibrinogen is a precursor of fibrin, an essential component of the blood clot (Manzi & Wasco 2000).

2.4.8.7   Elevated homocysteine and low vitamin B_6 status

Elevated total homocysteine levels have been found in RA patients and may be associated with the elevated cardiovascular mortality seen in such patients (Roubenoff et al. 1997; Hernanz et al. 1999). The situation appears to be exacerbated after ingestion of a quantity of methionine, the precursor of homocysteine, such as may occur after a meal or in a test situation.

A number of B vitamins are required for the metabolism of homocysteine including vitamin B_6, which has been found to be deficient in RA patients (Chiang et al. 2003). The metabolic pathways involved are shown in Figure 2.7. Vitamin B_6 is required by the enzyme cystathionine β-synthase (CBS) which irreversibly converts homocysteine to cystathionine. In a study that challenged 37 RA patients with a methionine load, Chiang and colleagues found that the increase in homocysteine correlated significantly with markers of inflammation such as erythrocyte sedimentation rate, C-reactive protein level, disability score, degree of pain and fatigue, number of painful joints, and number of swollen joints. They ascribed the increase in homocysteine to deficiency of vitamin B_6, since markers of vitamin B_6 status in this patient group correlated inversely with disease activity, severity, synovial burden, and pain. They concluded that the abnormal vitamin B_6 status in rheumatoid arthritis is inherent to the disease itself, as it is not caused by lower intake or excessive catabolism of vitamin B_6 but is likely to result from the inflammatory process that reduces circulating and hepatic levels of vitamin B_6.

2.4.8.8   Elevated homocysteine and impaired sulphur metabolism

There is an alternative explanation for elevated homocysteine in RA patients which relates to their impaired sulphur metabolism, as demonstrated in the following study by Hernanz and colleagues (1999). Plasma concentrations of thiol compounds, including methionine as a precursor of homocysteine, were studied in 38 women with RA and compared to levels in 25 normal controls. Significantly higher levels of total plasma homocysteine {mean (SD); 17.3 (7.8) *vs.* 7.6 (1.9); $p < 0.001$}, cysteine {293 (61) *vs.* 201 (45); $p < 0.001$}, cysteinylglycine {32.7 (8.3) *vs.* 22.3 (4.7); $p < 0.001$} and methionine {25 (9) *vs.* 18 (3); $p < 0.01$} were found. Importantly, levels of folate and vitamin B_{12}, also required for homocysteine metabolism, were similar in the RA and control subjects. Hernanz and colleagues (1999) concluded that impaired metabolism of thiols was responsible. The build up of methionine, homocysteine and cysteine can be explained by the RA patients having reduced ability for methyltransfer by the enzyme thiol methyltransferase (EC 2.1.1.9, Bradley et al. 1991) and to oxidise cysteine by cysteine dioxygenase (Bradley

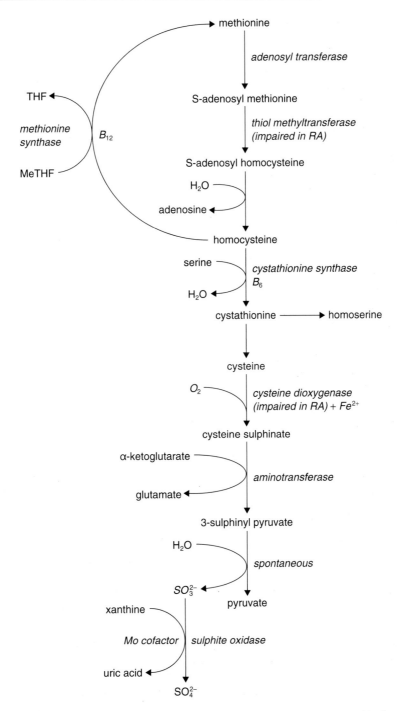

Figure 2.7 Metabolic pathways in homocysteine and sulphur amino acid metabolism (adapted from Salway 1994).

et al. 1994) (see the relevant metabolic pathways in Figure 2.7). An additional effect of these low enzyme activities is significantly reduced levels of both plasma and synovial fluid sulphate in RA (Bradley et al. 1994). Sulphate is an important component of connective tissues as will be explained further in 11.5.

2.4.8.9 *Insulin resistance*

RA patients have basal hyperinsulinaemia and insulin resistance, both abnormalities correlating with the degree of inflammation (Paolisso et al. 1991; Hallgren & Berne 1983). Cytokines such as TNF-α can directly impede insulin mediated glucose uptake in skeletal muscle while both IL-6 and TNF-α can stimulate lipolysis, increasing the movement of free fatty acids: fatty acid flux is known to be important in the pathophysiology of insulin resistance (Sattar et al. 2003).

2.4.9 Angiogenesis

Angiogenesis is central to the development and perpetuation of rheumatoid synovitis. Without angiogensesis, leucocyte entry to the inflammatory pannus could not occur (Koch 2000). The hyperplasia of the synovium requires new blood vessels to nourish and oxygenate the tissue (Paleolog & Miotla 1998). If angiogenesis does not keep pace with synovial proliferation, regions of hypoperfusion and hypoxia will develop (Paleolog & Miotla 1998). Vascular endothelial growth factor (VEGF), one of the main mediators of angiogenesis, is found in the synovial fluid and serum of patients with RA, and its expression is correlated with disease severity (Clavel et al. 2003). VEGF secretion by RA synovial membrane cells is uregulated by cytokines and hypoxia (Paleolog & Miotla 1998). The importance of angiogenesis in RA is shown by the fact that angiogenesis inhibition by the novel VEGF receptor tyrosine kinase inhibitor, PTK787/ZK222584, caused significant anti-arthritic effects in mouse and rat models of RA (Grosios et al. 2004).

VEGF is not the only player, however. One of the key events required for successful angiogenesis is extracellular proteolysis where a rate-limiting step is the activity of the matrix metalloproteinase (MMP) family of enzymes involved in extracellular matrix remodelling (Moses 1997). MMPs are a large family of zinc-containing, calcium-dependent enzymes that include within their subgroups collagenases (MMP-1, -8, -13), stromelysins (MMP-3, 10, -11), gelatinases (MMP-2, -9), and membrane type MMPs (MMP-14 to -17, -24, -25) (Murphy et al. 2002). The activity of MMPs is normally balanced by that of tissue inhibitor of MMP (TIMP). During angiogenesis, endothelial cells must degrade at least two distinct barriers, the microvascular basement membrane and the interstitium: the gelatinases are vital during these stages (Jackson et al. 2001). Accordingly, both *in vivo* and *in vitro*, MMP-1, MMP-2 (gelatinase A), and/or MMP-9 (gelatinase B) have been found to be upregulated in angiogenesis (Kolb et al. 1999).

Another MMP, MMP-19 appears to play a different role: small synovial capillaries in acutely inflamed tissues of early arthritis strongly express MMP-19 along with the VEGF-receptor, VEGF-R2, and without TIMP-1 (Kolb et al. 1999). After the first events of angiogenesis, the enzymatic activity (MMP) appears to be held in check by the co-expression of TIMP (Kolb et al. 1999).

2.4.10   Osteoporosis

The balance between the activity of osteoclasts (destructive) and osteoblasts is altered in favour of net bone loss in RA (Mikuls 2003). The elevated levels of pro-inflammatory cytokines produced in RA have been implicated in the dysregulation of bone and cartilage remodelling. Both IL-1 and TNF-α have been shown to upregulate the production of the receptor activator of NF-κB ligand, which acts to enhance osteoclastic bone resorption (Goldring 2003). TNF-α stimulates differentiation of osteoclast progenitors into mature osteoclasts and IL-1 acts directly on osteoclasts to increase their bone resorbing capacity (Goldring 2003). IL-1 and TNF-α also adversely affect cartilage remodelling. Secretion of IL-1 by macrophages stimulates both synoviocytes and chondrocytes to release proteases, stimulating cartilage matrix degradation: IL-1 can also promote bone resorption by inhibiting the synthesis of type II collagen and proteoglycans (Halliwell & Gutteridge 1999; Goldring 2003). The use of glucocorticoids in RA further exacerbates bone loss by a number of mechanisms, not the least of which is the inhibition of new bone formation (Mikuls 2003).

2.5   Assessment of severity of RA and OA

As the following chapters will describe interventions in arthritic subjects, the reader needs to be familiar with outcome measures used to assess disease status from which any improvement can be gauged. Such outcome measures have been clearly set out by Symmons (1994) in a paper on the Arthritis Research Campaign (ARC) website from which the following section is largely derived, except where otherwise specified. One measure that applies to both OA and RA is non-steroidal anti-inflammatory drug (NSAID) or analgesic dosage and the extent to which that alters with an intervention.

2.5.1   Outcome measures for RA (largely taken from Symmons 1994, with permission)

2.5.1.1   Patient's global assessment

The patient's wellbeing can be quantified by using a 10 cm Visual Analogue Scale (VAS). Although a rather subjective measurement, it is a useful instrument. Patients indicate their current perception of pain, stiffness etc. on a 10 cm line, ranging from no pain at one end to extreme pain at the other. A mark at 6.5 cm, for example, would indicate a VAS score of 65% (ARC for Research, 1995). Improvement is thus reflected by a falling score.

2.5.1.2   Pain

A pain score is valuable in all patients with RA and in the assessment of all antirheumatic therapies. Many methods have been devised for quantifying pain but the most commonly used are a 10 cm VAS and a five-point descriptive (Likert) scale. The assessment of pain is a very sensitive measure in short-term drug trials in RA. Its value in longitudinal studies has not been assessed. Preliminary work suggests that the pain score plateaus or even improves with time. This is a situation where the more relevant measure of disease outcome is the area under the curve.

2.5.1.3   Disability

It has been suggested that a self-report functional questionnaire is the single most useful tool in the quantitative assessment of the rheumatoid patient. The one in most widespread use is the validated Stanford Health Assessment Questionnaire (HAQ), which has been modified and validated for use in the UK. The HAQ lists 20 everyday tasks such as dressing/grooming, waking, eating, walking, hygiene, reach, grip and activities, and asks the patient to rate their difficulty in performing these tasks on a four point scale. The HAQ is sensitive to change and is able to discriminate between therapies in short term studies. Current disability is the strongest predictor of a premature death in RA.

2.5.1.4   Swollen and tender joint counts

A count of the number of swollen joints is the closest the clinician comes to quantifying the bulk of inflamed tissue. Joint tenderness is another way of assessing pain. The correlation between joint swelling and tenderness is not as high as might be expected, which is why both need to be assessed. There is no consensus on a single standardised method of assessing joint involvement. The methods available vary in the number of joints assessed, whether these joints are weighted according to size, and whether the joint abnormality is scored on a linear scale or simply as being normal or abnormal. A joint count is obtained when the number of abnormal joints is recorded. A joint score is obtained when the abnormality is graded. Joint counts are more reproducible than joint scores.

The Ritchie articular index (Ritchie et al. 1968) is a way in which joint tenderness is widely measured. Pressure is applied around the joint. Tenderness is assessed by passive movement. The individual is scored from 0 to 3 at each joint following pressure. A score of 0 would indicate no reaction (not tender), 1 would be a complaint of pain (tender), 2 tender and wincing and 3 tender, wincing and withdrawal of the limb. The index is the sum of all marks for all joints (David &

Lloyd, 1999). A 28-joint index (which includes 10 metacarpophalangeal, 10 proximal interphalangeal and two shoulder, elbow, wrist and knee joints) performs as well as the 80-joint count recommended by the ACR.

2.5.1.5 Acute phase reactants

Recent research suggests that circulating levels of cytokines may be a more direct indication of inflammatory activity. However, no routine assays are available to detect these substances. The erythrocyte sedimentation rate (ESR), a measure of erythrocytes that settle in unclotted blood, and C-reactive protein (CRP), which increases as acute phase proteins are produced in response to inflammation, remain the two most widely used laboratory tests to assess inflammation in RA. They are closely correlated so there is no need to measure both when assessing progress. In patients with long-standing RA (more than 20 years) the ESR may be persistently elevated with no clinical evidence of inflammation and in this situation the CRP is the better measure. Both the ESR and the CRP are sensitive to change in the short term. Neither has any value in assessing the long-term damage caused by RA. Although initial rheumatoid factor titre is of prognostic significance, serial measurements are not useful in assessing progress.

2.5.1.6 RA quality of life index

This measures pain and fatigue alongside other disease-specific criteria. It is a questionnaire that is able to provide quantitative information from the answers given.

2.5.1.7 Radiological assessment

Unlike all the measures described above, the radiograph records *only* what has happened in the past. There is only a modest correlation between the radiological score and self-reported function. There is a variety of methods for quantifying radiological findings. The preferred system in Europe is that proposed by Larsen (1977) whose method involves comparing the patient's films with a set of standard radiographs graded on a 0–5 scale. The MCP and PIP joints are scored individually and the wrist is scored as a whole and then weighted by multiplying by 5. Although Larsen's method is most commonly used to score hand and feet X-rays, standard films are also available for other joints. Radiological scores rise progressively with disease duration. A number of longitudinal studies have shown a plateauing of radiological score with time, which has led to the suggestion that most radiological damage occurs early in disease. However, this observation may be an artifact of a scoring system that has a built in ceiling effect (i.e. it is not possible to deteriorate within the highest grade). The involvement of previously unaffected joints may be a more relevant outcome measure when it comes to judging the efficacy of treatment.

2.5.2 Some outcome measures for OA (reproduced, with permission, from Symmons 1994)

2.5.2.1 Patient global assessment

As with RA, this provides a valuable insight into how the patient views their own progress.

2.5.2.2 Pain score

Whereas in RA the pain score usually relates to the total amount of pain experienced by the patient, in OA it is useful to distinguish between use-related pain, pain at rest, and pain which disturbs sleep.

2.5.2.3 New joint score

The Doyle index is an adaptation of the Ritchie index for use in OA. It assesses joint tenderness on pressure or movement in 48 joints or joint groups. It provides a total score but it may be more useful to keep the result disaggregated. The natural history of OA is the slow accumulation of new sites, thus progress can by quantified by measuring new sites clinically and radiographically.

2.5.2.4 Severity score

Lequesne and Samson (1991) have developed indices of severity for knee and hip OA. The Lequesne questionnaires consist of 10–12 doctor-administered questions, which cover pain at rest, duration of morning and inactivity stiffness, walking distance and appropriate activities of daily living. The Lesquesne indices have not been fully validated. It is unlikely that they will prove sufficiently sensitive to change to be of use in the trial situation. However, they are already being used in the epidemiologically based needs assessment for joint replacement and are likely to be helpful in quantifying cumulative damage in the individual patient.

2.5.2.5 Disability

The HAQ is useful in assessing disability in patients with OA in multiple joints. However patients with OA in a single joint often have almost normal HAQ scores. Bellamy et al. (1988) have developed a validated 24-item self-administered questionnaire for use in the assessment of knee and hip OA, called the Western Ontario and McMaster Universities (WOMAC) Osteoarthritis index, which covers three domains: pain, stiffness and physical function. The score for each domain is calculated separately. Each of the 24 questions is graded either on a five point Likert scale or a 100 mm visual analogue scale (VAS) ranging from 'no or 0' to 'extreme or 100'. This index is progressively becoming the most widely used instrument for assessment of OA-specific health status in Europe and is now available in a number of languages. The French Canadian version is given below as Table 2.4 (Faucher et al. 2002).

Table 2.4   The WOMAC (Western Ontario and McMaster Universities) index for assessment of OA (adapted from Bellamy et al. 1988).

Grade the amount of pain you feel when:
- walking on a flat surface
- going up or down stairs
- at night while in bed
- sitting or lying
- standing upright

Grade how stiff you feel after:
- first awakening in the morning
- sitting, lying or resting later in the day

Grade the degree of difficulty you feel when:
- descending stairs
- ascending stairs
- rising from sitting
- standing
- bending to floor
- walking on flat
- getting in/out of car
- going shopping
- putting on socks/stockings
- rising from bed
- taking off socks/stockings
- lying in bed
- getting in/out of bath
- sitting
- getting on/off toilet
- heavy domestic duties
- light domestic duties

2.5.2.6   Radiological assessment

Progress in OA has traditionally been assessed radiologically despite the poor correlation between X-ray findings and symptoms. The method introduced by Kellgren and Lawrence in the 1950s (Kellgren & Lawrence 1977) remains the gold standard. This involves comparing the patient's films with a set of standardised X-rays graded from 0 (normal) to 4 (severe OA). The system has been shown to be reproducible but it is not sensitive to change and, as with some of the systems used to score RA, it has a ceiling effect. Standardised measures of joint space narrowing are more sensitive to change but less reproducible. The rate of progression in OA is highly variable and non-linear.

References

Alavi A, Axford J, Pool AJ (2004) Serum galactosyl transferase isoform changes in rheumatoid arthritis. *Journal of Rheumatology* 31, 1513–20.

Albani S, Carson DA (1996) A multistep molecular mimicry hypothesis for the pathogenesis of rheumatoid arthritis. *Immunology Today* 17(10), 466–70.

Altman R, Alarcon G, Appelrouth D, Bloch D, Borenstein D, Brandt K, et al. (1991) The American College of Rheumatology criteria for the classification and reporting of osteoarthritis of the hip. *Arthritis and Rheumatism* 34, 505–14.

Altman R, Asch E, Bloch D, Bole G, Borenstein D, Brandt K, et al. (1986) The American College of Rheumatology criteria for the classification and reporting of osteoarthritis of the knee. *Arthritis and Rheumatism* 29, 1039–49.

ARC (Arthritis Research Campaign) for Research. (1995) Collected reports on the Rheumatic diseases.

Aust SD, Morehouse LA, Thomas CE (1985) Role of metals in oxygen radical reactions. *Journal of Free Radical Biology & Medicine* 1(1), 3–25.

Axford JS (1999) Glycosylation and rheumatic disease. *Biochimica et biophysica acta* 8, 1455(2–3), 219–29.

Axford JS, Cunnane G, Fitzgerald O, Bland M, Bresnihan B, Frears E (2003) Rheumatic disease differentiating using immunoglobulin G sugar printing by high density electrophoresis. *Journal of Rheumatology* 30, 2540–46.

Bathon JM (1998–2005) Rheumatoid Arthritis Pathophysiology, Johns Hopkins www.hopkins-arthritis.som.jhmi.edu/rheumatoid/rheum_clin_path.htmlread

Bellamy N, Buchanan WW, Goldsmith CH, Campbell J, Stitt LW (1988) Validation study of WOMAC: a health status instrument for measuring clinically important patient relevant outcomes to antirheumatic drug therapy in patients with osteoarthritis of the hip or knee. *Journal of Rheumatology* 15, 1833–40.

Beth Israel (2005) Deaconess Medical Center Boston MA 02115, website. Image used with permission of Dr. Deborah Burstein, Associate Professor of Radiology http://bidmc.harvard.edu/display.asp?leaf_id=5578

Blake DR, Merry P, Unsworth J, Kidd BL, Outhwaite JM, Ballard R, Morris CJ, Gray L, Lunec J (1989) Hypoxic reperfusion injury in the inflamed human joint. *The Lancet* 11, 1(8633), 289–93.

Blake DR, Merry P, Stevens C, Dabbagh A, Sahinoglu T, Allen R, Morris C (1990) Iron-free radicals and arthritis. *Proceedings of the Nutritional Society* 49(2), 239–45.

Bobkov VA, Brylenkova TN, Kopilov EI, Mitskaia SG, Kazakova NI (1999) Changes in the acid-base status of the synovial fluid in rheumatoid arthritis patients. *Terapevticheski arkhiv* 71, 20–22.

Bonnet CS, Walsh DA (2005) Osteoarthritis, angiogenesis and inflammation. *Rheumatology* 44(1), 7–16.

Bradley H, Waring RH, Emery P (1991) Reduced thiol methyl transferase activity in red blood cell membranes from patients with rheumatoid arthritis. *Journal of Rheumatology* 18(12), 1787–89.

Bradley H, Gough A, Sokhi RS, Hassell A, Waring R, Emery P (1994) Sulfate metabolism is abnormal in patients with rheumatoid arthritis. Confirmation by *in vivo* biochemical findings. *Journal of Rheumatology* 21(7), 1192–96.

Caughey GE, Mantzioris E, Gibson RA, Cleland LG, James MJ (1996) The effect of human tumor necrosis factor a and interleukin 1b production of diets enriched in n-3 fatty acids from vegetable oil or fish oil. *American Journal of Clinical Nutrition* 63, 116–22.

Chevalier X (1993) Fibronectin, cartilage, and osteoarthritis. *Seminars in Arthritis and Rheumatism* 22(5), 307–18.

Chiang EP, Bagley PJ, Selhub J, Nadeau M, Roubenoff R (2003) Abnormal vitamin B(6) status is associated with severity of symptoms in patients with rheumatoid arthritis. *American Journal of Medicine* 114(4), 283–87.

Clavel G, Bessis N, Boissier MC (2003) Recent data on the role for angiogenesis in rheumatoid arthritis. *Joint Bone Spine* 70(5), 321–26.

Cordain L, Toohey L, Smith MJ, Hickey MS (2000) Modulation of immune function by dietary lectins in rheumatoid arthritis. *British Journal of Nutrition* 83(3), 207–17.

Corsaro MM, Pietraforte D, Di Lorenzo AS, Minetti M, Marino G (2004) Reaction of peroxynitrite with hyaluronan and related saccharides. *Free Radical Research* 38(4), 343–53.

Creamer P, Hochberg MC (1997) Osteoarthritis. *The Lancet* 350, 503–8.

Darlington LG, Ramsey NW (1993) Clinical Review – review of dietary therapy for rheumatoid arthritis. *British Journal of Rheumatology* 32, 507–14.

Das A, Hammad TA (2000) Efficacy of a combination of FCHG49 glucosamine hydrochloride TRH122 low molecular weight sodium chondroitin sulphate and manganese ascorbate in the management of knee osteoarthritis. *Osteoarthrits and Cartilage* 8(5), 343–50.

David C, Lloyd J (1999) Rheumatological Physiotherapy. London, Mosby pp. 3–9, 55–61, 65–81 and 83–96.

Day JS, Van Der Linden JC, Bank RA, Ding M, Hvid I, Sumner DR, Weinans H (2004) Adaptation of subchondral bone in osteoarthritis. *Biorheology* 41(3–4), 359–68.

Devereux G (2002) The immune system: an overview. In: *Nutrition and Immune Function.* (PC Calder, CJ Field, HS Gill, eds). Frontiers in Nutritional Science No. 1. Wallingford, Cabi Publishing.

Dorner T, Egerer K, Feist E, Burmester GR (2004) Rheumatoid factor revisited. *Current Opinion in Rheumatology* 16(3), 246–53.

Ebringer A, Ptaszynska T, Corbett M, Wilson C, Macafee Y, Avakian H, Baron P, James DC (1985) Antibodies to proteus in rheumatoid arthritis. *The Lancet* 10, 2(8450), 305–7.

Eyre DR (2004) Collagens and cartilage matrix homeostasis. *Clinical Orthopaedics & Related Research* 427(S), S118–22.

Farrell AJ, Blake DR, Palmer RM, Moncada S (1992) Increased concentrations of nitrite in synovial fluid and serum samples suggest increased nitric oxide synthesis in rheumatic diseases. *Annals of the Rheumatic Diseases* 51, 1219–22.

Faucher M, Poiraudeau S, Lefevre-Colau MM, Rannou F, Fermanian J, Revel M (2002) Algofunctional assessment of knee osteoarthritis: comparison of the test–retest reliability and construct validity of the Womac and Lequesne indexes. *Osteoarthritis and Cartilage* 10, 602–610.

Freed DL (1999) Do dietary lectins cause disease? *British Medical Journal* 17, 318 (7190), 1023–24.

Gerli R, Lunardi C, Pitzalis C (2002) Unmasking the anti-inflammatory cytokine response in rheumatoid synovitis. *Rheumatology* 41(12), 1341–45.

Goldring SR (2003) Pathogenesis of bone and cartilage destruction in rheumatoid arthritis. *Rheumatology* 42, Suppl 2:ii11–6.

Gonzalez-Gay MA, Gonzalez-Juanatey C, Ollier WE (2004) Endothelial dysfunction in rheumatoid arthritis: influence of HLA-DRB1 alleles. *Autoimmunity Reviews* 3(4), 301–4.

Grosios K, Wood J, Esser R, Raychaudhuri A, Dawson J (2004) Angiogenesis inhibition by the novel VEGF receptor tyrosine kinase inhibitor, PTK787/ZK222584, causes significant antiarthritic effects in models of rheumatoid arthritis. *Inflammation Research* 53(4), 133–42.

Hal Scofield R (2004) Autoantibodies as predictors of disease. *The Lancet* 363, 1544–46.

Hallgren R, Berne C (1983) Glucose intolerance in patients with chronic inflammatory diseases is normalized by glucocorticoids. *Acta Medica Scandinavica* 213(5), 351–55.

Halliwell B, Gutteridge JMC (1999) *Free Radicals. Biology and Medicine,* 3rd edition. Oxford, Oxford University Press.

Hernanz A, Plaza A, Martin-Mola E, De Miguel E (1999) Increased plasma levels of homocysteine and other thiol compounds in rheumatoid arthritis women. *Clinical Biochemistry* 32(1), 65–70.

Howell WM, Calder PC, Grimble RF (2002) Gene polymorphisms, inflammatory diseases and cancer. *Proceedings of the Nutrition Society* 61(4), 447–56.

Jackson C, Nguyen M, Arkell J, Sambrook P (2001) Selective matrix metalloproteinase (MMP) inhibition in rheumatoid arthritis – targetting gelatinase A activation. *Inflammation Research* 50, 183–86.

Kellgren JH, Lawrence JS (1957) Radiological assessment of osteoarthritis. *Annals of the Rheumatic Diseases* 16, 494–502.

Kidd P (2003) Th1/Th2 balance: the hypothesis, its limitations, and implications for health and disease. *Alternative Medicine Review* 8(3), 223–46.

Kjeldsen-Kragh J (1999) Rheumatoid arthritis treated with vegetarian diets. *American Journal of Clinical Nutrition* 70 (suppl), 594S–600S.

Koch A (2000) The role of angiogenesis in rheumatoid arthritis: recent developments. *Annals of the Rheumatic Diseases* 59, Suppl 1:I, 65–71.

Kolb C, Mauch S, Krawinkel U, Sedlacek R (1999) Matrix metalloproteinase-19 in capillary endothelial cells: expression in acutely, but not in chronically, inflamed synovium. *Experimental Cell Research* 10, 250(1), 122–30.

Kus ML, Fairburn K, Blake D, Winyard PG (1995) A vascular basis for free radical involvement in inflammatory joint disease. In: *Immunopharmacology of Free Radical Species*, D Blake, PG Winyard, eds. London, San Diego, Academic Press.

Lajeunesse D (2004) The role of bone in the treatment of osteoarthritis. *Osteoarthritis Cartilage* 12 Suppl A, S34–8.

Larsen A, Dale K, Eek M (1977) Radiographic evaluation of rheumatoid arthritis and related conditions by standard reference films. *Acta Radiologica* (Diagnosis) 18, 481–91.

Lequesne MG, Samson M (1991) Indices of severity in osteoarthritis for weightbearing joints. *Journal of Rheumatology* 18 (suppl 27), 16–18.

McAlindon T (2001) Glucosamine for osteoarthritis: dawn of a new era? *The Lancet* 357, 247–48.

Malhotra R, Wormald MR, Rudd PM, Fischer PB, Dwek RA, Sim RB (1995) Glycosylation changes of IgG associated with rheumatoid arthritis can activate complement via the mannose-binding protein. *Nature Medicine* 1(3), 237–43.

Manzi S, Wasko MC (2000) Inflammation-mediated rheumatic diseases and atherosclerosis. *Annals of the Rheumatic Diseases* 59(5), 321–25.

Martin JA, Klingelhutz AJ, Moussavi-Harami F, Buckwalter JA (2004) Effects of oxidative damage and telomerase activity on human articular cartilage chondrocyte senescence. *The Journals of Gerontology Series A, Biological Sciences and Medical Sciences* 59(4), 324–37.

Matei L, Matei I (2000–2001) Lectin-binding profile of serum IgA in women suffering from systemic autoimmune rheumatic disorders. *Romanian Journal of Internal Medicine* 38–39, 73–82.

Matsumoto AK (2005) Johns Hopkins Arthritis, Rheumatoid Arthritis Clinical Presentation, www.hopkins-arthritis.som.jhmi.edu/rheumatoid/rheum_clin_pres.htmllabo

Mikuls TR (2003) Co-morbidity in rheumatoid arthritis. *Best Practice & Research Clinical Rheumatology* 17, 729–52.

Morris CJ, Earl JR, Trenam CW, Blake DR (1995) Reactive oxygen species and iron – a dangerous partnership in inflammation. *International Journal of Biochemistry and Cell Biology* 27(2), 109–22.

Moses MA (1997) The regulation of neovascularization of matrix metalloproteinases and their inhibitors. *Stem Cells* 15(3), 180–89.

Murphy G, Knauper V, Atkinson S, Butler G, English W, Hutton M, Stracke J, Clark I (2002) Matrix metalloproteinases in arthritic disease. *Arthritis Research* 4, Suppl 3, S39–49.

Nuki G (2002) Osteoarthritis: risk factors and pathogenesis. *Rheumatic Disease Topical Reviews*, September 2002, Number 9, Arthritis Research Campaign www.arc.org.uk/about_arth/med_reports/series4/tr/6609/6609.htm

Otero M, Lago R, Lago F, Casanueva FF, Dieguez C, Gomez-Reino JJ, Gualillo O (2005) Leptin, from fat to inflammation: old questions and new insights. *FEBS Letters* 17, 579(2), 295–301.

Paleolog EM, Miotla JM (1998) Angiogenesis in arthritis: role in disease pathogenesis and as a potential therapeutic target. *Angiogenesis* 2(4), 295–307.

Paolisso G, Valentini G, Giugliano D, Marrazzo G, Tirri R, Gallo M, Tirri G, Varricchio M, D'Onofrio F (1991) Evidence for peripheral impaired glucose handling in patients with connective tissue diseases. *Metabolism* 40(9), 902–7.

Pasceri V, Yeh ET (1999) A tale of two diseases: atherosclerosis and rheumatoid arthritis. *Circulation* 23, 100(21), 2124–26.

Peltonen R, Nenonen M, Helve T, Hanninen O, Toivanen P, Eerola E (1997) Faecal microbial flora and disease activity in rheumatoid arthritis during a vegan diet. *British Journal of Rheumatology* 36(1), 64–68.

Reginster JY, Deroisy R, Rovati LC, Lee RL, Lejeune E, Bruyere O, Giacovelli G, Henrotin Y, Dacre JE, Gossett C (2001) Long-term effects of glucosamine sulphate on osteoarthritis progression: a randomized, placebo-controlled trial. *The Lancet* 357, 251–56.

Reines BP (2004) Is rheumatoid arthritis premature osteoarthritis with fetal-like healing? *Autoimmunity Reviews* 3(4), 305–11.

Ritchie DM, Boyle JA, McInnes JM, Jasani MK, Dalakos TG, Grieveson P (1968) Clinical studies with an articular index for the assessment of joint tenderness in patients with rheumatoid arthritis. *Quarterly Journal of Medicine* 37, 393–406.

Rizzo R, Grandolfo M, Godeas C, Jones KW, Vittur F (1995) Calcium, sulfur, and zinc distribution in normal and arthritic articular equine cartilage: a synchrotron radiation-induced X-ray emission (SRIXE) study. *Journal of Experimental Zoology* 1, 273(1), 82–86.

Roubenoff R, Dellaripa P, Nadeau MR, Abad LW, Muldoon BA, Selhub J, Rosenberg IH (1997) Abnormal homocysteine metabolism in rheumatoid arthritis. *Arthritis and Rheumatism* 40(4), 718–22.

Roy RS, McCord JM (1983) Superoxide and ischemia: conversion of xanthine dehydrogenase to xanthine oxidase. In: *Oxy Radicals and their Scavenger Systems, Vol. II: Cellular and Medical Aspects*, RA Greenwald, G Cohen, eds. New York, Elsevier Science, pp. 145–53.

Rudd PM, Elliott T, Cresswell P, Wilson IA, Dwek RA (2001) Glycosylation and the immune system. *Science* 23, 291(5512), 2370–76.

Sakurai H, Kohsaka H, Liu MF, Higashiyama H, Hirata Y, Kanno K et al. (1995) Nitric oxide production and inducible nitric oxide synthase expression in inflammatory arthritides. *Journal of Clinical Investigation* 96(5), 2357–63.

Salway JG (1994) *Metabolism at a Glance*. Oxford, Blackwell Scientific Publications.

Sattar N, McCarey DW, Capell H, McInnes IB (2003) Explaining how 'high-grade' systemic inflammation accelerates vascular risk in rheumatoid arthritis. *Circulation* 16, 108(24), 2957–63.

Sauerland K, Plaas AH, Raiss RX, Steinmeyer J (2003) The sulfation pattern of chondroitin sulfate from articular cartilage explants in response to mechanical loading. *Biochimica et Biophysica Acta* 30, 1638(3), 241–48.

Siassi M, Riese J, Steffensen R, Meisner M, Thiel S, Hohenberger W, Schmidt J (2005) Mannanbinding lectin and procalcitonin measurement for prediction of postoperative infection. *Critical Care* 9, R483–R489.

Situnayake RD, Thurnham DI, Kootathep S, Chirico S, Lunec J, Davis M, McConkey B (1991) Chain breaking antioxidant status in rheumatoid arthritis: clinical and laboratory correlates. *Annals of the Rheumatic Diseases* 50, 81–86.

Stryer L (1988) *Biochemistry*, 3rd edition. New York, WH Freeman and Co, p. 276.

Sutton BJ, Corper AL, Sohi MK, Jefferis R, Beale D, Taussig MJ (1998) The structure of a human rheumatoid factor bound to IgG Fc. *Advances in Experimental Medicine and Biology* 435, 41–50.

Symmons D (1994) Quantifying progress in arthritis. *Topical Reviews* Series 3, Arthritis Research Campaign (ARC) www.arc.org.uk/about_arth/med_reports/series3/tr/6401/6401.htm

Symmons D, Mathers C, Pfleger B (2003a) *The Global Burden of Rheumatoid Arthritis in the Year 2000*. Geneva, World Health Organization. www3.who.int/whosis/menu.cfm?path= evidence,burden,burden_gbd2000docs,burden_gbd2000docs_diseasedoc,burden_gbd2000docs_ diseasedoc_ra&language=English

Symmons D, Mathers C, Pfleger B (2003b) *Global Burden of Osteoarthritis in the Year 2000*. Geneva, World Health Organization. www3.who.int/whosis/menu.cfm?path= evidence,burden,burden_gbd2000docs,burden_gbd2000docs_diseasedoc,burden_gbd2000docs_ diseasedoc_oa&language=english

Toivanen P (2001) From reactive arthritis to rheumatoid arthritis. *Journal of Autoimmunity* 16, 369–71.

Toivanen P (2003) Normal intestinal microbiota in the aetiopathogenesis of rheumatoid arthritis. *Annals of the Rheumatic Diseases* 62(9), 807–11.

van der Kraan PM, Vitters EL, de Vries BJ, van den Berg WB (1990) High susceptibility of human articular cartilage glycosaminoglycan synthesis to changes in inorganic sulfate availability. *Journal of Orthopaedic Research* 8(4), 565–71.

West S (2002) (ed) *Rheumatology Secrets*, 2nd edition. Philadelphia, Hanley & Belfus.

Williams RC (1992) Rheumatoid factors: historical perspective, origins and possible role in disease. *Journal of Rheumatology* Suppl 32, 42–45.

Yudoh K, Nguyen T, Nakamura H, Hongo-Masuko K, Kato T, Nishioka K (2005) Potential involvement of oxidative stress in cartilage senescence and development of osteoarthritis: oxidative stress induces chondrocyte telomere instability and downregulation of chondrocyte function. *Arthritis Research & Therapy* 7(2), R380–91.

3 Aetiology and risk factors for osteoarthritis and rheumatoid arthritis

3.1 Introduction

Both rheumatoid arthritis (RA) and osteoarthritis (OA) are multifactorial diseases with significant genetic elements. Non-genetic factors involved in the aetiology include endogenous factors such as age, gender, malalignment and obesity and environmental factors such as trauma, diet and cigarette smoking. It is likely that a series of events or triggers in an arthritis-prone genetic context is required before the development of disease. There is some overlap between risk factors for the two conditions, as can be seen from Figure 3.1, which shows the recognised risk factors for OA and RA. These will be expanded upon in the sections below.

3.2 Genetic risk factors

The comparison between concordance rates of RA in monozygotic twins and the prevalence in the respective populations shows that about 50% of the variation in

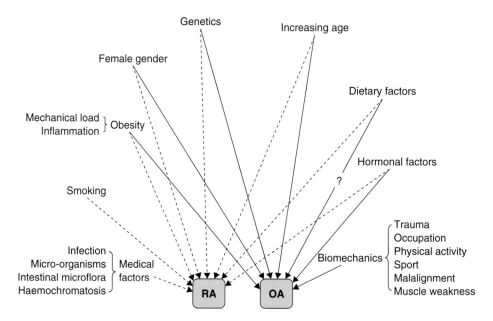

Figure 3.1   Risk factors for OA and RA.

disease occurrence is caused by genetic factors (Huizinga 2003). Genes definitely implicated in RA susceptibility are immune response genes encoding human leucocyte antigen (HLA) molecules, the job of which is to present processed peptides (antigens) to T-cell receptor molecules on the surface of T-cells (Howell et al. 2002). These are located within the major histocompatibility complex (MHC) on chromosome 6 and are highly polymorphic, resulting in functional amino acid substitutions in the HLA molecules expressed (Howell et al. 2002). Though multiple genes are likely to be involved in susceptibility to RA, no gene other than HLA-DRB1 has been clearly demonstrated to be involved in the disease (Howell et al. 2002; Newton et al. 2004). While several HLA-DRB1 alleles contribute to RA susceptibility, each contains identical nucleotide sequences encoding amino acids 67–74 of the DRβ1 chain. This identical sequence is referred to as the 'shared epitope' where the encoded amino acids form two of the pockets in the peptide-binding groove of the HLA-DR molecule that presents antigens to T-cell receptors (Howell et al. 2002). These amino acids may favour the binding and presentation of molecules that cause an arthritic response. The presence of the HLA-DR4 allele gives a relative risk of 9 for RA in those carrying the allele compared to those not carrying the allele (Howell et al. 2002).

There is some evidence that genetic factors may be more important in determining disease severity than disease susceptibility (Huizinga 2003; Symmons & Harrison 2000). Findings from a number of studies, including that of the Norfolk Arthritis Register (NOAR) cohort, suggest that HLA genes are more useful in predicting the clinical course of disease (for instance whether severe erosive disease will develop or not) rather than risk of occurrence (Symmons & Harrison 2000). In 337 UK patients with RA, homozygosity for the HLA-DRB1 shared epitope was associated with a significantly higher level of an enzyme that can degrade cartilage matrix, pro-matrix metalloproteinase-3 (proMMP-3) (Cheung et al. 2000). Levels of proMMP-3 were significantly though weakly correlated with disease activity and severity as measured by radiographic damage (Larsen score), Health Assessment Questionnaire score, and C-reactive protein (CRP) levels (Cheung et al. 2000). In the near future, it is likely that a large number of genetic risk factors will be identified which will allow identification of patients who could benefit from early timing of treatment (Huizinga 2003).

In addition to the polymorphisms mentioned above in the HLA-DRB1 alleles, those in the promoter regions of certain cytokine genes are also thought to be relevant to RA risk and severity e.g. TNF-α, IL-10 and IL-2 polymorphisms. TNF-α has a broad range of pro-inflammatory and immunostimulatory actions and is thought to play a pivotal role in RA (Brinkman et al. 1997). A significant association between the −238GA polymorphism of the TNF-α gene and decreased radiologically detectable progression of RA, in terms of erosions, was found in a case control study in 283 RA patients and 116 healthy controls (Brinkman et al. 1997). However, results of a later study implied that the polymorphism might be serving as a marker for additional polymorphisms in a neighbouring locus or gene linked to disease severity (Kaijzel et al. 1998). Of interest, cytokine genotype may interact with dietary factors in modulating pro-inflammatory immune response (Howell et al. 2002).

Table 3.1 Genes implicated in OA in association studies (reproduced with permission from Spector & MacGregor 2004).

VDR (vitamin D receptor)	CRTL (cartilage link protein)
COL2A	A1ACT
AGC1	COL9A1
IGF-1	COL11A1
ER alpha	COL1A1
TGF beta	ANK
CRTM (cartilage matrix protein)	

According to Cerhan and colleagues (2002), genetic epidemiology studies also suggest that genetic factors may play a relatively larger role in younger onset RA than in later onset RA, where non-genetic risk factors appear to be more important.

OA also has a complex hereditary component, the nature of which has been excellently reviewed by Spector & MacGregor (2004). Twin studies have shown that genetic factors are responsible for between 39% and 65% of OA in the hand and knee in women, about 60% in OA of the hip and about 70% in OA of the spine (Spector & MacGregor 2004). These figures suggest that around half the susceptibility to OA in the population is explained by genetic factors (Spector & MacGregor 2004). Linkage studies implicated chromosomes 2q, 9q, 11q and 16p in OA: candidate genes on these chromosomes include:

'... those encoding for fibronectin, a glycoprotein present in the extracellular matrix of normal cartilage; the alpha-2 chain of collagen type V, a major constituent of bone; the interleukin 8 receptor, important in the regulation of neutrophil activation and chemotaxis within the 2q23–25 region of chromosome 2; and the so-called high bone mass locus and the matrix metalloproteinase (MMP) gene cluster on chromosome 11q' (Spector & MacGregor 2004).

Female hip OA has been linked to the type IX collagen gene COL9A1 on chromosome 6q (Mustafa et al. 2000). Type IX collagen is critical for cartilage stability (Creamer & Hochberg 1997). Genes implicated in OA from association studies are shown in Table 3.1 (Spector & MacGregor 2004). A large Japanese study has also implicated the collagen gene, COL9A3, in knee OA (Ikeda et al. 2002). Different genes are involved in different disease features, e.g. bone formation or cartilage loss, and may also operate differently in males and females and at different body sites (Spector & MacGregor 2004).

Apart from collagen, the other major component of cartilage is proteoglycan, mainly present as the macromolecule, aggrecan. An association has been shown between a polymorphism in this gene and OA of the hand in elderly men (Creamer & Hochberg 1997). Other inherited disorders of joints and bones may also predispose to development of OA.

3.3 Age

Almost 80% of people will have changes in at least one joint that are visible on X-ray by the age of 60 (Loeser 2004). Increasing age is the strongest determinant of

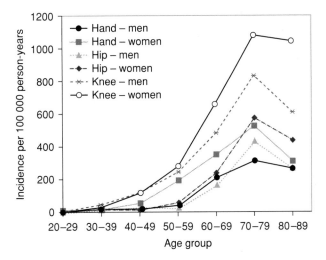

Figure 3.2 Incidence of OA of the hand, hip and knee in members of the Fallon Community Health Plan, 1991–92, by age and sex (reproduced with permission from Oliveria et al. 1995).

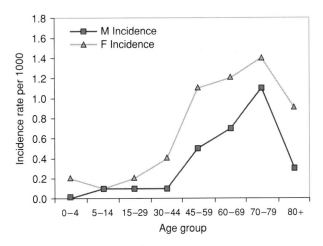

Figure 3.3 Male and female RA incidence rates in Rochester USA, according to age group (from Symmons et al. 2003).

risk of OA (Creamer & Hochberg 1997). In women, the prevalence of OA in the hand, hip and knee increases rapidly after age 50 (Felson & Nevitt 1998). Figure 3.2 demonstrates the increase in risk of severe OA that occurs with increasing age as measured by age at total hip replacement due to OA (Karlson et al. 2003). The incidence of new OA declines in both sexes after the age of 80 (Nuki 2002).

Although RA is often considered as a disease of middle-aged women, its incidence increases in women until age 70 (Cerhan et al. 2002) with a pronounced shoulder in the perimenopausal years. It is rare before menarche (Symmons & Harrison 2000). Figure 3.3 shows the incidence rate of RA in males and females as measured in the Rochester 1955–1985 study in the USA (Symmons et al. 2003).

There are a number of changes that occur with ageing that increase susceptibility to OA and contribute to joint vulnerability in RA without being a direct cause. Sarcopaenia (muscle wasting), loss of proprioception and balance and increased joint laxity all increase mechanical stress on ageing joints (Nuki 2002; Loeser 2004). The effect of ageing on cartilage is particularly relevant. Articular cartilage is unusual in that chondrocytes and most of the extracellular matrix proteins experience very little turnover, resulting in a tissue that must withstand many years of use and can also accumulate years of ageing-associated changes (Loeser 2004). Age-related changes in articular cartilage matrix in individuals with OA who experience progressive cartilage destruction are different to those in individuals without OA (Nuki 2002). A number of changes occur in aged cartilage that affect its structure and function as outlined below.

- The most striking age-related change in articular cartilage is the accumulation of advanced glycation end products (AGEs), such as pentosidine (Loeser 2004). The amount of pentosidine, which can cross link collagen molecules, is directly proportional to donor age in human cartilage. Pentosidine is associated with collagen stiffness, altered cartilage biomechanics and reduced proteoglycan (see section 2.3.2) synthesis (Loeser 2004).
- Decreased cartilage mitotic and synthetic activity and decreased responsiveness to anabolic growth factors occurs with ageing (Martin and Buckwalter 2002; Loeser 2004). The capacity of chondrocytes to synthesise normal matrix proteins decreases (Nuki 2002).
- Aggrecan, the major cartilage proteoglycan (see section 2.3.2) decreases in size and is altered in structure owing to modification of the core protein and changes in the length and abundance of the attached glycosaminoglycan chains (Martin and Buckwalter 2002; Loeser 2004). The water content also falls, reducing resilience (Loeser 2004). The result is decreased ability to maintain and repair tissue and loss of matrix tensile strength and stiffness (Martin & Buckwalter 2002).
- Oxidative stress in cartilage increases with age (Loeser 2004). Nitrotyrosine (a product of interaction between peroxynitrite and protein) formation increases with age and is particularly prominent in OA cartilage (Loeser 2004). Oxidative stress increases the ratio of oxidised to reduced glutathione, making chondrocytes more susceptible to oxidant mediated cell death (Carlo & Loeser 2003). Dead chondrocytes are unlikely to be replaced (Loeser 2004).
- Cartilage calcification increases with age (Loeser 2004).
- Age is associated with some degree of cartilage thinning (Loeser 2004).

3.4 Gender

OA is more prevalent in women than men (Creamer & Hochberg 1997). Female gender is an independent risk factor for knee OA as shown in a large Finnish study of more than 6000 farmers that found an odds ratio of 4.8 (95% CI 2.4, 9.3) for women developing bilateral knee OA (Nuki 2002). The situation for hip OA is not so clear cut (Nuki 2002). Postmenopausal women are more likely to suffer from OA than men of a similar age and premenopausal women (Creamer & Hochberg 1997). Oestrogen deficiency after the menopause has been suggested to be an important factor (see section 3.11).

Female gender is also a risk factor for RA, which is more common in women than in men, especially in the premenopausal age groups. In the UK the condition occurs 2.6 times as commonly in women as in men (Symmons et al. 2002).

3.5   Biomechanical factors as risk factors for OA

3.5.1   Occupation, sport and physical activity

Occupations involving physical activity and repetitive mechanical stress such as kneeling, squatting, climbing stairs, heavy lifting and pinch gripping (e.g. farming, firefighting, construction working and textile working) are associated with higher rates of knee and hip OA (Creamer & Hochberg 1997; Nuki 2002). In one study of 518 patients listed for surgical treatment of knee OA *vs.* sex and age matched controls, after adjustment for body mass index (BMI), history of knee injury and the presence of Herberden's nodes, the risk of OA was significantly associated with prolonged kneeling or squatting (odds ratio {OR} 1.9; 95% confidence interval {CI} 1.3, 2.8), walking more than two miles per day (OR 1.9; 95% CI 1.4, 2.8) or regularly lifting weights of at least 25 kg (OR 1.7; 95% CI 1.2, 2.6) while at work (Coggon et al. 2000). The risks associated with kneeling or squatting were greatly increased in those with a BMI {weight (kg)/height (m^2)} greater than 30. Similar conclusions were drawn from the Framingham study where heavy physical activity was found to be an important risk factor for the development of OA in the elderly, especially among obese individuals where the risk was 13 times greater in those carrying out three hours or more per day of heavy physical activity: light to moderate activity did not increase risk (McAlindon et al. 1999).

Participation in sport is also associated with risk of lower limb OA, notably in former élite runners, footballers, weightlifters and tennis players (Creamer & Hochberg 1997; Cooper et al. 1998, 2000; Nuki 2002). Activities such as jogging and even marathon running do not seem to confer excess risk as long as the joints being stressed are biomechanically normal (Creamer & Hochberg 1997; Nuki 2002).

3.5.2   Joint trauma and surgery

Major trauma to a joint or previous joint surgery is also associated with increased risk of developing OA in that joint. Meniscus injury predisposes to OA: nearly 50% of patients have knee OA 21 years after open meniscectomy, while the average time to develop secondary hip OA following fracture dislocation is seven years (Nuki 2002). In a UK study of 611 patients listed for hip replacement, OA of the hip was strongly associated with hip injury (OR 4.3; 95% CI 2.2–8.4) (Cooper et al. 1998).

Unilateral hip osteoarthritis can also result from congenital dislocation of the hip, acetabular dysplasia, Perthes disease and slipped capital epiphysis (Harris 1986).

3.5.3   Load distribution and malalignment

Alterations in the mechanical environment of the joint adversely affect load distribution (Felson et al. 2000). Limb malalignment, both static (standing) and dynamic (moving), is an important factor in joint space loss, the latter being more predictive of progression (Lohmander et al. 2004). Varus and valgus alignments have shown association with fourfold increases in medial and lateral compartment knee OA respectively over an 18-month period (Nuki 2002). Knee laxity, displacement or rotation of the tibia with respect to the femur, also predisposes to disease development as does poor proprioception, which is critical to the maintenance of joint stability in motion (Felson et al. 2000).

3.5.4   Muscle weakness

Quadriceps muscle weakness not only results from disuse atrophy associated with painful knee OA but pre-existing quadriceps weakness is a risk factor for structural damage to the joint (Felson et al. 2000). A relatively small increase in quadriceps strength (20–25%) was predicted to result in a 20–30% decrease in the odds of having OA of the knee (Felson et al. 2000).

3.6   Obesity

Obesity is a clear risk factor for OA, in particular OA of the knee and hip. For each one pound increase in weight, the overall force across the knee in a single leg stance increases by two to three pounds (Felson et al. 2000).

A number of case control and prospective studies of the effect of obesity of OA risk have been carried out by a group in Southampton, UK. Obesity was found to be a significant independent risk factor (OR 1.7; 95% CI 1.3, 2.4) for hip OA in 611 patients listed for hip replacement (Cooper et al. 1998). When 525 patients listed for knee replacement were compared with matched controls, the risk of knee OA was found to increase progressively with body mass index (BMI) (Coggon et al. 2001). A prospective study in 354 men and women assessed by radiographs at baseline and five-year follow-up, showed that the risk of incident knee OA was increased more than 18-fold in those in the top third of BMI at baseline compared to those in the bottom third (Cooper et al. 2000).

North American studies have come to similar conclusions. A Canadian study showed a significantly elevated odds ratio for obesity (1.6) in association with subsequent arthritis in both men and women (Wilkins 2004). Data from the US National Health and Nutrition Examination Survey (NHANES) showed that men and women with a BMI of 30–35 kg/m^2 had a fourfold increase in knee OA compared with normal weight controls (Nuki 2002). Women from the Nurses' Health

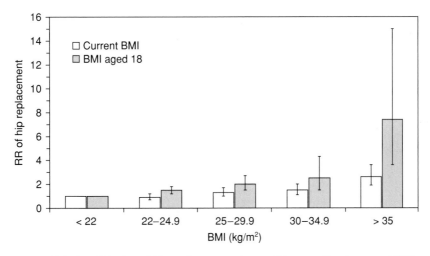

Figure 3.4 Relative risk of total hip replacement due to OA according to current BMI and BMI aged 18 (drawn by Alexander Thompson using data from Karlson et al. 2003a).

study with a BMI over 35 kg/m^2 had a significantly greater (twofold) risk of hip replacement, due to OA, than those with a BMI of 22 kg/m^2 (Karlson et al. 2003a). The same study found that those who were in the highest category of BMI at age 18 years, had a more than fivefold increased risk, suggesting that the risk for hip osteoarthritis is established early in life (see Figure 3.4).

Weight loss can be beneficial in reducing the risk of OA. Observational data from the Framingham OA study suggested that obesity precedes the development of knee OA with a 40% increase in risk (RR 1.4, 95% CI 1.1, 1.8) for every 5 kg (11 lb) gain in weight (Nuki 2002), or alternatively expressed, weight loss of approximately 5 kg will reduce a person's risk of development of knee OA over the subsequent 10 years by 50% (Felson et al. 1992).

There is evidence that obesity is also a risk factor for RA: a case control study of 349 cases and 1457 controls, showed that women in the highest quartile of BMI had a higher relative risk of RA compared to individuals with the lowest BMI (RR 1.4; 95% CI 1.0, 2.0) (Voigt et al. 1994). However, the US Nurses' Health Study found no association between BMI and RA (Hernandez-Avila et al. 1990). Similarly, a study of risk factors for RA in a cohort of 31 336 older women which also examined a series of anthropometric factors – height, weight, BMI and body fat distribution – found no association of any of these factors with RA (Cerhan et al. 2002). The NOAR study of 165 case control sets showed that the association for both genders was with obesity rather than overweight: having a BMI greater than or equal to 30 kg/m^2 was associated with an adjusted odds ratio (OR) of 3.7 (95% CI 1.1, 12.3) for developing RA. The association with obesity but not overweight may perhaps help to explain some of the discrepancy between study results.

To confuse the issue, however, slight overweight among RA patients is associated with less rapid destruction of joints and slower disease progression (Kaufmann et al. 2003). This is probably because pro-inflammatory cytokines such as TNF-α and IL-1 play a key role both in inflammation-mediated loss of weight and joint destruction (Kaufmann et al. 2003). Thus low BMI was found to be associated with faster disease progression as shown by radiological joint damage in RA patients (Kaufmann et al. 2003).

Clearly the increased mechanical load on weightbearing joints such as the hip, knee or feet resulting from obesity is likely to put extra strain on these joints. However, increase in adiposity is also associated with worsening symptoms in non-weightbearing joints such as the hand (Creamer & Hochberg 1997). This association is probably explained by the fact that adipose tissue itself functions as an endocrine organ (Hauner 2005). Obesity increases endogenous oestrogen production, particularly in postmenopausal women (Voigt et al. 1994), which may be associated with positive or negative consequences (see section 3.11). More importantly perhaps, it has recently been recognised that adipose tissue is highly reactive metabolically, secreting a variety of factors with inflammatory and other effects (Hauner & Hochberg 2002; Hauner 2005). As expressed by Conway and Rene (2004):

> *'The adipocyte not only stores lipid, but also acts as an endocrine cell. It releases the hormone leptin, TNF-α, resistin and other cytokines, complement proteins such as adipsin, adiponectin, prothrombic agents, substrates (free fatty acids, glycerol), enzymes such as aromatase (which synthesises oestrogen) and angiotensin.'*

Angiotensin II, for instance, stimulates the production of IL-6 and IL-8, and promotes the expression of leptin, contributing to chronic inflammation (Hauner 2005). Convincing evidence also exists that obesity is associated with the accumulation of macrophages in adipose tissue (Hauner 2005). Macrophages are responsible for almost all the adipose tissue TNF-α expression and the production of major amounts of other inflammatory markers (Hauner 2005).

Thus high BMI is associated not only with the accumulation of magrophages and production of the pro-inflammatory cytokines, IL-6 and TNF-α, and other inflammatory proteins in adipose tissue, but also with decreased production of the anti-inflammatory adiponectin, inducing low grade systemic inflammation in persons with excess body fat (Visser et al. 1999; Hauner & Hochberg 2002; Hauner 2005). This has been confirmed by the finding of a significant increase in C-reactive protein (CRP), a marker of inflammation, in overweight or obese subjects compared to normal weight subjects in the Third National Health and Nutrition Examination Survey (NHANES) in the US (Visser et al. 1999). Thus the chronic inflammation associated with high BMI may account for at least some of the excess risk of RA and OA in these subjects. The good news is that weight reduction is accompanied with an improvement in the inflammatory secretory pattern (Hauner 2005).

3.7 Smoking

Smoking, known to be associated with the production of rheumatoid factor, has been found to be a risk factor for RA in men (Heliövaara et al. 1993; Uhlig et al. 1999; Krishnan 2003) though less consistently so in women. A large Finnish prospective study on 24 445 women and 28 364 men in whom 512 incident cases of RA developed, showed the relative risk of RF-positive RA to be 2.6 (95% CI 1.3, 5.3) in male ex-smokers and 3.8 (95% CI 2.0, 6.9) in current male smokers compared to men who had never smoked (Heliövaara et al. 1993). Smoking did not predict RF-positive RA in women nor RF-negative RA in either men or women (Heliövaara et al. 1993). In a later Finnish study of 1095 RA patients and 1530 controls, a past history of smoking was associated with increased risk of RA overall in men (OR 2.0; 95% CI 1.2, 3.2) but not in women (Krishnan 2003). Among men, the effect was only seen in those with rheumatoid factor-positive RA and indeed the association between smoking and RF-positive RA is recognised as meeting the Bradford Hill criteria for causation (Krishnan 2003). In an associated US study with 644 RA cases and 1509 geographically matched controls, ever having smoked was found to be a significant risk factor for RA (OR 2.31; 95% CI 1.36, 3.94) with an increasing gradient of risk as exposure to smoking increased (Krishnan 2003). The risk of RA associated with smoking in this study seemed also to be linked to the gender of the individual, being greater in men. Similar results were obtained in the UK where RA was found to be associated with ever having smoked cigarettes (OR 1.7; 95% CI 1.0, 3.7) in the NOAR cohort (Symmons & Harrison 2000).

An effect was found in women in a population-based case control study of 349 US women with RA and 1457 controls: women with 20 or more pack years of smoking had one and a half times the risk of RA of those who had never smoked (Voigt et al. 1994). In the large prospective Nurses' Health Study (Hernandez-Avila et al. 1990), current and former cigarette smokers showed a non-significant increased risk of RA while in a UK study (Vessey et al. 1987), the rate of referral of women to hospital for RA was strongly associated with cigarette smoking. In contrast to these results, one study in the Netherlands comparing 135 young women with RA to 378 controls with OA or soft tissue rheumatism found smoking to be protective: the adjusted risk of RA in women who smoked at least one cigarette per day compared to those who did not smoke was 0.61 (95% CI 0.42, 0.89) (Hazes et al. 1990).

A number of the studies described above suggest the presence of an underlying gender-specific factor that modifies the association between smoking, production of RF and RA. This factor may well be hormonal as suggested by the fact that in women only cohorts, an association between smoking and RA appeared to be dependent on menopausal status of participants (Krishnan et al. 2003).

Symmons and Harrison (2000) have suggested that it is possible that factors associated with smoking, such as a poor diet, may actually be responsible for the development of RA.

3.8   Dietary factors

Any study of prevalent cases of arthritis will be confounded by changes in eating habits subsequent to disease onset (Symmons & Harrison 2000) so ideally, prospective studies are required to investigate the role of dietary factors in the aetiology of arthritis. Unfortunately, relatively few of the studies carried out have been prospective studies. Furthermore, the methodology used in assessing dietary intake is prone to error, and at best, rather inaccurate. In addition, food frequency questionnaires are not always validated. These factors must be borne in mind when drawing conclusions from the data presented below.

Though there is little evidence for an effect of dietary factors on susceptibility to OA, there is considerably more evidence for an effect in RA. The role of diet in susceptibility to RA has been systematically reviewed by Pattison and colleagues (2004a). Results from 14 studies that examined dietary intake or biological markers prior to the onset of RA were included. There was evidence of a protective effect of higher consumption of olive oil, fish, fruit, cooked vegetables, β-cryptoxanthin (a carotenoid) and vitamin C. However, the authors concluded that though there was evidence that diet may play a role in the aetiology of RA, the evidence was inconclusive owing to the small number of studies available and the heterogeneity of study design. Studies looking at various dietary factors are summarised below. As vitamin D is obtained from the action of sunlight on the skin as well as from the diet, it is treated separately from purely dietary factors (see section 3.9).

3.8.1 Olive oil

Two Greek studies, neither of which was prospective, found a strong negative association between greater olive oil consumption and RA risk (see Pattison et al. 2004a). The odds of developing RA were 0.38 (95% CI 0.17, 0.85) for those in the highest quartile of intake compared to those in the lowest quartile of intake (Linos et al. 1999).

3.8.2 Fish and n-3 polyunsaturated fatty acid (PUFA)

High fish consumption also seems to be protective: more than two servings of broiled or baked fish per week compared to less than one serving gave a significantly reduced risk of developing RA (OR 0.57; 95% CI 0.35, 0.93) in a population case-control study (Shapiro et al. 1996). Shapiro and colleagues suggested that the beneficial effect of fish intake was related to the n-3 PUFA content of the fish and indeed, for RF-positive RA, they found a significant protective trend with increasing quartiles of n-3 PUFA intake. In contrast to the Greek studies, no protective effect of olive oil was seen.

3.8.3 Meat

An ecological study that compared data for RA prevalence in up to 15 countries with components of the national food supply found that there was a strong association (r^2 0.88, $p < 0.001$) with intake of fat from meat and offal and a slightly weaker association with meat and offal themselves (Grant 2000). Grant suggests that meat fat, iron and nitrite may contribute to the association. While such a study design can be criticised, a later prospective study also found an association with red meat and meat product consumption (Pattison et al. 2004b). A nested case control study in the UK EPIC–Norfolk cohort identified 88 cases of inflammatory polyarthritis, defined as a history of having two or more swollen joints lasting for four weeks or more and known to be a potential precursor of RA. Subjects in the highest third of intake of red meat and meat products combined had more than twice the risk (OR 2.3; 95% CI 1.1, 4.9) of developing inflammatory polyarthritis than those in the lowest third of intake (Pattison et al. 2004b). However, Pattison and colleagues point out that meat may act as a marker for a group of persons with an increased risk from other lifestyle causes.

3.8.4   Fruit and vegetables

Two studies found a weak negative association between fruit intake and risk of RA (Cerhan et al. 2003; Shapiro et al. 1996) while one found an effect of composite fruit and vegetable consumption (Pattison et al. 2004c). A significant inverse association was found between the highest category of vegetable intake and arthritis (type unspecified, but probably any musculoskeletal condition reported) in a study using data from the Italian Multipurpose Household survey (La Vecchia et al. 1998; Pattison et al. 2004d). In a Greek case control study, higher intakes of cooked vegetables were significantly associated with a reduced risk of RA: those in the highest quartile of intake had only one-quarter of the risk of those in the lowest quartile (Linos et al. 1999). Data from the prospective Iowa Women's Health Study showed a nearly significant protective effect of intake of cruciferous vegetables in those eating more than 11 servings per month compared with those eating fewer than six servings per month (RR 0.65; 95% CI 0.42, 1.01; p = 0.07) (Cerhan et al. 2003).

3.8.5   Antioxidants

Two prospective nested case-control Finnish studies and one US study of serum antioxidants (see sections 8.3.2, 8.4.3 and Pattison et al. 2004a) showed lower concentrations of α-tocopherol, β-carotene, retinol and selenium in samples collected before RA disease onset, though the difference only reached significance for β-carotene (Comstock et al. 1997) and selenium, the latter being significant only in RF-negative subjects (RR 0.16; 95% CI 0.04, 0.69) (Knekt et al. 2000). In one of the Finnish studies, a significantly higher risk of RA was observed in the lowest tertile of antioxidant index compared with the highest tertile. There appears to be no evidence for a protective effect of antioxidant micronutrients against OA development despite the production of damaging ROS by human chondrocytes. Though the Framingham Knee OA Cohort Study showed that vitamin C retarded the progression of OA, there was no evidence for a reduction in the risk of incident RA by vitamin C, β-carotene or α-tocopherol (McAlindon et al. 1996).

3.8.6   Vitamin C

The association of intake of vitamin C and risk of inflammatory polyarthritis was investigated in a nested case control study in the UK EPIC–Norfolk cohort mentioned above where 73 cases were identified (Pattison et al. 2004c). The study showed that people in the lowest category of vitamin C intake compared with the highest, had a greater than threefold risk of developing inflammatory polyarthritis (OR 3.3, 95% CI 1.4, 7.9). Intakes of less than 56 mg/d formed the lowest category of vitamin C intake in this study yet 56 mg/d is above the current UK RNI of 40 mg/d. Pattison and colleagues (2004c) point out, however, that vitamin C may be a marker of intake of fruit, which has many more protective constituents.

3.8.7 β-Cryptoxanthin

β-cryptoxanthin is present in only a few commonly eaten fruit, notably oranges, some tropical fruit and bell peppers (Pattison et al. 2005). The prospective Iowa Women's Health Study found that intake of β-cryptoxanthin protected against the development of RA (RR 0.59; 95% CI 0.39, 0.90; p = 0.01) (Cerhan et al. 2003). This was supported by a later prospective study in the EPIC–Norfolk cohort that identified 88 incident cases of inflammatory polyarthritis (Pattison et al. 2005). The mean daily intake of zeaxanthin was 20% lower and that of β-cryptoxanthin 40% lower in the 88 cases than in 176 age and sex matched controls. The β-cryptoxanthin intake in this cohort was attributed mainly to the consumption of oranges, orange juice and satsumas. The association with β-cryptoxanthin was significant after adjustments for total energy and protein intake and for cigarette smoking were made: for the highest third *vs.* lowest third of intake, the risk of developing RA was reduced by almost 60% (OR 0.42; 95% CI 0.20, 0.88; p for trend 0.02). Owing to the strong correlation between the intakes of β-cryptoxanthin and vitamin C, when adjustment for vitamin C intake was made, the association with β-cryptoxanthin, though of similar magnitude, no longer reached significance. Pattison and colleagues point out that the difference between the top and bottom thirds of β-cryptoxanthin intake represents just one glass of freshly squeezed orange juice per day.

3.9 Vitamin D

Vitamin D appears to protect against both RA and OA susceptibility. Vitamin D may come from the diet (vitamin D_2 in foods of plant origin, vitamin D_3 in foods of animal origin) or from the action of sunlight (UVB) on the skin (vitamin D_3) (see section 8.7). It is converted into the active hormone, calcitriol (1,25-dihydroxyvitamin D_3), by hydroxylation reactions in the liver and kidneys (see Figure 8.2).

Low vitamin D status has been implicated in the aetiology of autoimmune diseases such as RA, probably because vitamin D has a role in the development of self-tolerance (Cantorna and Mahon 2004). Vitamin D and 1,25-dihydroxy vitamin D_3 regulate T-helper cell (Th1) development by inhibiting Th1 and inducing other $CD4^+$ T-cell populations including regulatory T-cells and Th-2 cells. If there is inadequate vitamin D, the immune system tends towards the development of self-reactive Th-1 cells and autoimmunity (Cantorna & Mahon 2004). Polymorphisms in the vitamin D receptor have been correlated with increased susceptibility to RA (for references, see Cantorna & Mahon 2004). The association of supplemental

Table 3.2 Relative risks and 95% confidence intervals (CI) for RA according to vitamin D intake from foods and supplements: data from the Iowa Women's Health Study 1986–97 (adapted from Merlino et al. 2004).

Vitamin D intake, IU/D (μg/d)			Cases of RA	RR (95% CI)	P for trend
Total	< 221	(< 5.5)	64	1.00 (referent)	
	221–468	(5.5–11.7)	42	0.67 (0.45, 1.01)	
	≥ 468	(≥ 11.7)	46	0.67 (0.44, 1.00)	0.05
Dietary	< 169	(< 4.2)	59	1.00 (referent)	
	169–290	(4.2–7.3)	50	0.87 (0.58, 1.29)	
	≥ 290	(≥ 7.3)	43	0.72 (0.46, 1.14)	0.16
Supplemental	Nonusers		109	1.00 (referent)	
	< 400	(< 10)	13	0.65 (0.36, 1.15)	
	≥ 400	(≥ 10)	30	0.66 (0.43, 1.00)	0.03

and dietary vitamin D and RA risk was investigated in a prospective cohort of 29 368 women, aged 55–59 (the Iowa Women's Health study), with no history of RA at baseline (Merlino et al. 2004). Both dietary (food frequency questionnaire) and supplemental vitamin D were inversely associated with RA risk in these older women (see Table 3.2).

Vitamin D might also be expected to influence the development of OA, as chondrocytes in osteoarthritic cartilage can develop vitamin D receptors (Felson et al. 2000). Data from Keen and colleagues (1997) showed a significant association between a Taq I polymorphism of the vitamin D receptor gene on chromosome 12 and early knee OA (OR 2.82; 95% CI 1.16, 6.85, for the 'T' compared to the 't' allele), while high levels of vitamin D were found to protect against both incident and progressive hip OA (Lane et al. 1999; Felson et al. 2000). The effect of vitamin D was investigated within the Framingham OA Cohort study. Two measures of vitamin D status were assessed – dietary intake and serum 25-hydroxyvitamin D. Though vitamin D appeared to reduce disease progression, it did not have any effect on the risk of new onset OA, nor was any link found with the vitamin D receptor polymorphism at the Bsm I site and OA occurrence (McAlindon & Felson 1997; Baldwin et al. 2002).

Low vitamin D status is widespread at northern latitudes in the general population: levels of UVB irradiation at these latitudes is low, there is an age related decline in the ability of vitamin D to be synthesised in the skin after exposure to UVB light and the vitamin D content of most foods is low (see section 8.7).

3.10 Beverage consumption

3.10.1 Coffee and tea

Suggestive associations between the risk of RA and the consumption of coffee, decaffeinated coffee and tea have been found, but the data are inconsistent (Karlson et al. 2003b). Among the 31 336 women included in the Iowa Women's Health Study, a prospective cohort study, 158 cases of RA were identified (Mikuls et al. 2002). Decaffeinated coffee intake (≥ 4 cups per day) was shown to be positively and independently associated with RA onset (RR, 2.58; 95% CI 1.63, 4.06), while tea intake (> 3 cups per day) was shown to have an inverse association with disease risk (RR 0.39, 95% CI 0.16, 0.97). There was no association with caffeinated coffee. In contrast, a Finnish study found that an intake of four or more cups of 'regular' coffee per day increased the risk of developing RF-positive RA but not RF-negative RA (Heliövaara et al. 2000). The authors have suggested that coffee consumption may be related to risk of RA through mechanisms contributing to the production of RF (Heliövaara et al. 2000).

A third study came to a different conclusion from both of these. In the Nurses' Health Study, a prospective longitudinal study, the influence of coffee, decaffeinated coffee, total coffee, tea and overall caffeine consumption on the risk of RA were investigated by means of food frequency questionnaires completed at baseline (1980) and every four years thereafter until 1998 (Karlson et al. 2003b). Of 83 124 women who completed the questionnaires at baseline, 480 were later diagnosed with RA. No significant associations were found between any of the beverages studied and RA risk (Karlson et al. 2003b). The strength of this study is that information on beverage intake and potential confounders was revised every four years. The authors suggest that previous studies that found a positive association between RA and coffee drinking may have been confounded by smoking, noting that in their own study, coffee drinkers were found to be 25% less likely to stop smoking over the follow up period than non-coffee drinkers (Karlson et al. 2003b). However, this cannot account for the different results found for caffeinated and decaffeinated coffee drinkers in the Iowa Women's Health Study (Mikuls et al. 2002).

3.10.2 Alcohol

In the study by Hazes and colleagues (1990) described above (3.7), the possible association between RA risk and alcohol intake was also investigated. They found alcohol intake to be protective: the risk of RA in women who consumed alcohol at least once per day compared to non-drinkers was 0.52 (95% CI 0.33, 0.84). However, information was only gathered at the time of first visit to the rheumatology clinic and not at the onset of RA symptoms, which may have influenced the results: it is not known whether onset of RA would alter an individual's behaviour in terms of alcohol consumption. These findings are supported by those of another study: Voigt and colleagues (1994), comparing 349 cases of RA and 1457 controls found that postmenopausal women who consumed over 14 alcoholic drinks per week were at decreased risk of RA compared to non-drinkers (RR, 0.5; 95% CI 0.2, 1.7). However, in a cohort of older American women (the Iowa Women's Health Study), Cerhan and colleagues (2002) found no effect of alcohol use on RA risk.

3.11 Hormones, OA and RA

The presence of oestrogen receptors in cartilage suggests a role there for oestrogen. This may be mediated by cytokines: oestrogens inhibit the production of Th1 pro-inflammatory cytokines such as IL-12, TNF-α and IFNγ whereas they stimulate the production of Th2 anti-inflammatory cytokines such as IL-10, IL-4 and TGF-β (Salem 2004). IL-1 and TNF-α, which can be produced by both cartilage and synovium, potentiate the synthesis and activation of enzymes (such as matrix metalloproteinases) that degrade cartilage matrix (Felson & Nevitt 1998). Oestrogen also has complex effects on the growth hormone–growth factor axis that can result in synthesis and repair of cartilage matrix through the action of IGF-1 and TGF-β (Felson & Nevitt 1998). Thus the effects of oestrogen are not straightforward. As endogenous oestrogen production increases with obesity, particularly among postmenopausal women (Voigt et al. 1994), obesity must be treated as a confounding factor in hormonal studies.

Evidence suggests that age at menarche, oral contraceptive use, termination of pregnancy, lactation and short fertile period are possible hormonal risk factors for RA (Krishnan 2003). When compared with women who experienced menarche at age 13 years, the age adjusted relative risk of RA among women with early menarche was 1.9 (95% CI 0.9–2.4) (Hernandez-Avila et al. 1990). The Nurses' Health Study similarly reported a higher risk of RA associated with early menarche and with irregular menstrual cycles (Karlson et al. 2004). Breastfeeding for between 12 and 23 months was inversely related to the risk of RA (RR 0.8, 95% CI 0.6, 1.0) with a significant trend (P = 0.001) towards lower risk with longer duration of breastfeeding (Karlson et al. 2004). Women have a reduced susceptibility to RA during pregnancy though an increased susceptibility in the immediate postpartum period (Symmons & Harrison 2000). Studies suggest that an adverse pregnancy outcome, either spontaneous or iatrogenic, may be a risk factor for subsequent development of RA (Symmons & Harrison 2000).

During the menopause, a dramatic reduction in circulating oestrogen occurs. While some studies have shown a peak in the incidence of RA in the perimenopausal years, others, notably the Norfolk Arthritis Register (NOAR) case control study, have found no link between menopausal status and the onset of RA (Symmons & Harrison 2000).

OA is more prevalent in women than men, its incidence increasing dramatically in the years after the menopause, suggesting a connection with hormonal alterations, in particular oestrogen deficiency (Reginster et al. 2003). In women, the prevalence of OA in the hand, hip and knee increases rapidly after age 50 (Felson & Nevitt 1998). For instance, menopausal arthritis, a rapidly progressing OA that affects the hand, occurs at the time of the menopause (Felson & Nevitt 1998). Despite these findings, overall the evidence for a role of oestrogen in OA is conflicting (Felson & Nevitt 1998; Nuki 2002).

Hormone replacement therapy (HRT) or oestrogen replacement therapy (ERT) can counterbalance the effects of oestrogen deprivation after the menopause, but its benefits in OA and RA are much debated. High bone mass and bone density are linked with OA. Oestrogen therapy reduces bone turnover and thus could help stabilise OA by slowing subchondral bone remodelling (Felson & Nevitt 1998). Women on ERT have a lower than expected risk of radiographic OA of the knee and hip (Felson & Nevitt 1998). However, the evidence for using HRT to prevent or treat OA and RA is limited mainly to observational studies. While most observational trials have suggested a protective effect of HRT on the prevalence of OA and on its long-term structural progression (Reginster et al. 2003), some have observed an increased risk (Felson & Nevitt 1998). Randomised trials of HRT or ERT are required to clarify the situation.

3.12   Medical risk factors for RA

3.12.1   Infection and micro-organisms

It has been suggested that infections with certain organisms could lead to the development of antibodies that recognise self-HLA molecules. For instance, the Epstein–Barr virus has an amino acid sequence in its glycoprotein B that also occurs in the HLA-DR molecule (Howell et al. 2002). *Escherichia (E.) Coli* and *Proteus* infections, in addition to parvovirus and rubella have also been linked to the development of RA in some cases (Howell et al. 2002; Symmons & Harrison 2000).

Arthritis, not otherwise explained, has been noted in 2% to 20% of subjects infected with hepatitis C virus, which has the characteristics of RA in two-thirds of those affected (Rosner et al. 2004). Rubella, tetanus and influenza immunisations have also been known to trigger RA in some susceptible hosts, though such individuals make up only a tiny fraction of RA cases (Symmons & Harrison 2000).

Carty and colleagues (2004) reviewed studies that investigated the possible role of infection in the aetiology of RA. They concluded that there was no overwhelming evidence to link any single known infectious agent with RA but pinpointed mycoplasmas and a human retrovirus (HRV-5) as being worthy of closer study.

Toivanen (2003) has suggested that normal intestinal microbiota in some people, which to a certain extent are genetically regulated, may induce arthritis. Patients with early RA have intestinal microflora significantly different to those of controls. Cell walls of several bacterial species representing normal human intestinal microbiota are arthritogenic in animal experiments and certain peptidoglycans, crucial components of bacterial cell walls, are known to stimulate rheumatoid factor production and severe chronic arthritis (Toivanen 2003). This hypothesis could go some way to explaining why clinical improvement has been linked in some people to a change to a vegan or vegetarian diet which caused changes in the intestinal microflora (Toivanen 2003).

3.12.2   Blood transfusions

A previous history of blood transfusions has shown opposite effects on risk of RA in two studies. In the NOAR cohort study, which had 165 case control pairs, RA was significantly positively associated with a history of blood transfusion (OR 4.83, 95% CI 1.29, 18.07) (Symmons & Harrison 2000). In an American cohort study of older women (the Iowa Women's Health Study) in which 158 cases of RA developed over 10 years, a history of blood transfusion was inversely associated with RA (multivariate RR 0.72; 95% CI 0.48, 1.08) particularly RF-positive RA (Cerhan et al. 2002). Further studies are clearly necessary to clarify the situation.

3.12.3 Haemochromatosis

Arthritis symptoms are common in individuals with the iron overload disease, haemochromatosis, characterised by increased iron absorption and tissue deposition (Jordan 2004). Several studies have shown a higher frequency of homozygous or heterozygous HFE mutations in individuals with various types of arthritis, compared with unselected populations (Jordan 2004). This may relate to the ability of free iron to catalyse oxidative stress in the joint.

References

Baldwin CT, Cupples LA, Joost O, Demissie S, Chaisson C, McAlindon T, Myers RH, Felson D (2002) Absence of linkage or association for osteoarthritis with the vitamin D receptor/type II collagen locus: the Framingham Osteoarthritis Study. *Journal of Rheumatology* **29**(1), 161–65.

Brinkman BMN, Huizinga TWJ, Kurban SS, Van der Velder EA, Schreuder GM, Hazes JMW, Breedveld FC, Verweij CL (1997) Tumor necrosis factor alpha gene polymorphisms in rheumatoid arthritis: association with susceptibility to, or severity of, disease? *British Journal of Rheumatology* **36**, 516–21.

Cantorna MT, Mahon BD (2004) Mounting evidence for vitamin D as an environmental factor affecting autoimmune disease prevalence. *Experimental Biology and Medicine* **229**(11), 1136–42.

Carlo MD Jr, Loeser RF (2003) Increased oxidative stress with aging reduces chondrocyte survival: correlation with intracellular glutathione levels. *Arthritis and Rheumatism* **48**(12), 3419–30.

Carty S, Snowden N, Silman A (2004) Should infection still be considered as the most likely triggering factor for rheumatoid arthritis? *Annals of the Rheumatic Diseases* **63**(Suppl II), ii46–ii49.

Cerhan JR, Saag KG, Criswell LA, Merlino LA, Mikuls TR (2002) Blood transfusion, alcohol use, and anthropometric risk factors for rheumatoid arthritis in older women. *Journal of Rheumatology* **29**(2), 246–54.

Cerhan JR, Saag KG, Merlino LA, Mikuls TR, Criswell LA (2003) Antioxidant micronutrients and risk of rheumatoid arthritis in a cohort of older women. *American Journal of Epidemiology* **15**, 157(4), 345–54.

Cheung NT, Dawes PT, Poulton KV, Ollier WE, Taylor DJ, Mattey DL (2000) High serum levels of pro-matrix metalloproteinase-3 are associated with greater radiographic damage and the presence of the shared epitope in patients with rheumatoid arthritis. *Journal of Rheumatology* **27**(4), 882–87.

Coggon D, Croft P, Kellingray S, Barrett D, McLaren M, Cooper C (2000) Occupational physical activities and osteoarthritis of the knee. *Arthritis and Rheumatism* **43**, 1443–9.

Coggon D, Reading I, Croft P, McLaren M, Barrett D, Cooper C (2001) Knee osteoarthritis and obesity. *International Journal of Obesity Related Metabolic Disorders* **25**, 622–7.

Comstock GW, Burke AE, Hoffman SC, Helzlsouer KJ, Bendich A, Masi AT, Norkus EP, Malamet RT, Gershwin (1997) Serum concentrations of alpha tocopherol, beta carotene and retinol preceding the diagnosis of rheumatoid arthritis and systemic lupus erythematosus. *Annals of the Rheumatic Diseases* **56**(5), 323–25.

Conway B, Rene A (2004) Obesity as a disease: no lightweight matter. *Obesity Reviews* 5(3), 145–51.

Cooper C, Inskip H, Croft P, Campbell L, Smith G, McLaran M, Coggon D (1998) Individual risk factors for hip osteoarthritis: obesity, hip injury, and physical activity. *American Journal of Epidemiology* 147(6), 516–22.

Cooper C, Snow S, McAlindon TE, Kellingray S, Stuart B, Coggon D, Dieppe PA (2000) Risk factors for the incidence and progression of radiographic knee osteoarthritis. *Arthritis and Rheumatism* 43(5), 995–1000.

Creamer P, Hochberg MC (1997) Osteoarthritis. *The Lancet* 350, 503–8.

Felson DT, Zhang Y, Anthony JM, Naimark A, Anderson JJ (1992) Weight loss reduces the risk for symptomatic knee osteoarthritis in women. The Framingham Study. *Annals of Internal Medicine* 1, 116(7), 535–39.

Felson DT, Nevitt MC (1998) The effects of estrogen on osteoarthritis. *Current Opinion in Rheumatology* 10(3), 269–72.

Felson DT, Lawrence RC, Dieppe PA, Hirsch R, Helmick CG, Jordan JM, Kington RS, Lane NE, Nevitt MC, Zhang Y, Sowers M, McAlindon T, Spector TD, Poole AR, Yanovski SZ, Ateshian G, Sharma L, Buckwalter JA, Brandt KD, Fries JF (2000) Osteoarthritis: new insights. Part 1: the disease and its risk factors. *Annals of Internal Medicine* 133, 635–46.

Grant WB (2000) The role of meat in the expression of rheumatoid arthritis. *British Journal of Nutrition* 84(5), 589–95.

Harris WH (1986) Aetiology of osteoarthritis of the hip. *Clinical Orthopaedics* 213, 20–33.

Hauner H, Hochberg Z (2002) Endocrinology of adipose tissue. *Hormone and Metabolic Research* 34(11–12), 605–6.

Hauner H (2005) Secretory factors from human adipose tissue and their functional role. *Proceedings of the Nutrition Society* 64, 163–69.

Hazes JM, Dijkmans BA, Vandenbroucke JP, de Vries RR, Cats A (1990) Lifestyle and the risk of rheumatoid arthritis: cigarette smoking and alcohol consumption. *Annals of the Rheumatic Diseases* 49(12), 980–82.

Heliövaara M, Aho K, Aromaa A, Knekt P, Reunanen A (1993) Smoking and risk of rheumatoid arthritis. *Journal of Rheumatology* 20(11), 1830–35.

Heliövaara M, Aho K, Knekt P, Impivaara O, Reunanen A, Aromaa A (2000) Coffee consumption, rheumatoid factor, and the risk of rheumatoid arthritis. *Annals of the Rheumatic Diseases* 59(8), 631–35.

Hernandez Avila M, Liang MH, Willett WC, Stampfer MJ, Colditz GA, Rosner B, Roberts WN, Hennekens CH, Speizer FE (1990) Reproductive factors, smoking, and the risk for rheumatoid arthritis. *Epidemiology* 1(4), 285–91.

Howell WM, Calder PC, Grimble RF (2002) Gene polymorphisms, inflammatory diseases and cancer. *Proceedings of the Nutrition Society* 61(4), 447–56.

Huizinga T (2003) Genetics in rheumatoid arthritis. *Best Practice and Research Clinical Rheumatology* 17, 703–16.

Ikeda T, Mabuchi A, Fukuda A, Kawakami A, Ryo Y, Yamamotos, Miyoshi K, Haga N, Hiraoka H, Takatori Y, Kawaguchi H, Nakamura K, Ikegawa S (2002) Association analysis of single nucleotide polymorphisms in cartilage-specific collagen genes with knee and hip osteoarthritis in the Japanese population. *Journal of Bone and Mineral Research* 17, 1290–96.

Jordan JM (2004) Arthritis in hemochromatosis or iron storage disease. *Current Opinion in Rheumatology* 16(1), 62–66.

Kaijzel EL, van Krugten MV, Brinkman BM, Huizinga TW, van der Straaten T, Hazes JM, Ziegler-Heitbrock HW, Nedospasov SA, Breedveld FC, Verweij CL (1998) Functional analysis of a human tumor necrosis factor alpha (TNF-alpha) promoter polymorphism related to joint damage in rheumatoid arthritis. *Molecular Medicine* 4, 724–33.

Karlson EW, Mandl LA, Aweh GN, Sangha O, Liang MH, Grodstein F (2003a) Total hip replacement due to osteoarthritis: the importance of age, obesity, and other modifiable risk factors. *American Journal of Medicine* 114, 93–98.

Karlson EW, Mandl LA, Aweh GN, Grodstein F (2003b) Coffee consumption and risk of rheumatoid arthritis. *Arthritis and Rheumatism* 48(11), 3055–60.

Karlson EW, Mandl LA, Hankinson SE, Grodstein F (2004) Do breast-feeding and other reproductive factors influence future risk of rheumatoid arthritis? Results from the Nurses' Health Study. *Arthritis and Rheumatism* 50, 3458–67.

Kaufmann J, Kielstein V, Kilian S, Stein G, Hein G (2003) Relation between body mass index and radiological progression in patients with rheumatoid arthritis. *Journal of Rheumatology* 30, 2350–55.

Keen RW, Hart DJ, Lanchbury JS, Spector TD (1997) Association of early osteoarthritis of the knee with a Taq I polymorphism of the vitamin D receptor gene. *Arthritis and Rheumatism* 40(8), 1444–9.

Knekt P, Heliövaara M, Aho K, Alfthan G, Marniemi J, Aromaa A (2000) Serum selenium, serum alpha-tocopherol, and the risk of rheumatoid arthritis. *Epidemiology* 1(4), 402–5.

Krishnan E (2003) Smoking, gender and rheumatoid arthritis – epidemiological clues to etiology. Results form the behavioural risk factor surveillance system. *Joint Bone Spine* 70(6), 496–502.

Lane NE, Gore LR, Cummings SR, Hochberg MC, Scott JC, Williams EN, Nevitt MC (1999) Serum vitamin D levels and incident changes of radiographic hip osteoarthritis: a longitudinal study. Study of Osteoporotic Fractures Research Group. *Arthritis and Rheumatism* 42(5), 854–60.

La Vecchia C, Decarli A, Pagano R (1998) Vegetable consumption and risk of chronic disease. *Epidemiology* 9(2), 208–10.

Linos A, Kaklamani VG, Kaklamani E, Koumantaki Y, Giziaki E, Papazoglou S, Mantzoros CS (1999) Dietary factors in relation to rheumatoid arthritis: a role for olive oil and cooked vegetables? *American Journal of Clinical Nutrition* 70(6), 1077–82. Erratum in: *American Journal of Clinical Nutrition* (2000) 71(4), 1010.

Loeser R (2004) Aging cartilage and osteoarthritis: what's the link? *Science of Aging Knowledge Environment* 29, 31.

Lohmander LS, Felson D (2004) Can we identify a 'high risk' patient profile to determine who will experience rapid progression of osteoarthritis? *Osteoarthritis Cartilage* 12, Suppl A, S49–52.

Martin JA, Buckwalter JA (2002) Articular cartilage chondrocyte senescence and osteoarthritis. *Biogerontology* 3(5), 257–64.

McAlindon TE, Jacques P, Zhang Y, Hannan MT, Aliabadi P, Weissman B, Rush D, Levy D, Felson DT (1996) Do antioxidant micronutrients protect against the development and progression of knee osteoarthritis? *Arthritis and Rheumatism* 39(4), 648–56.

McAlindon TE, Felson DT (1997) Nutrition: risk factors for osteoarthritis. *Annals of the Rheumatic Diseases* 56, 397–402.

McAlindon TE, Wilson PW, Aliabadi P, Weissman B, Felson DT (1999) Level of physical activity and the risk of radiographic and symptomatic knee osteoarthritis in the elderly: the Framingham study. *American Journal of Medicine* 106(2), 151–57.

Merlino LA, Curtis J, Mikulus TR, Cerhan JR, Criswell LA, Saag KG (2004) Vitamin D intake is inversely associated with rheumatoid arthritis: results from the Iowa Women's Health Study. *Arthritis and Rheumatism* 50(1), 72–77.

Mikuls TR, Cerhan JR, Criswell LA, Merlino L, Mudano AS, Burma M, Folsom AR, Saag KG (2002) Coffee, tea and caffeine consumption and risk of rheumatoid arthritis: results from the Iowa Women's Health Study. *Arthritis and Rheumatism* 46(1), 83–91.

Mustafa Z, Chapman K, Irven C, Carr AJ, Clipsham K, Chitnavis J, Sinsheimer JS, Bloomfield VA, McCartney M, Cox O, Sykes B, Loughlin J (2000) Linkage analysis of candidate genes as susceptibility loci for osteoarthritis-suggestive linkage of COL9A1 to female hip osteoarthritis. *Rheumatology* 39(3), 299–306.

Newton JL, Harney SM, Wordsworth BP, Brown MA (2004) A review of the MHC genetics of rheumatoid arthritis. *Genes and Immunity* 5(3), 151–7.

Nuki G (2002) Osteoarthritis: risk factors and pathogenesis. In: *Rheumatic Disease Topical Reviews*, September 2002, Number 9, (A Adebajo, ed). Chesterfield, Arthritis Research Campaign.

Oliveria S, Felson D, Reed J, Cirillo P, Walker A (1995) Incidence of symptomatic hand, hip and knee osteoarthritis among patients in a health maintenance organisation. *Arthritis and Rheumatism* 38, 1134–41.

Pattison D, Harris A, Symmons DP (2004a) The role of diet in susceptibility to rheumatoid arthritis: a systematic review. *Journal of Rheumatology* **31**(7), 1310–19.

Pattison DJ, Symmons DP, Lunt M, Welch A, Luben R, Bingham SA, Khaw KT, Day NE, Silman AJ (2004b) Dietary risk factors for the development of inflammatory polyarthritis: evidence for a role of high level of red meat consumption. *Arthritis and Rheumatism* **50**, 3804–12.

Pattison DJ, Silman AJ, Goodson NJ, Lunt M, Bunn D, Luben R, Welch A, Bingham S, Khaw KT, Day N, Symmons DP (2004c) Vitamin C and the risk of developing inflammatory polyarthritis: prospective case-control study. *Annals of the Rheumatic Diseases* **63**, 843–47.

Pattison DJ, Symmons DP, Young A (2004d) Does diet have a role in the aetiology of rheumatoid arthritis? *Proceedings of the Nutrition Society* **63**, 137–43.

Pattison DJ, Symmons DP, Lunt M, Welch A, Bingham SA, Day NE, Silman AJ (2005) Dietary beta-cryptoxanthin and inflammatory polyarthritis: results from a population-based prospective study. *American Journal of Clinical Nutrition* **82**, 451–55.

Reginster JY, Kvasz A, Bruyere O, Henrotin Y (2003) Is there any rationale for prescribing hormone replacement therapy (HRT) to prevent or to treat osteoarthritis? *Osteoarthritis and Cartilage* **11**(2), 87–91.

Rosner I, Rozenbaum M, Toubi E, Kessel A, Naschitz JE, Zuckerman E (2004) The case for hepatitis C arthritis. *Seminars in Arthritis and Rheumatism* **33**(6), 375–87.

Salem ML (2004) Estrogen, a double-edged sword: modulation of TH1- and TH2-mediated inflammations by differential regulation of TH1/TH2 cytokine production. *Current Drug Targets: Inflammation and Allergy* **3**(1), 97–104.

Shapiro JA, Koepsell TD, Voigt LF, Dugowson CE, Kestin M, Nelson JL (1996) Diet and rheumatoid arthritis in women: a possible protective effect of fish consumption. *Epidemiology* **7**(3), 256–63.

Spector TD, MacGregor AJ (2004) Risk factors for osteoarthritis: genetics. *Osteoarthritis Cartilage* **12**, S39–44.

Symmons D, Harrison B (2000) Early inflammatory polyarthritis: results from the Norfolk Arthritis Register with a review of the literature. I. Risk factors for the development of inflammatory polyarthritis and rheumatoid arthritis. *Rheumatology* **39**(8), 835–43.

Symmons D, Turner G, Webb R, Asten P, Barrett E, Lunt M, Scott D, Silman A (2002) The prevalence of rheumatoid arthritis in the United Kingdom: new estimates for a new century. *Rheumatology* **41**, 793–800.

Symmons D, Mathers C, Pfleger B (2003) *The Global Burden of Rheumatoid Arthritis in the Year 2000.* Geneva, World Health Organization. www3.who.int/whosis/menu.cfm?path= evidence,burden,burden_gbd2000docs,burden_gbd2000docs_diseasedoc,burden_ gbd2000docs_diseasedoc_ra&language=english

Toivanen P (2003) Normal intestinal microbiota in the aetiopathogenesis of rheumatoid arthritis. *Annals of the Rheumatic Diseases* **62**(9), 807–11.

Uhlig T, Hagen KB, Kvien TK (1999) Current tobacco smoking, formal education, and the risk of rheumatoid arthritis. *Journal of Rheumatology* **26**(1), 47–54.

Vessey MP, Villard-Mackintosh L, Yeates D (1987) Oral contraceptives, cigarette smoking and other factors in relation to arthritis. *Contraception* **35**(5), 457–64.

Visser M, Bouter LM, McQuillan GM, Wener MH, Harris TB (1999) Elevated C-reactive protein levels in overweight and obese adults. *Journal of the American Medical Association* **8**, 282(22), 2131–5.

Voigt LF, Koepsell TD, Nelson JL, Dugowson CE, Daling JR (1994) Smoking, obesity, alcohol consumption and the risk of rheumatoid arthritis. *Epidemiology* **5**, 525–32.

Wilkins K (2004) Incident arthritis in relation to excess weight. *Health Reports* **15**(1), 39–49.

4 Current management of osteoarthritis and rheumatoid arthritis

As there is no cure for osteoarthritis (OA) or rheumatoid arthritis (RA), treatment is aimed at management of symptoms and delaying of disease progression (Martin 1998).

Drug treatment has changed and evolved in recent years: previously, a treatment regimen known as the therapeutic pyramid was commonly used in RA. This used non-steroidal anti-inflammatory drugs (NSAIDs) (analgesia) for initial, first line, conservative management, often for many years, followed by introduction of disease modifying antirheumatic drugs (DMARDs) as second line treatment once joint erosions became apparent. Glucocorticoids were also commonly used, though not for initial treatment.

Partly as a result of research published in the 1980s, the treatment approach of the therapeutic pyramid has been rejected as inadequate for the following reasons (Pipitone & Choy 2003):

- RA is now recognised as causing substantial morbidity and mortality.
- Delayed DMARD treatment has been shown to lead to more damage.
- DMARDs are more effective in relieving symptoms than NSAIDs.
- DMARDs are more potent yet have a better safety profile.

Early institution of DMARD treatment is now widely advocated (Pipitone & Choy 2003). Addition of anti-cytokine (TNF-α blockers) therapy is an additional option for patients who have not responded to DMARDs (Pipitone & Choy 2003).

Treatment regimens should be tailored to individual patients. West (2002) gives the following advice for RA medication in clinical practice:

- Initial use of methotrexate (a DMARD), unless contraindicated.
- If this is unsuccessful, combination therapy should be tried using hydroxy-chloroquine, sulfasalazine or leflunomide (DMARDs) along with methotrexate.
- Improvement in symptoms and radiographic evidence of disease have been shown when etanercept or infliximab (anti-TNF-α drugs) are added alongside methotrexate, but effects of the long-term usage of these anti-TNF-α drugs are not known.

There are no disease modifying drugs available for OA, therefore treatment is aimed at symptom management (namely pain). Treatment is normally based on a

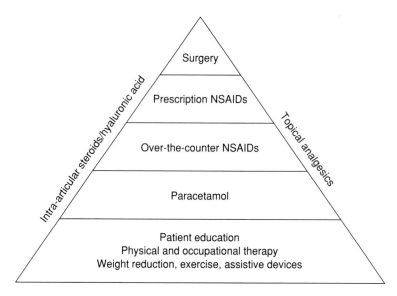

Figure 4.1 Pyramid approach to the management of OA (reproduced with permission from Creamer & Hochberg 1997).

pyramid approach as shown in Figure 4.1 – initially patient education, physical and occupational therapy, weight reduction and exercise, followed by full dose paracetamol (an analgesic) if pain becomes an issue. If patients are unresponsive to these simple analgesics, NSAID treatment may be started.

More detail on current medications available for OA and RA (analgesics, NSAIDs, DMARDs, biological agents and glucocorticoids) together with information on surgical management, physiotherapy and occupational therapy is given in the following sections.

4.2 Medication

4.2.1 Analgesia

Analgesic treatment is of primary importance for OA and RA sufferers as their condition may be severe and painful. Analgesics can be classified as non-opioid, such as paracetamol and low-dose aspirin (higher doses of aspirin have anti-inflammatory effects and are therefore classed as NSAIDs), or opioid analgesics, such as tramadol, morphine and dihydrocodeine (see Table 4.1, BNF 2005a). Opioid analgesics are far stronger than non-opioids and accordingly have greater side effects and adverse reactions. Dependency may also occur and thus in a long-term disease, such as RA or OA, they may not be appropriate (Hill 1998; West 2002).

Table 4.1 Opioid and non-opioid analgesics (adapted from BNF 2005a).

Non-opioid analgesics	aspirin
	paracetamol
	nefopam hydrochloride
Opioid analgesics	buprenorphine
	codeine phosphate
	diamorphine hydrochloride
	dihydrocodeine tartrate
	dipipanone hydrochloride
	fentanyl
	hydromorphone hydrochloride
	meptazinol
	methadone hydrochloride
	morphine salts
	nalbuphine hydrochloride
	oxycodone hydrochloride
	papaveretum
	pentazocine
	pethidine hydrochloride
	tramadol hydrochloride

4.2.2   Non-steroidal anti-inflammatory drugs (NSAIDs)

NSAIDs are prescribed for both OA and RA. They are able to suppress the classical features of inflammation (swelling, warmth, erythema, tenderness and loss of function) and:

> 'are indicated in situations where joint or soft tissue inflammation causes pain, stiffness and swelling.' (ARC for Research 1995).

Though they suppress the symptoms, they do not prevent disease progression (Wakley et al. 2001). NSAIDs inhibit cyclo-oxygenases (Cox), the enzymes that convert arachidonic acid to prostaglandins. Many prostaglandins are pro-inflammatory, so a fall in their level relieves inflammation and painful symptoms but there is also a downside.

It is now known that there are at least three forms of Cox (Loeser 2003). While Cox-2 produces the prostaglandins that mediate the inflammatory response, Cox-1 produces protective prostaglandins that mediate gastric protection and renal perfusion and reduce platelet aggregation (Wakley et al. 2001). Thus, while NSAIDs that inhibit Cox-1 or are non-specific in their action may provide effective relief from symptoms, serious gastrointestinal complications can occur with their use including abdominal pain, diarrhoea, nausea, vomiting, ulcers, perforations and bleeds (Deeks 2002). Many of the older NSAIDs appear to inhibit Cox-1 to a physiological degree, thereby explaining their well recognised gastrointestinal tract toxicity (McKenna 2000).

Up to a third of patients cannot tolerate NSAIDs because of dyspepsia, and there is a significant morbidity and mortality from the development of ulcers and

Table 4.2 Classification of NSAIDs and their ability to inhibit Cox-1 or Cox-2 action (adapted from West 2002).

Nomenclature	NSAIDs in this classification
Cox-1 selective/specific Cox non-selective/non-specific Cox-2 selective/preferential* Cox-2 highly selective/specific	low-dose aspirin ibuprofen, naproxen, meclomen, indomethacin etodolac, diclofenac, nabumetone, meloxicam celecoxib, rofecoxib, valdecoxib

* preferential – drugs that are partially selective for Cox-2

Table 4.3 NSAIDs and risk of serious upper GI side effects (adapted from BNF 2005b).

Level of risk	NSAID
Highest risk Intermediate risk Lowest risk	azapropazone piroxicam, ketoprofen, indometacin (indomethacin), naproxen, diclofenac sodium ibruprofen

their complications (McKenna 2000). The combination of NSAID and low dose aspirin may also increase the risk of gastrointestinal side effects. In 2002, Deeks estimated that there were between 2000–2500 deaths annually in the United Kingdom attributable to the use of NSAIDs.

Understanding of the different effects of Cox-1 and Cox-2 has led to the production of drugs that can be selective in their inhibition of a particular form of Cox (Table 4.2). Cox-1 is inhibited by the non-selective NSAIDs (such as ibuprofen), Cox-2 by both the non-selective and the Cox-2-selective inhibitors produced specifically for use in inflammatory arthritis (such as celecoxib, rofecoxib and valdecoxib) and Cox-3 by the non-selective inhibitors and some other analgesics such as acetaminophen (Loeser 2003).

However, even preferential Cox-2 inhibitors (e.g. etodolac) and highly selective Cox-2 inhibitors (e.g. rofecoxib and celecoxib) still have associated risks of gastrointestinal side effects and are contraindicated in people with a history of peptic ulcer, perforation or bleeding (Wakley et al. 2001). The level of risk associated with various NSAIDs is shown in Table 4.3 (BNF 2005b).

NSAID use is associated with a myriad of other side effects including acute renal failure, cardiac failure, liver toxicity, rashes, neutropenia and haemolytic anaemia and these drugs have a number of contraindications (BNF 2005b). The market leaders in Cox-2 inhibitors, rofecoxib (Vioxx, Merck) and celecoxib (Celebrex, Pharmacia, Pfizer) have been found to be associated with serious adverse effects. People taking Vioxx had a 34% higher chance of acute myocardial infarction than those taking other NSAIDs such as ibuprofen and aspirin and a 300% greater risk if taking a dose greater than 25 mg/d (Graham et al. 2005). Vioxx was estimated as having caused between 88 000 and 140 000 excess cases of serious heart disease (Graham et al. 2005). It was withdrawn in September 2004. Celebrex, used by 600 000 people in the UK, was found to have increased the risk of acute myocardial infarction and stroke 2.5-fold in patients taking 400 mg daily and 3.4-fold in those taking 800 mg daily in the course of a trial for the prevention of colorectal adenoma – the APC trial (Solomon et al. 2005). (In consequence, the APC trial was halted by the US National Cancer Institute.) The question then quite properly arose as to whether all Cox-2 inhibitors should be withdrawn. In February 2005, a Food and Drug Administration (FDA) advisory committee recommended that Cox-2 inhibitors should stay on the market but with stricter warnings on their labels about cardiovascular side effects (*The Economist* 2005). The committee also recommended tighter restrictions on consumer advertising of Cox-2 medicines. Patients and their doctors will have to assess the risks very carefully on an individual basis before taking Cox-2 inhibitors for relief of pain and inflammation: in all cases, the lowest effective dose should be used.

UK NICE (National Institute for Health and Clinical Excellence) guidelines (NICE 2001) for patients with OA and RA state that Cox-2 selective inhibitors should:

- Not be used routinely in the management of patients with these conditions.
- Be used in preference to standard NSAIDs only where clearly indicated, i.e. in patients at 'high risk' of gastroduodenal ulcers/perforation or GI bleeding.
- Not be used in preference to standard NSAIDs in patients with CVD.

The NICE guidelines on Cox-2 selective inhibitors are currently being reviewed in the light of the recent evidence of adverse cardiovascular events.

The influence that NSAIDs have on cartilage is unknown: some have been suggested to hasten joint damage (Rainsford et al. 1997); therefore in OA for example, simple analgesics should be considered first. If NSAID treatment is necessary, a low dose should initially be used.

Topical creams based upon NSAIDs or capsaicin are also on the market and may be used either on their own or in addition to analgesics. Though these are popular, they may not be of great value, and should not be used in the long term as they may cause local skin sensitivity and may lead to systemic side effects (Deal et al. 1991; Lin et al. 2004).

4.2.3   Disease-modifying antirheumatic drugs (DMARDs)

Though there is no cure for RA, its course may be altered with the aid of DMARDs, immunosuppressive agents. DMARDs are used as a monotherapy or combination therapy and have more recently been introduced alongside NSAIDS when RA is diagnosed. A DMARD is classified by having one of the following actions: over a period of at least one year, improvement in physical function, decreased inflammatory synovitis and prevention or slowing of structural joint damage (West 2002). There are many DMARDs in use (Table 4.4) including methotrexate, intramuscular and oral gold, hydroxychloroquine, sulfasalazine, D-penicillamine and leflunomide (West 2002). They normally take six weeks to six months to achieve significant improvements.

Currently the most widely prescribed DMARD is a weekly low dose of methotrexate used as a monotherapy: 7.5–25 mg of methotrexate is prescribed per week,

Table 4.4 DMARDS used, dosage and side effects (West 2002; White & Cooper 2002; Pipitone & Choy 2003).

	Indications	Dosage*	Time to benefit	Side effects*	Assessment/monitoring*
Auranofin (oral gold)	Active progressive RA	3–9 mg/day	4–6 months	Diarrhoea – most common (reduced with bulking agents), Leucopenia, Proteinuria, Rashes and pruritus, Nausea, Taste disturbances, Mouth ulcers	FBC Urine analysis U & Es LFTs
Gold therapy (IM)	Active progressive RA	25–50 mg weekly until improvement	3 months	Mouth ulcers, Skin reactions, Skin pigmentation, Proteinuria, Blood disorders, Severe reactions (occasionally fatal) in up to 5% of patients	FBC U & Es Urine dipstick Serum creatinine LFTs
Azathioprine	RA, where disease has not responded to other DMARDs	1–3 mg/kg/d	2–3 months	Dose-related bone marrow suppression, Hypersensitivity reactions, Cholestatic jaundice, Hair loss, Colitis, Increased susceptibility to infection, Liver impairment	FBC U & Es Creatinine LFTs
Cyclosporin	Severe active RA when conventional 2nd line therapy is ineffective/inappropriate	2.5–4 mg/kg/d	6 weeks to 3 months	Dose-dependent increase in serum creatinine, Renal structural changes, Hypertrichosis, Headaches, Tremor, Hypertension, Hepatic dysfunction, Fatigue, Gingival hypertrophy, GI disturbances, Burning sensation in hands/feet	FBC U & Es LFTs Serum creatinine Blood pressure

Drug	Indication	Dose		Side effects	Monitoring
Hydroxy-chloroquine sulphate	Active RA	200–400 mg/d (< 6.5 mg/kg ideal body weight)	3–6 months	GI disturbance, Headaches, Skin reactions	Ophthalmic exam every 6–12 months
Leflunomide	Moderate-severe active RA	10–20 mg/d	4 weeks to 6 months	Diarrhoea, Nausea, Vomiting, Anorexia, Oral mucosal disorders, Abdominal pain, Weight loss, Increase in blood pressure, Headache, Dizziness, Asthenia, Paraesthesia, Tenosynovitis, Alopecia, Eczema, Dry skin, Rash, Pruritus, Leucopenia	FBC LFTs Blood pressure
Methotrexate	Moderate-severe active RA	7.5–25 mg per week. 1–5 mg of folic acid should be given	6 weeks to 3 months	Side effects of cytotoxic drugs: Oral mucositis, Hyperuricaemia, Nausea and vomiting, Bone marrow suppression, Alopecia, Reproductive function	FBC U & Es Creatinine LFTs Chest X-ray
Penicillamine	Severe active RA	125–1000 mg/d	3–6 months	Nausea, Anorexia, Fever, Skin reactions, Blood disorders, Loss of taste, Haemolytic disorders, Nephrotic syndrome	Monthly FBC Urine dipstick
Sulfasalazine	Active RA	1–3 g/d	3 months	Rashes, GI intolerance, Leucopenia, Neutropenia, Thrombocytopenia, Hypersensitivity reactions, Loss of appetite, Fever, Blood disorders, Lung complications, Ocular complications, Stomatitis	FBC LFTs

* For complete information please refer to the latest edition of the British National Formulary (BNF)
FBC, full blood count; U & Es, urea and electrolytes; LFTs, liver function tests

often with folic acid (1–5 mg per day) as methotrexate is a known folate antagonist. The addition of folic acid reduces potential side effects such as gastrointestinal intolerance, and may prevent neutropenia. Folic acid supplementation does not appear to reduce the effectiveness of methotrexate (Griffith et al. 2000; Whittle & Hughes 2004). This drug treatment is effective and well tolerated and is now used when RA is diagnosed, unless contraindicated. Disease activity should be measured routinely to check the effectiveness of therapy and patients should be monitored for adverse effects that may indicate toxicity. Table 4.4 shows the recommended dosage, side effects and suggested monitoring indices of DMARDs used, including methotrexate (West 2002; White & Cooper 2002; Pipitone & Choy 2003).

4.2.4 Biological agents

According to the UK National Institute for Clinical Excellence (NICE) and The British Society for Rheumatology, patients with highly active disease who have failed to respond to at least two DMARDs (including methotrexate) are eligible for anti-TNF-α therapy (Pipitone & Choy 2003).

Anti-TNF-α biological response modifiers are relatively new to the treatment of RA. As TNF-α along with IL-1 are key cytokines in inflammatory synovitis and destruction of bone and cartilage, drugs able to block TNF-α or IL-1 are of great interest (Pipitone & Choy 2003). Etanercept and infliximab are two examples of anti-TNF-α drugs that have shown significant benefit in RA in terms of quality of life, functional status and general wellbeing. They have also been shown to have a better gastrointestinal safety profile than NSAIDs though they have been associated with infections, sometimes severe, including tuberculosis and septicaemia and other side effects (BNF 2005b). Also recently licensed in the UK is the IL-1 receptor antagonist, anakinra, which has shown remarkable efficacy in clinical trials and appears to be well tolerated (Pipitone & Choy 2003) though it is not recommended for routine management of RA (BNF 2005b). Two new biological agents that work in a completely different way have been submitted for licence – rituximab, which depletes B-cells, and abatacept, which inhibits T-cell co-stimulatory pathways (Emery 2006).

4.2.5 Glucocorticoids

Glucocorticoids or corticosteroids are potent medications used in the management of rheumatological disease. They may be given systemically or by injection (intramuscular, intravenous or intra-articular). They are able to suppress the inflammatory cascade and modify the immune response, inhibiting both cytokines and Cox-2. At low doses, steroids (i.e. prednisolone) may be used to control early RA inflammation (Hill 1998; West 2002).

Care must be taken with the use of corticosteroids as they have many documented side effects, including glucose intolerance, cataract formation, peptic ulcer disease, obesity, mental disturbance, muscle weakness and osteoporosis (BNF 2005c).

Oral corticosteroids should be avoided wherever possible and similar benefits can be obtained with intra-articular delivery. Patients with OA may benefit from corticosteroid injection therapy (West 2002). Injections of corticosteroids and hyaluronic acid are widely used to relieve severe local pain and inflammation in the short term, most frequently in knee joints. It is advised that these injections be given no more than 3–4 times per year in the same joint or tendon sheath, as the long-term effects are as yet unclear (West, 2002; Dorfman 2004).

In order to minimise complications and side effects, when patients receive corticosteroids they should (West 2002):

- Receive the lowest dose for the shortest time period
- Be encouraged to exercise
- Be involved in a falls prevention programme
- Be prescribed a calcium supplement to ensure overall intake is at least 1500 mg/d
- Receive at least 400 IU Vitamin D per day
- Receive education on the side effects of the therapy

4.2.6 Side effects of arthritis medication likely to affect nutritional status

Medication for arthritis is associated with nutritional and metabolic side effects. Vitamin and mineral status can be affected most notably by methotrexate treatment, which reduces folate status. Known side effects are shown in Table 4.5 (also see section 5.6).

4.3 Surgical management

There are two main indications for surgical intervention (joint replacement) in RA and OA:

(1) Severe pain unresponsive to medical therapy, i.e. the patient wakes frequently in the night due to pain
(2) Loss of joint function, i.e. cannot walk moderate distances and unable to climb stairs

Surgical treatments may be classified as preventative, preservative, corrective or salvage (David & Lloyd 1999).

4.3.1 Preventative

Arthroscopic debridement: often indicated in early OA, yet may also reduce pain in those with advanced OA.

Table 4.5 Nutritional and other side effects of arthritis medications (X indicates an effect; data from Dorfman 2004).

Side effects	Salicylates	NSAIDs	Anti-malarials	D-penicillamine	Corticosteroids	Immunosuppressive agents	Gold
Affecting nutritional status							
Anorexia			X				
Stomatitis		X		X		X	X
Nausea	X	X	X	X	X	X	
Vomiting	X	X	X	X		X	X
Gastritis	X			X			X
Duodenal ulcer		X			X		
Peptic ulcer	X						
Constipation		X					
Gastrointestinal bleeding	X	X					
Diarrhoea		X*	X	X		X	X
Altered taste				X		X	
Metabolic							
Glucose intolerance					X		
Proteinuria				X			X
Negative nitrogen balance					X		X
Altered serum K	X						
Oedema		X**			X		
Anaemia	X	X		X	X		
Decreased vitamin or mineral							
Ascorbic acid	X						
Folate	X					X***	
Zinc				X			
Copper				X			
Calcium					X	X	
Iron				X			

* Meclomen only, ** May occur with pre-existing oedema, *** Methotrexate only

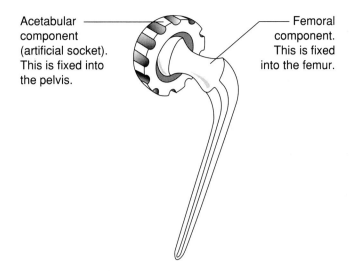

Acetabular component (artificial socket). This is fixed into the pelvis.

Femoral component. This is fixed into the femur.

Figure 4.2 Artificial hip joint (reproduced with permission from Fisher 2004).

4.3.2 Preservative

Surgical or radiation synovectomy: this is indicated where there is excess synovium proliferation within one or two affected joints, most commonly in the knee or wrist joints. This procedure is normally performed on individuals with no erosions or minimal erosions. Though the synovium removed does regenerate, normally within three months, there is long-lasting pain relief and restoration of function in the joint. Surgical synovectomy of the knee may provide effective pain relief in around 70% of patients up to 10 years after the procedure.

4.3.3 Corrective

Excision or replacement arthroplasty (joint replacement): this procedure involves either excision (removal of the end of the affected bone joint) or replacement of a joint, the aim of which is to decrease pain as well as to improve function (ARC for Research 1995). Total joint arthroplasty (replacement) commonly involves the knee or hip joints (Figures 4.2 and 4.3) and is often used to alleviate OA problems.

> 'Total joint replacement is an excellent treatment for OA and has been responsible for a dramatic improvement in the quality of life of individuals with moderate-severe lower-limb OA in the past 20 years' (Creamer & Hochberg 1997).

Currently over 50 000 total hip replacements and over 30 000 knee joint operations are undertaken annually in the UK (Fisher 2004).

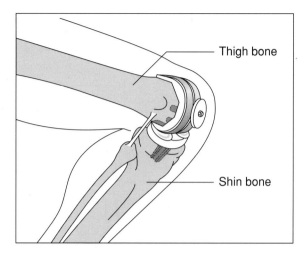

Figure 4.3   Artificial knee joint *in situ* (reproduced with permission from Fisher 2004).

4.3.4 Salvage

Arthrodesis: this is an uncommon procedure but aimed at reducing pain and increasing stability in severely damaged joints. It may be the only option for failed joint replacements. It involves the surgical fusion of the hips, knees or ankles in a position for optimum function. This procedure will lead to a considerable restriction in mobility in one or more joints.

4.4 Physiotherapy and occupational therapy management

4.4.1 Physiotherapy

Physiotherapists can be of tremendous help in the management of OA and RA. Main roles include teaching exercises and supervising activities, making splints to rest joints, applying soothing measures (such as short wave ultrasound) and applying mobilisation and manipulation to restore mobility.

Exercise and rest: There is no evidence to support the use of bed rest in the treatment of acute or chronic arthritis. Bed rest will actually reduce muscle strength (by 5–10% in one week), and in the longer term, inactivity can lead to poor cardiovascular fitness (West 2002). However, according to David and Lloyd (1999), bed rest should not be totally discouraged because it will help with the inflammatory response. Rest can be classified into three categories (West 2002):

(1) Local rest, using splinting techniques
(2) Systemic rest – used for periods of up to four weeks if NSAIDs and rehabilitation management are ineffective

(3) Short rest periods, which are increasingly being used in RA, i.e. short breaks of 30 minutes as a preventative and proactive way of preventing inflammation and fatigue

According to David and Lloyd (1999), daily exercises through the available range of joint movement are necessary, even with only minimal repetitions to maintain range of movement and avoid atrophy and contractures. While exercise may be painful in the early stages, over time it will improve arthritic symptoms.

There have been a number of clinical trials designed to look at the efficacy of exercise in improving symptoms and quality of life. Da Costa and colleagues (2003) found that both moderate and higher intensity leisure time physical activity was associated with less generalised distress in individuals with rheumatic conditions. In a randomised two-year trial of high intensity, weightbearing exercise compared with usual care in 309 patients with RA, those undergoing the exercise programme developed less radiological damage of the hands and feet (de Jong et al. 2004).

Strong evidence for the efficacy of muscle conditioning and aerobic exercise in lessening symptoms in OA of the knee exists (Felson et al. 2000). In a randomised controlled study, Hughes et al. (2004) found that in OA patients, those who exercised benefited greatly compared to those who did not exercise: lower extremity stiffness and pain at two and six months improved. In ADAPT (Arthritis, Diet and Activity Promotion Trial), 316 sedentary overweight individuals with OA were randomly assigned to one of four groups (Messier et al. 2004):

- Healthy lifestyle control
- Dietary weight loss (aim 5% of total body weight in 18 months)
- Structured exercise (aerobic and strength training for 60 minutes three times per week, group or home-based)
- Combined exercise and dietary weight loss (aim 5% of total body weight in 18 months)

In the combined exercise and dietary weight loss group, significant improvements in self-reported physical function ($P < 0.05$), 6 minute walk distance ($P < 0.05$), stair climb time ($P < 0.05$), and knee pain ($P < 0.05$) were observed relative to the healthy lifestyle group and weight loss groups. Better overall improvements were seen compared to weight loss or exercise interventions alone. A number of trials investigating the impact of exercise on individuals with OA are ongoing.

Current recommendations for physical activity and exercise: Recommendations should be individually tailored to take into account the patient's stage of disease, extent of inflammation and deformity, general health and activities enjoyed in order to aid compliance (West 2002). Recommendations from the Work Group on Exercise and Physical Activity Conference at St Louis, Missouri are given below (Minor et al. 2003).

(1) Aerobic exercise for people with hip/knee OA:
   - Accumulate 30 minutes of moderate intensity (50–70% maximal heart rate), physical activity or exercise on at least three days a week.

- Tailor the type of aerobic activity and venue to individual needs.
- If overweight, reduce weight and combine activity/exercise with diet modification.
- Incorporate self-management education into activity/exercise recommendations and programmes.

(2) Neuromuscular rehabilitation for people with knee OA:
- A lower extremity exercise programme should combine strengthening, coordination/balance and functional exercise.
- Recommended programmes will progress in duration, intensity and complexity and be tailored to the individual needs, abilities and preferences; move from clinical supervision to self-directed community setting; be periodically reviewed, revised and reinforced.

(3) Conditioning exercises for cardiovascular and neuromuscular fitness in adults with RA:
- Initial assessment of fitness to determine safety and dose
- Supervised or self-directed settings
- Periodic review, revision and reinforcement
- Cardiovascular recommendations: Intensity: 60–85% maximal heart rate, progressively adjusted; Frequency: 2–3 times per week; Duration: 30–60 minutes; Mode: whole body, dynamic (walk, dance, water, stationary cycle)
- Neuromuscular recommendations: Intensity: 50–80% of maximal load, progressively adjusted; Frequency 2–3 times per week; Volume: 8–10 exercises; 8–12 repetitions; 1–2 sets; Mode: dynamic (static) (Minor et al. 2003)

Hydrotherapy: Used in the management of individuals with OA and RA where the buoyancy may be valuable in reducing the acute pain of exercise. Hydrotherapy is also used for strengthening purposes as exercises can be graded using turbulence and buoyancy to strengthen weakened muscles gradually without stressing the joints (David & Lloyd 1999). Hydrotherapy treatment is contraindicated for patients who are immunosuppressed or who have systemic manifestations.

4.4.2 Occupational therapy

Occupational therapists assess and provide practical solutions to everyday problems encountered by individuals who are affected by arthritis. Advice may be given on alternative working methods, use of specialist equipment (electric tin opener, stairlift or bath seat) and they may also make splints to allow patients to rest joints for varying time periods.

4.5 Acupuncture

'Acupuncture relieves pain through activation of the gate-control system in which large nerve fibres are stimulated and suppress small fibres that transmit signals *in the dorsal horn of the spinal cord or through the release of neurochemicals in the CNS' (Felson et al. 2000).*

Several clinical trials have been conducted in the US and Europe on the effectiveness of acupuncture for OA and have shown some effect on pain (Felson et al. 2000).

The longest and largest randomised controlled phase III clinical trial of acupuncture ever conducted was carried out on 570 patients with osteoarthritis of the knee proven by X-ray (Berman et al. 2004). The study, funded by the National Center for Complementary and Alternative Medicine (NCCAM) and the National Institute of Arthritis and Musculoskeletal and Skin Diseases (NIAMS), both components of the National Institutes of Health, was published in the *Annals of Internal Medicine* in December 2004. Patients received either 23 sessions of acupuncture or sham acupuncture (needles inserted but not at special points) over 26 weeks (twice a week during the first 8 weeks then down to once a month by the 14th week), or arthritis education. After 8 weeks, patients in the acupuncture group had greater improvement in function, but not pain, compared with patients in the sham acupuncture group. Among patients who remained in the study, those in the acupuncture group had greater improvements in both pain and function after 26 weeks compared with the other groups. However, by week 26, 25% of participants from each acupuncture group had dropped out which introduces some uncertainty in the 26-week results. Less intensive acupuncture treatment might not have produced the same results. Acupuncture seems to provide improvement in function and pain relief as an adjunctive therapy for osteoarthritis of the knee when compared with credible sham acupuncture and education control groups.

References

ARC (Arthritis Research Campaign) for Research. (1995) *Collected reports on the Rheumatic Diseases.* Pages 3–10, 20–43, 49–51, 168–77, 186–97, 218–21, 229–35, 245–55.

Berman BM, Lao L, Langenberg P, Lee WL, Gilpin AM, Hochberg MC (2004) Effectiveness of acupuncture as adjunctive therapy in osteoarthritis of the knee: a randomized, controlled trial. *Annals of Internal Medicine* 21, 141(12), 901–10.

BNF 50 (2005a) *British National Formulary.* British Medical Association, Royal Pharmaceutical Society of Great Britain, Section 4.7.

BNF 50 (2005b) *British National Formulary.* British Medical Association, Royal Pharmaceutical Society of Great Britain, Section 10.1.

BNF 50 (2005c) *British National Formulary.* British Medical Association, Royal Pharmaceutical Society of Great Britain, Section 6.3.

Creamer P, Hochberg MC (1997) Osteoarthritis. *The Lancet* 350, 503–8.

Da Costa D, Lowensteyn I, Dritsa M (2003) Leisure-time physical activity patterns and relationship to generalized distress among Canadians with arthritis or rheumatism. *Journal of Rheumatology* 30(11), 2299–301.

David C, Lloyd J (1999) *Rheumatological Physiotherapy.* London, Mosby, pp. 3–9, 55–61, 65–81 and 83–96.

Deal CL, Schnitzer TJ, Lipstein E, Seibold JR, Stevens RM, Levy MD, Albert D, Renold F (1991) Treatment of arthritis with topical capsaicin: a double-blind trial. Clinical Therapeutics 13(3), 383–95.

Deeks JJ, Smith LA, Bradley MD (2002) Efficacy, tolerability, and upper gastrointestinal safety of celecoxib for treatment of osteoarthritis and rheumatoid arthritis: a systematic review of randomised controlled trials. *British Medical Journal* 325, 619–23.

de Jong Z, Munneke M, Zwinderman AH, Kroon HM, Ronday KH, Lems WF, Dijkmans BA, Breedveld FC, Vliet Vlieland TP, Hazes JM, Huizinga TW (2004) Long-term high intensity exercise and damage of small joints in rheumatoid arthritis. *Annals of the Rheumatic Diseases* **63**, 1399–1405.

Dorfman L (2004) Medical nutrition therapy for rheumatic disorders. In: *Krause's Food, Nutrition and Diet Therapy*, 11th edition, LK Mahan and S Escott-Stump, eds. Philadelphia, WB Saunders, pp. 1121–42.

The Economist (2005) Special report: the drugs industry. *The Economist* March 19–25, pp. 89–91.

Emery P (2006) Treatment of rheumatoid arthritis. *British Medical Journal* **332**, 152–5.

Felson DT, Lawrence RC, Hochberg MC, McAlindon T, Dieppe PA, Minor MA, Blair SN, Berman BM, Fries JF, Weinberger M, Lorig KR, Jacobs JJ, Goldberg V. NIH conference (2000) Osteoarthritis: new insights. Part 2: Treatment approaches. *Annals of Internal Medicine* **133**, 726–37.

Fisher J (2004) Surgery for arthritis. Total hip and knee joint replacement. *Topical Reviews* (Arthritis Research Campaign) Series 5, No 3.

Graham DJ, Campen D, Hui R, Spence M, Cheetham C, Levy G, Shoor S, Ray WA (2005) Risk of acute myocardial infarction and sudden cardiac death in patients treated with cyclo-oxygenase 2 selective and non-selective non-steroidal anti-inflammatory drugs: nested case-control study. *The Lancet* **5**, 365(9458), 475–81.

Griffith SM, Fisher J, Clarke S, Montgomery B, Jones PW, Saklatvala J, Dawes PT, Shadforth MF, Hothersall TE, Hassell AB, Hay EM (2000) Do patients with rheumatoid arthritis established on methotrexate and folic acid 5 mg daily need to continue folic acid supplements long term? *Rheumatology* **39**, 1102–9.

Hill J (1998) *Rheumatology, a creative approach*. Edinburgh, Churchill Livingstone.

Hughes SL, Seymour RB, Campbell R, Pollak N, Huber G, Sharma L (2004) Impact of the fit and strong intervention on older adults with osteoarthritis. *Gerontologist* **44**, 217–28.

Lin J, Zhang W, Jones A, Doherty M (2004) Efficacy of topical non-steroidal anti-inflammatory drugs in the treatment of osteoarthritis: meta-analysis of randomised controlled trials. *British Medical Journal* **7**, 329(7461), 324.

Loeser RF (2003) A stepwise approach to the management of osteoarthritis. Bulletin on the Rheumatic Diseases 52 (5). Arthritis Foundation. www.arthritis.org/research/bulletin/vol52no5/introduction.asp

Martin RH (1998) The role of nutrition and diet in rheumatoid arthritis. *Proceedings of the Nutrition Society* **57**, 231–34.

McKenna F (2000) The relevance of Cox-2 specificity. *Rheumatic Disease in Practice* January, No 1.

Messier SP, Loeser RF, Miller GD, Morgan TM, Rejeski WJ, Sevick MA, Ettinger WH Jr, Pahor M and Williamson JD (2004) Exercise and dietary weight loss in overweight and obese older adults with knee osteoarthritis: the Arthritis, Diet and Activity Promotion Trial. *Arthritis and Rheumatism* **50**(5), 1501–10.

Minor M, Stenstrom CH, Klepper SE, Hurley M, Ettinger WH (2003) Work group recommendations: 2002 Exercise and Physical Activity Conference, St Louis, Missouri. Session V: evidence of benefit of exercise and physical activity in arthritis. *Arthritis and Rheumatism* June **49**(3), 453–54.

NICE (2001) Guidance on the use of cyclo-oxygenase (Cox) II selective inhibitors, celecoxib, rofecoxib, meloxicam and etodolac for osteoarthritis and rheumatoid arthritis. *Technology Appraisal Guidance* **27**, July 2001. www.nice.org.uk

Pipitone N, Choy E (2003) Treatment of rheumatoid arthritis. *Rheumatic Disease Topical Reviews* (A Adebajo. ed). January 2003 No **10**. Chesterfield, Arthritis Research Campaign.

Rainsford KD, Ying C, Smith FC (1997) Effects of meloxicam, compared with other NSAIDs, on cartilage proteoglycan metabolism, synovial prostaglandin E2, and production of interleukins 1, 6 and 8, in human and porcine explants in organ culture. *Journal of Pharmacy and Pharmacology* **49**(10), 991–98.

Solomon SD, McMurray JJ, Pfeffer MA, Wittes J, Fowler R, Finn P, Anderson WF, Zauber A, Hawk E, Bertagnolli M (2005) Adenoma Prevention with Celecoxib (APC) Study Investigators. Cardiovascular risk associated with celecoxib in a clinical trial for colorectal adenoma prevention. *New England Journal of Medicine* **17**, 352(11), 1071–80.

Wakley G, Chambers R, Dieppe P (2001) *Musculoskeletal Matters in Primary Care*. Oxford, Radcliffe Publishing.

West SG (ed) (2002) *Rheumatology Secrets*, 2nd edition, Philadelphia, Hanley and Belfus.

White C, Cooper R (2002) Prescribing and monitoring of disease-modifying anti-rheumatic drugs (DMARDs) for inflammatory arthritis. *Rheumatic Disease in Practice* (J Dickson, ed). May 2002, No **8**. Chesterfield, Arthritis Research Campaign.

Whittle SL, Hughes RA (2004) Folate supplementation and methotrexate treatment in rheumatoid arthritis: a review. *Rheumatology* **43**, 267–71.

5 Nutritional status and adequacy of the diet in rheumatoid arthritis and osteoarthritis

5.1 Introduction

Nutritional status is frequently poor in those suffering from serious and debilitating arthritis, particularly if they suffer from RA. Though OA sufferers are more likely to be overweight (see 3.6), inflammatory joint disease has long been recognised to be associated with weight loss and this can be profound in some people, particularly when associated with more severe disease (Munro & Capell 1997). Weight loss in RA is likely to result not only from lower food intake owing to decreased ability to shop and prepare food, but also from poorer appetite and muscle wasting as a result of diminished physical activity, and the metabolic burden of the inflammatory process (Munro & Capell 1997). It is likely that in the case of RA, the severity of the disease adversely affects nutritional status (Helliwell et al. 1984).

5.2 Body mass index (BMI)

A mean value of BMI {weight (kg)/height (m^2)} in a group of RA patients is not a very useful measure as it disguises the fact that some subjects are underweight – probably those with the most severe disease (see 5.2.1) – while some are overweight, partly because of reduced physical activity. Results from three studies illustrate the point. A Danish study found the BMI of 81 RA patients with active disease to be 21.5–25.5 kg/m^2, no different from that of healthy Danes i.e. 22.5–24.5 kg/m^2 (Hansen et al. 1996) while average BMI (kg/m^2) of 48 New Zealand RA patients was 25.9 kg/m^2, similar to that of the general population and slightly higher than the ideal range (Stone et al. 1997). However, in a study of 79 RA patients in the south east of the US, 60% had a BMI of less than 25 kg/m^2, 10% of the group were moderately underweight and 4% were severely underweight (Morgan et al. 1997). By contrast, 40% of the patients were overweight, of whom 30% had a BMI between 25 and 25.9 kg/m^2 and 10% had a BMI of 30 kg/m^2 or over.

5.2.1 Low BMI and rheumatoid cachexia

Numerous authors have documented impaired nutritional status and inadequate nutrient intake patterns in RA patients (for references, see Morgan et al. 1997).

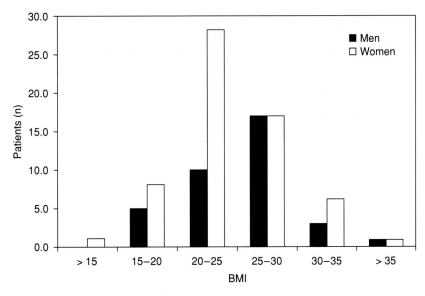

Figure 5.1 Distribution of Body Mass Index (BMI) in patients with RA (reproduced with permission from Munro & Capell 1997).

Low BMI, often indicative of poor nutritional status, may be associated with the phenomenon of 'rheumatoid cachexia' that has been described in patients with RA. It is characterised by increased catabolism and resting energy expenditure, muscle wasting and anorexia and is associated with the production of the pro-inflammatory cytokines IL-1β and TNF-α (Roubenoff et al. 1994). IL-6 may also be systemically released in RA (Munro & Capell 1997). IL-1β may cause reduced appetite while IL-6 participates in the production of acute phase reactants by the liver (Munro & Capell 1997). TNF can cause protein degradation: higher serum TNF concentrations have been detected in RA patients with cachexia experiencing a flare-up in their disease than in patients without a cachectic flare (Munro & Capell 1997). Increased TNF production in RA is associated with increasing resting energy expenditure. Thus these cytokines play a key role in inflammation mediated loss of appetite, weight and joint destruction (Kaufmann et al. 2003).

In a Scottish study, Munro and Capell (1997) investigated the prevalence of low BMI in 96 patients with RA, comparing weight at study entry to weight when diagnosed. Various anthropometric measurement indices were used (knee height, triceps skinfold thickness, upper-arm circumference, mid-arm muscle circumference and waist circumference) and fat mass was calculated. BMI averaged 26 kg/m² (21.3–28.4) in men and 23.5 kg/m² (21.5–26.9) in women, at study entry. BMI distribution in these patients is shown in Figure 5.1. Of these patients, seven, all females, had had a weight loss of > 15% since referral.

Age and sex matched, 13% of this group of RA patients (both male and female) were in the lowest fifth centile of the general population for BMI. Taking the cut-off as the lowest fifth centile of the reference population, one in eight patients with RA were underweight compared with one in 20 people in the general population.

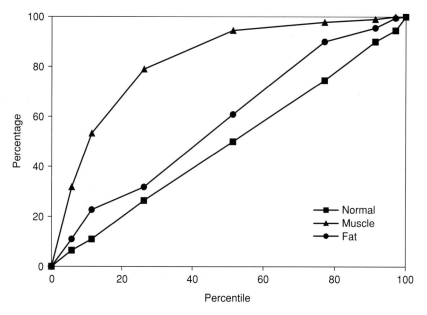

Figure 5.2 Percentage distribution of upper arm muscle and fat areas in RA patients compared with that in normal controls. While the distribution of upper arm fat area is very similar to that of the normal population, that of muscle mass is skewed to the left with 50% of the RA group falling into the lowest tenth centile of the reference population (reproduced with permission from Munro & Capell 1997).

Reduction in body mass was greatest for lean tissue (muscle) while fat mass was comparatively well maintained (see Figure 5.2). 50% of the RA group fell into the lowest tenth centile for muscle mass of the reference population. In female patients, there was a significant correlation between reduced lean tissue mass and the acute phase response {erythrocyte sedimentation rate (ESR), p = 0.016; C-reactive protein (CRP), p = 0.003}. Thus the conclusion from this study was that weight loss is a significant problem in female patients with RA, and is greatest in those patients with the highest acute phase response to their disease (Munro & Capell 1997).

A study by Kaufmann and colleagues (2003) also suggested a relationship between low BMI and more severe disease. A BMI < 27 kg/m^2 at the beginning of disease was found to be significantly associated with severely progressive joint damage [Odds ratio (OR) 7.69; p = 0.003] (Kaufmann et al. 2003). The authors have suggested that low BMI at diagnosis could be used as a predictive factor for severe joint damage in RA.

5.2.2 High BMI

There is evidence that obesity is associated with OA, in particular of the knee and hip, and obesity is also common in RA patients (see 5.2). The evidence for an association between high BMI and the risk of both these conditions is discussed fully in section 3.6.

Those with joint disease of the lower limbs are likely to have lower energy expenditure as a consequence of reduced mobility and pain associated with exercise, resulting in the risk of weight gain. Though change in weight was not found to be related to disease activity in RA subjects (Morgan et al. 1997), according to McAlindon and Felson (1997), weight reduction may decrease the risk for the development and progression of OA. However, if a weight reducing programme is followed, it is vital that an appropriate regime including moderate physical training is followed in order to preserve lean body mass as far as possible (Englehart et al. 1996; Work Group Recommendations 2002). A patient with significant disease must have professional support so that micronutrient status is maintained during the course of any weight reducing diet. Ideally, the advice of a dietitian should be sought.

5.3   Malnutrition and malnutrition screening

A nutritional assessment of 50 RA patients compared to 50 controls showed that 26% of them could be classified as malnourished (Helliwell et al. 1984): these patients had more active disease. BMI and triceps skinfold thickness values were significantly reduced in patients of both sexes when compared with controls (Helliwell et al. 1984). Biochemical determinants of nutritional status – serum albumin, transferrin, retinal binding protein, thyroxine binding prealbumin, zinc and folate – were also significantly lower in the RA group (Helliwell et al. 1984).

Given the prevalence of poor nutritional status associated with arthritis, health professionals need to be able to identify those who are malnourished or at risk of malnutrition, undernutrition or obesity so that appropriate action can be taken. A simple screening tool can be used for this purpose. In the UK, the Malnutrition Universal Screening Tool (MUST, see Appendix 2) is used (Malnutrition Advisory Group 2003). This and similar tools are useful to identify, and subsequently treat, malnutrition, rheumatoid cachexia and OA related obesity. The MUST consists of five steps:

(1)   BMI is first measured. A score is then attributed to the measured BMI (e.g. a BMI under 18 kg/m^2 would give a score of 2 while a BMI of 19–20 kg/m^2 would score 1 point). If the BMI cannot be obtained, clinical impression – thin, acceptable weight or overweight – should be used or the measurement of mid-upper-arm circumference, which can then be used to estimate the BMI category.

(2)   Noting percentage unintentional weight loss. (A weight loss of 5–10% would score 1 point). If this information is unavailable, unplanned weight loss can be assessed by asking the individual several questions including whether clothes have become looser, food intake decreased, or appetite reduced.

(3)   Establishing an acute disease effect (if the patient is acutely ill and there has been, or is likely to be, no food intake for five or more days, the score given is 2).

(4) Add up the scores gained from 1, 2 and 3 to identify the overall risk of malnutrition.

(5) Consult management and referral guidelines:

Score 0   Low risk of malnutrition. Routine clinical care.

Score 1   Medium risk. Observe patient, i.e. in the community at least every 2–3 months.

Score 2+   High risk. Refer to dietitian or nutrition support team. Review monthly in a community setting.

5.4 Macronutrient intake

Poor nutrient status in RA patients has been reported in observational studies, with reduced intake from carbohydrates, low fibre intake and high consumption of saturated fat (Kremer & Bigaouette 1996; Morgan et al. 1997).

A Korean study of 97 RA patients and 97 matched controls found a lower mean calorie intake and a lower intake of fat among the RA patients (Bae et al. 2003). In a US study, both men and women with RA were found to ingest significantly less carbohydrate and more fat than the recommended level of 30% (36.8 and 35.2% of total energy intake in women and men respectively) (Kremer & Bigaouette 1996). Women ate significantly more saturated and monounsaturated fat than the US recommended dietary allowance (RDA) and significantly less polyunsaturated fatty acid (PUFA) and fibre. Men ingested significantly less carbohydrate, PUFA and fibre and significantly more protein than the RDA. However, according to Kremer and Bigaouette (1996) these intakes were not significantly different from the typical American diet. Morgan and colleagues (1997) in a subsequent US study similarly found that RA subjects consumed 38% of their energy from fat and only 46% from carbohydrate rather than the recommended 55%.

5.5 Micronutrient intake and deficiency in RA

Many patients with RA and OA are at least marginally inadequate in selected micronutrients some of which might contribute to disease perpetuation (Kowsari et al. 1983). Not all studies have found such differences; however, Honkanen and colleagues (1991) found recorded seven day dietary intakes of copper and zinc in 40 RA patients to be comparable with the ordinary Finnish diet.

A number of studies have looked at the adequacy of dietary intake of those with RA by analysis of diet diaries or diet histories (Kremer & Bigaouette 1996; Hansen et al. 1996; Bigaouette et al. 1987; Stone et al. 1997; Morgan et al. 1997; New et al. 1997; Goff & Barasi 1999). It is difficult to compare the results of these studies as they evaluated intakes according to different recommended criteria for adequacy. To overcome this problem, we have taken the raw results from the individual studies and compared them to the UK reference nutrient intake (RNI). (A list of UK RNI and US RDA values can be found in Appendix 3). We have used the RNI values recommended for the over 50 age category as the ages of patients involved in the studies were as follows: a mean of 59 years (Hansen et al. 1996);

mean 55 years (Bigaouette et al. 1987); mean 64.5 years (Stone et al. 1997); mean 53.2 years (Morgan et al. 1997) age range 58–67 years (New et al. 1997) and mean 57 years (Goff & Barasi 1999). Findings from the studies are shown in Table 5.1. Not all studies measured all of the nutrients tabulated.

Patients met the RNI for vitamin C in all seven studies but only did so for the other vitamins – folate, B_6, D and E – in half of the studies. Mean intake levels of potassium and magnesium were below the RNI in two-thirds of the studies and for calcium in half. With respect to the trace minerals, the intakes of iron, zinc and copper only met the RNI in around half the studies that measured them. Selenium and iodine intakes were below the RNI in all studies that measured them. The failure to meet the UK RNI for selenium in the two UK studies is in line with data on UK intake generally (Rayman 2000). New Zealand intakes of selenium were also notably low at the time measured, i.e. 1997.

In fact, looking only at mean or median values in comparison with the RNI can give an overoptimistic picture of intake, as it does not reveal the number of people who fall far below the RNI. For example, in their study results, Stone and colleagues (1997) also reported the percentage of RA patients achieving 100% of the Australian RDI (recommended dietary intake, similar to US RDA values), an amount advised for 'patients at risk'. This revealed that only 46% of patients achieved the RDI for folate, 29% for vitamin E, 27% for magnesium, 23% for calcium, 10% for zinc, 6% for selenium and 4% for copper.

It is hard to know what, if any, conclusion to draw from these studies: nutrient intake is notoriously difficult to measure precisely and a three day diet diary/diet history, as used in three of these studies, is unlikely to give an accurate estimate of nutrient consumption. The number of subjects providing such data was small – as few as 20 in one of the UK studies. Overall, however, there is an indication that intake of some micronutrients is likely to be inadequate in RA sufferers. Interestingly, and perhaps not surprisingly, the quality of the diet in RA patients is strongly influenced by whether they think that diet affects their disease. Goff and Barasi (1999) compared intake in two groups of subjects – those who believed that diet had some effect on their condition or symptoms and those who believed it had no effect. The nutrient intake of the two study groups differed significantly, with the 'diet believers' having a more nutrient dense, well balanced, and healthier diet than the group that believed diet had no effect.

With regard to nutritional status, deficient vitamin and mineral status has been found in RA patients (Giordano et al. 1984; Helliwell et al. 1984; Roubenoff et al. 1995; Morgan et al. 1997). Low plasma levels of pyridoxal-5-phosphate, the metabolically active form of vitamin B_6, have been measured in RA patients as have low concentrations of vitamins B_{12}, C, E and β-carotene (Helliwell et al. 1984; Roubenoff et al. 1995; Morgan et al. 1997). Low serum zinc has also been reported (Helliwell et al. 1984) though this could partly be a result of the acute phase response associated with RA (Halliwell & Gutteridge 1999) rather than low dietary intake. While iron deficiency anaemia is commonly associated with RA, this may also be a consequence of the disease process (see section 8.6) or its medication, rather than a reflection of low dietary intake (Giordano et al. 1984).

Table 5.1 Mean micronutrient intake in RA patients: failure to meet UK RNI.

Study	Kremer & Bigaouette (1996)		Hansen et al. (1996)	Bigaouette et al. (1987)		Stone et al. (1997)	Morgan et al. (1997)	New et al. (1997)	Goff & Barasi (1999)
Country	USA		Denmark	USA		New Zealand	USA	UK	UK
No. patients	n = 41		n = 81	n = 52		n = 48	n = 79	n = 20	n = 25
Measure	3-d diet diary		Food diary	3-d diet history		5-d diet diary	5 × 24 h recall	7-d diet diary	3-d diet diary
Gender	M	F	M & F	M	F	M & F	M & F	M & F	M & F
Vitamin B₆	X	X	—	✓	✓	✓	X	—	✓
Folate	X	✓	—	✓	✓	✓	X	—	✓
Vitamin C	✓	✓	✓	✓	✓	✓	✓	✓	✓
Vitamin D	—	—	✓	—	—	—	—	✓	X
Vitamin E	✓	✓	✓	✓	✓	X	X	—	X
Potassium	X	X	—	—	—	X	—	—	✓
Magnesium	X	X	—	X	X	X	X	✓	✓
Calcium	✓	✓	—	✓	✓	X	X	✓	✓
Iron	✓	✓	—	✓	✓	X	X	✓	X
Zinc	X	X	—	✓	✓	X	X	✓	X
Copper	✓	✓	—	—	—	X	X	✓	✓
Selenium	—	—	—	—	—	X	—	X	X
Iodine	—	—	X	—	—	—	—	—	X

n Number of subjects providing dietary intake information
— Not estimated
X Mean intake lower than UK RNI
✓ Mean intake above UK RNI

The finding of inadequate intake or status of some nutrients in RA patients has to be seen within the context of dietary intake in the general population. In the UK National Diet and Nutrition Survey of adults aged 19–64, riboflavin status was found to be low in about 50% and vitamin D low in around 15% of both men and women while plasma iron was below the lower limit of the normal range (13 µmol/l) in one-third of the women (Henderson et al. 2002). In the corresponding survey of the elderly (Finch et al. 1998), the percentage of subjects with biochemical indices suggesting deficiency was 35% for riboflavin, 15% for serum folate, 14% for vitamin C and 10% for iron in the free living, while for those in institutions, the corresponding values were 41%, 39%, 40% and 45%. Intakes of vitamin D were less than recommended (< 10 µg/d) in 95% of the elderly, with 8% of the free living and 37% of those in institutions showing biochemical indices of deficiency (Finch et al. 1998). The risk of poor bone health resulting from inadequate vitamin D intake is likely to be exacerbated by poor vitamin K status, which was found to be low compared to intakes and plasma levels in other population groups (Finch et al. 1998).

It is clear, however, that where there is a lower intake of food overall, a reduced intake of the micronutrients normally ingested with food is inevitable. Given the oxidative stress associated particularly with RA, it is important that health professionals should advise that nutrient dense foods must be consumed and if this is not possible, there is a case for recommending at least a multivitamin and mineral supplement at the RNI/RDA level to compensate for this deficient intake. Martin (1998) suggests that dietary supplementation with vitamin D, calcium, folic acid or multivitamins and minerals should be recommended if necessary while Kremer and Bigaouette (1996) recommend routine dietary supplementation with vitamins and minerals in the RA population.

5.6   Drug–nutrient interactions

Management of arthritis involves use of medication to reduce pain and inflammation. Some of these medications have known anti-nutrient properties (Bigaouette et al. 1987; see Table 4.5). For example, D-penicillamine chelates zinc, copper, cobalt and magnesium and inactivates pyridoxine; prednisolone increases urinary excretion of zinc, calcium and nitrogen; NSAIDs decrease iron stores through gastrointestinal erosion and chronic blood loss (Bigaouette et al. 1987). Methotrexate, a drug often used to manage RA, is a known folate antagonist, reducing hepatic folate stores by more than 80% (Bigaouette et al. 1987). The combination of poor initial folate status, poor folate intake and methotrexate therapy increases the risk of subsequent folate deficiency and toxicity from methotrexate therapy (Morgan et al. 1997). If patients are not supplemented with folic acid they may become folate deficient. A Cochrane review of seven trials found a case for low doses of folic acid supplement (< 5 mg/week) in RA patients treated with methotrexate (Ortiz et al. 2001). A high calcium intake should be encouraged for those on corticosteroids, and bone mineral density testing is advisable (Morgan et al. 1997). Vitamin D intake is also important for these individuals if insufficient sun exposure is likely.

5.7   Importance of individual assessment

The variable results of the studies quoted in 5.5 added to the drug nutrient interactions described in 5.6, show that it is difficult to identify specific nutrients that may be low in all patients with RA. Thus sweeping generalisations should not be made with respect to particular nutrient deficiencies in RA (or OA). Ideally, patients should have their individual dietary intake assessed by a qualified dietitian who can advise on dietary changes that may be necessary or on nutritional supplements that may be beneficial. Likely deficiencies in the diet of the population as a whole should be taken into account, as it may be even more important to address these in this particular group of subjects.

References

Bae SC, Kim SJ, Sung MK (2003) Inadequate antioxidant nutrient intake and altered plasma antioxidant status of rheumatoid arthritis patients. *Journal of the American College of Nutrition* 22(4), 311–15.

Bigaouette J, Timchalk MA, Kremer J (1987) Nutritional adequacy of diet and supplements in patients with rheumatoid arthritis who take medications. *Journal of the American Dietetic Association* 87(12), 1687–88.

Englehart M, Kondrup J, Hoie L, Andersen V, Kristensen J, Heitmann B (1996) Weight reduction in obese patients with rheumatoid arthritis, with preservation of body cell mass and improvement of physical fitness. *Clinical and Experimental Rheumatology* 14, 289–93.

Finch S, Doyle W, Lowe C, Bates CJ, Prentice A, Smithers G, Clarke PC (1998) *National Diet and Nutrition Survey*: People aged 65 years and over. Report of the diet and nutrition survey. London, The Stationery Office.

Giordano N, Floravanti A, Sancasciani S, Marcolongo R, Borghi C (1984) Increased storage of iron and anaemia in rheumatoid arthritis: usefulness of desferrioxamine. *British Medical Journal* 289, 961–62.

Goff LM, Barasi ME (1999) An assessment of diets consumed by people with rheumatoid arthritis. *Journal of Human Nutrition and Dietetics* 12, 93–102.

Halliwell B, Gutteridge JMC (1999) *Free Radicals in Biology and Medicine*, 3rd edition. London, Oxford University Press, p. 336.

Hansen GV, Nielsen L, Kluger E, Thysen M, Emmertsen H, Stengaard-Pedersen K, Hansen EL, Unger B, Andersen PW (1996) Nutritional status of Danish rheumatoid arthritis patients and effects of a diet adjusted in energy intake, fish meal and antioxidants. *Scandinavian Journal of Rheumatology* 25, 325–30.

Helliwell M, Coombes EJ, Moody BJ, Batstone GF, Robertson JC (1984) Nutritional status in patients with rheumatoid arthritis. *Annals of the Rheumatic Diseases* 43(3), 386–90.

Henderson L, Gregory J, Swan G (2002–2004) National Diet and Nutrition Survey: adults aged 19–64 years. Food Standards Agency, Department of Health, Office for National statistics, Medical Research Council Human Nutrition Research. The Stationery Office, Norwich 2003/ 04. www.food.gov.uk/science/101717/ndnsdocuments/

Honkanen V, Lamberg-Allaardt C, Vesterinen M, Lehto J, Westermarck T, Metsa-Ketela T, Mussalo-Rauhamaa M, Kontinnen Y (1991) Plasma zinc and copper concentrations in rheumatoid arthritis: influence of dietary factors and disease activity. *American Journal of Clinical Nutrition* 54, 1082–86.

Kaufmann J, Kielstein V, Kilian S, Stein G, Hein G (2003) Relation between Body Mass Index and radiological progression in patients with rheumatoid arthritis. *Journal of Rheumatology* 30, 2350–55.

Kowsari B, Finnie SK, Carter RL, Love J, Katz P, Longley S, Panush RS (1983) Assessment of the diet of patients with rheumatoid arthritis and osteoarthritis. *Journal of the American Dietetic Association* 82(6), 657–59.

Kremer JM, Bigaouette J (1996) Nutrient intake of patients with rheumatoid arthritis is deficient in pyridoxine, zinc, copper, and magnesium. *Journal of Rheumatology* 23(6), 990–94.

Malnutrition Advisory Group (2003) *Malnutrition Universal Screening Tool*. Redditch, BAPEN.

Martin RH (1998) The role of nutrition and diet in rheumatoid arthritis. *Proceedings of the Nutrition Society* 57(2), 231–34.

McAlindon T, Felson DT (1997) Nutrition: risk factors for osteoarthritis. *Annals of the Rheumatic Diseases* 56, 397–402.

Morgan S, Anderson A, Hood S, Matthews P, Lee J, Alarcün (1997) Nutrient intake patterns, body mass index and vitamin levels in patients with rheumatoid arthritis. *Arthritis Care and Research* 10, 9–17.

Munro R, Capell H (1997) Prevalence of low body mass in rheumatoid arthritis: association with the acute phase response. *Annals of the Rheumatic Diseases* 56, 326–29.

New SA, Terry AR, Williams EE, Behn AR, Gray RES (1997) Nutrient intake and food sensitivity in patients with rheumatoid arthritis. *Proceedings of the Nutrition Society* 57, 63A.

Ortiz Z, Shea B, Suarez A, Moher D, Wells G, Tugwell P (2001) Folic and folinic acid for reducing side effects of patients receiving methotrexate for rheumatoid arthritis. *The Cochrane Library* Update Software, 2.

Rayman MP (2000) The importance of selenium to human health. *The Lancet* 356, 233–41.

Roubenoff R, Roubenoff RA, Cannon JG, Kehayias JJ, Zhuang H, Dawson-Hughes B, Dinarello CA, Rosenberg IH (1994) Rheumatoid cachexia: cytokine-driven hypermetabolism accompanying reduced body cell mass in chronic inflammation. *Journal of Clinical Investigation* 93(6), 2379–86.

Roubenoff R, Roubenoff RA, Selhub J, Nadeau MR, Cannon JG, Freeman LM, Dinarello CA, Rosenberg IH (1995) Abnormal vitamin B_6 status in rheumatoid cachexia. Association with spontaneous tumor necrosis factor alpha production and markers of inflammation. *Arthritis and Rheumatism* 38, 105–9.

Stone J, Doube A, Dudson D, Wallace J (1997) Inadequate calcium, folic acid, vitamin E, zinc, and selenium intake in rheumatoid arthritis patients: results of a dietary survey. *Seminars in Arthritis and Rheumatism* 27(3), 180–5.

Work Group Recommendations (2002) Exercise and Physical Activity Conference, St Louis, Missouri (2003). *Arthritis and Rheumatism* 49, 453–54.

6 Popular dietary approaches

6.1 Introduction

Dietary modification is commonly tried by patients with RA and OA with the aim of reducing symptoms (Bigaouette et al. 1987; Darlington & Ramsey 1993; Martin 1998; Goff & Barasi 1999; Thomas 2001). Goff and Barasi (1999) investigated food intake in 54 mainly female patients with RA. The respondents were asked about their general diet and any supplements used: 52% of the respondents believed that diet did affect their condition. Other studies have reported figures of up to 75% (Garrett et al. 1993).

Modification most commonly involves food avoidance and the taking of supplements (Goff & Barasi 1999). There are many popular books on sale recommending diets that are claimed to help arthritic subjects. While some of these dietary approaches may be based upon sound nutritional principles, more often than not there is little or no evidence for their efficacy. Many self-imposed nutritional alterations have been described by Martin (1998) as *'fads, myths and quackery'*.

6.2 Well known popular diets

Darlington and Gamlin (1996) identified a number of popular diets that patients with RA and OA use to try to alleviate symptoms (see Table 6.1). All of these diets are based to some extent on food exclusion and may therefore be effective for some people if they eliminate foods to which they happen to be sensitive. While there are anecdotal reports of successful responses to these diets, none has shown efficacy on scientific testing: for instance, the Dong diet was subjected to a ten-week double-blind, randomised, placebo diet-controlled trial in 26 patients with RA (Panush et al. 1983). This diet, popular in the US, excludes meat, fruit, tomatoes, milk products, egg yolks, vinegar or other acid, pepper, most spices, alcohol, chocolate and anything containing additives. At the end of the ten-week period, 45% of the patients on the Dong diet had improved but so had 40% of those on the placebo diet, showing the power of the placebo effect. Two of the patients on the Dong diet were markedly better, suggesting that certain types of dietary manipulation may be beneficial for a subset of patients (Panush et al. 1983).

Many of the diets cannot work in the manner claimed and beneficial effects are more likely to result from food avoidance (fasting in the extreme case, which is known to reduce inflammation), increased fish intake (see Chapter 9), increased fruit and vegetable intake (see Chapter 8), favourable alteration in gut flora (see Chapter 7) or indeed as a result of the placebo effect (Darlington & Gamlin 1996).

Table 6.1 Popular diets recommended for OA and RA (adapted from Darlington & Gamlin 1996).

Nutritional approach	Description
The Dong Diet	*Avoidance of*: meat, fruit, tomatoes, milk products, egg yolks, vinegar (or other acid), pepper, most spices, alcohol, chocolate and anything containing additives. Occasional poultry is allowed.
Sister Hills Diet	*Avoidance of*: citrus fruits, high fat milk products (cream, butter and cheese), processed meats, alcoholic drinks, fried foods, white sugar, white bread, cream cakes, biscuits, fruit in syrup, duck, kidney, tinned fish and tomatoes. *Reduce*: salt intake, tea and coffee intake and eggs, three-four/week. *Supplements*: vitamin and mineral supplements, 1 tsp of honey and 1 dsp cider vinegar in hot water three times daily, 1 tsp molasses three times daily. Plenty of fish, fresh vegetables and salads.
Living Foods Diet	*Avoidance of*: Animal foods (vegan diet). Foods are eaten raw, although may be blended. *Restrictions*: Foods that cannot be eaten together, e.g. oranges and sunflower seeds, fruits and vegetables must not be combined, and melons can only be eaten alone. *Examples of drinks to include*: Rejuvelac – the liquid produced from soaked wheat grains allowed to ferment for two days. Another drink is made from young green leaves from wheat put through a juicer.
Norman F Childers Diet	*Avoidance of*: Plants from the Solanaceae (nightshade) family i.e. tomato, potato, aubergine (eggplant), peppers (bell peppers, capsicums), pimento and chilli peppers, white and black pepper, all spices made from such peppers, curry powder, foods that have vitamin A or D added.
Dr Campbell's Diet	*Day 1*: A complete fast for 24 hours. *Day 2*: Raw fruits and vegetables (not citrus), raw or lightly cooked with liver and non-homogenised unpasteurised milk. *Day 3*: Fresh (or frozen unprocessed) seafood added, heart, kidney, brain, sweetbread or tripe. This diet is maintained for three to ten days, after this one food is added each day, avoiding foods that cause stiffness. *Entirely forbidden*: flour, coffee, tea, soft drinks, alcohol, sugar, ice cream, puddings, jams, canned/processed food, frozen fruit and processed breakfast cereals. *Supplements*: cod liver oil (two tbsp per day), black molasses (one tbsp per day) and powdered brewers' yeast (one tbsp per day).
Fasting	Complete fast for a number of days (4–maximum of 7), or a juice fast when fruit and vegetable juices are allowed.

Many are unorthodox and extreme, risking the development of nutrient deficiencies, e.g. a complete fast, or the 'Living Foods Diet', the latter being effectively a vegan diet, containing no vitamin B_{12} and being very low in calcium (Thomas 2001; Darlington & Gamlin 1996).

6.3 Food avoidance

Vegetarian and vegan diets are one manifestation of food avoidance practised by some arthritics to reduce symptoms. Of 54 UK respondents with RA, 67% reported practising food avoidance (Goff & Barasi 1999). The most commonly avoided group of foods was citrus fruits followed by tomatoes, vinegar, red meat, and dairy products (Martin 1998; Goff & Barasi 1999). A similar percentage of RA subjects, 66%, reported food sensitivity in a UK study by New and colleagues (1997). Citrus fruits were highlighted as problem foods for 41.2% and dairy products by 15.2%. Other foods that were less problematical included other fruit (9.7%), meat (3.6%), fish (3%), alcohol (3%), additives (3%) and cereals (2.4%). Food exclusion will be discussed more fully in Chapter 7.

6.4 Supplements

Perhaps not surprisingly, as it shows an awareness of the importance of nutrition to health, supplement taking is associated with a healthier diet overall. Older adults who take supplements tend to eat healthier diets and individuals taking supplements tend to have diets higher in fibre, fruits and vegetables, and lower in percent energy from fat (Murphy 2003).

In a UK study of rheumatoid arthritic subjects, 50% reported taking supplements, cod liver oil being the most common (Goff & Barasi 1999). Evening primrose oil, iron, garlic, vitamin C, vitamins A, C and E, selenium, multivitamins, B-vitamin complex and calcium were among the others named by the questionnaire respondents. This is in line with findings from the UK National Diet and Nutrition Survey of those aged 65 or over (Finch et al. 1998) which showed that 29% of the free living took some kind of supplement, most commonly cod liver oil (17.8%), single vitamins (4.1%), vitamins and minerals (4.0%), and multivitamins (3.5%).

In a 1987 US study by Bigaouette and colleagues, supplements were taken by 46% of RA subjects at an average of four supplements each (range, one to seven): ascorbic acid was taken by 19% of participants, 15% took vitamin B-complex and 15% took vitamin E. Many other supplements were also taken. Somewhat more recent data, though not specific to RA sufferers, have been reported by Tucker (2003):

'Dietary supplement use is prevalent among older adults in the United States. Data from the NHANES III show that from 1988–1994, more than 40% of men and 50% of women aged 60 and above reported the use of at least one supplement during the past month.'

Furthermore, there has been an increasing trend in supplement use over the last 15 years so that the percentage of people taking supplements is now likely to be higher. Other studies of the US elderly have found a multivitamin/mineral preparation to be the most popular supplement followed by vitamin C, E and calcium. Eleven per cent of men and 14% of women reported using herbal or other supplements, including ginkgo biloba, garlic, saw palmetto, glucosamine and ginseng (Tucker 2003).

Other supplements used by arthritis sufferers include kelp, blackstrap molasses, yucca, alfalfa tablets, New Zealand green-lipped mussel (seatone), garlic, algal extracts, *Lactobacillus acidophilus*, cider vinegar, iron, calcium, glucosamine sulphate, chondroitin, honey, propolis, royal jelly and ginseng. We shall return to some of these in Chapter 11.

References

Bigaouette J, Timchalk MA, Kremer J (1987) Nutritional adequacy of diet and supplements in patients with rheumatoid arthritis who take medications. *Journal of the American Dietetic Association* 87(12), 1687–88.

Darlington LG, Ramsey NW (1993) Clinical Review – Review of dietary therapy for rheumatoid arthritis. *British Journal of Rheumatology* 32, 507–14.

Darlington G, Gamlin L (1996) *Diet and Arthritis. A comprehensive guide to controlling arthritis through diet.* London, Vermilion.

Finch S, Doyle W, Lowe C, Bates CJ, Prentice A, Smithers G, Clarke PC (1998) *National Diet and Nutrition Survey*: People aged 65 years and over. Report of the diet and nutrition survey. London, The Stationery Office.

Garrett SL, Kennedy LG, Calin A (1993) Patients' perceptions of disease modulation by diet in inflammatory (rheumatoid arthritis/ankylosing spondylitis) and degenerative joint disease. *British Journal of Rheumatology* 32, Suppl. 2, 24.

Goff LM, Barasi M (1999) An assessment of the diets of people with rheumatoid arthritis. *Journal of Human Nutrition and Dietetics* 12, 93–101.

Martin RH (1998) The role of nutrition and diet in rheumatoid arthritis. *Proceedings of the Nutrition Society* 57, 231–34.

Murphy SP (2003) *Ethnic, demographic and lifestyle determinants of dietary supplement use in the elderly*. NIH Office of Dietary Supplements, conference on Dietary Supplement Use in the Elderly, January 14–15, 2003, Bethesda, MD. http://ods.od.nih.gov/pubs/elderly.14jan03.abst.murphy.pdf

New SA, Terry AR, Williams EE, Behn AR, Gray RES (1997) Nutrient intake and food sensitivity on patients with rheumatoid arthritis. *Proceedings of the Nutrition Society* 57, 63A.

Panush R, Carter R, Katz P, Kowsari B, Longley S, Finnie S (1983) Diet therapy for rheumatoid arthritis. *Arthritis and Rheumatism* 26, 462–71.

Thomas B (2001) *The Manual of Dietetic Practice*, 3rd edition. Oxford, Blackwell Science, Chapter 4.32, 588–92.

Tucker KL (2003) *Evidence of use of dietary supplements by the elderly: current usage patterns: who and what?* NIH Office of Dietary Supplements, conference on Dietary Supplement Use in the Elderly, January 14–15, 2003, Bethesda. http://ods.od.nih.gov/pubs/elderly.14jan03.abst.murphy.pdf

7 Exclusion, vegetarian, vegan and other dietary approaches in rheumatoid arthritis

7.1 Introduction

There has always been an interest in the potential of foods or diet to affect arthritis. Panush (1991) has tabulated 49 studies dating back to 1928 that investigated the influence of nutritional factors in rheumatic diseases, a number of which showed beneficial effects resulting from dietary change. Perhaps not surprisingly, self-imposed dietary exclusion is common in arthritic subjects (see Chapter 6): in one study, as many as 67% of RA patients reported some form of food exclusion (Martin 1998).

Adverse reactions to food encompass classical IgE-mediated food allergy and a range of reactions to food that are less well categorised, which together can be referred to as food intolerance. Food intolerance has been implicated in a number of conditions, including RA, where avoidance of foods such as cereals, dairy produce, caffeine, yeast and citrus fruits has been reported to relieve symptoms (Hunter 1991). The following sections describe studies that have investigated the effects of different diets on RA and the conclusions that can be drawn from them. No such studies have been undertaken in OA, which is not primarily an inflammatory disease (but see section 7.6 and 7.7.5). The mechanisms by which these main dietary approaches – exclusion, elemental, vegan or vegetarian diets – may have their effects will be explored.

7.2 Exclusion diets

Many studies investigating dietary exclusion in RA are based upon anecdotal evidence i.e. individual case reports, and are therefore an insufficient basis from which to draw conclusions for the efficacy of particular dietary alterations. It is very difficult to carry out double-blind, controlled studies of dietary elimination. Rennie and colleagues (2003) assert that many studies reported as controlled were not rigorously or completely controlled and cannot therefore be considered as definitive.

The most extreme form of exclusion diet is a complete fast for which there is some evidence of effectiveness. Fasting is known to decrease mitogen and antigen-induced lymphocyte proliferative responses and to suppress IL-2 production and inflammation (Danao-Camara & Shintani 1999; Haugen et al. 1999). A seven-day fast in RA patients decreased $CD4^+$ lymphocyte activation and numbers, suggesting transient immunosuppression (Haugen et al. 1999). Indeed, a preliminary period of fasting may confound any reported improvement in symptoms in an elimination diet (Rennie et al. 2003). RA patients (n = 43) who consumed only water for one week, experienced significant improvement in measurements of arthritic activity (Kroker et al. 1984). In a further study, 15 RA patients who fasted for seven or ten days experienced decreased joint tenderness, pain and stiffness allowing them to reduce their intake of NSAIDs (Sköldstam & Magnusson 1991). One week after returning to their normal diets, no benefit of the fast remained. According to Darlington and Gamlin (1996) this strategy has been used by some RA patients in order to reduce symptoms for a special occasion, fasting from four days before the big event and eating on the day itself. Clearly, however, fasting is a risky strategy in a group of patients already at risk of malnutrition and cannot be recommended. Fasting is usually ineffective in osteoarthritis (Darlington 2002).

Early studies of dietary elimination in RA have been reviewed by Panush (1991) and by Darlington and Ramsey (1993). Though some success was seen in these studies, there was no significant effect between treatment groups in the only study that was double-blind, randomised and placebo diet-controlled (Panush et al. 1983), though this diet, the popular Dong diet, eliminated the same foods for all test subjects (see section 6.2), a strategy now believed to be flawed. However, in that study, two patients out of 11 on the experimental diet, having shown notable improvements, elected to remain on the diet and noted recurrence of symptoms when they deviated from it. Further studies by the same group showed induction or symptomatic exacerbation of arthritis on exposure to milk in both humans and certain rabbit strains while double-blind, encapsulated food challenges pro-voked rheumatologic symptoms in three out of 16 patients that claimed to have food-related arthritis (Panush 1991). Panush suggests that probably fewer than 5% of rheumatic disease patients have immunological sensitivity to foods (Panush 1991).

A more individualised approach was used in the successful study of Darlington and colleagues (1986) who carried out a blinded, placebo-controlled study of the influence of food elimination in 53 rheumatoid patients. All subjects followed an exclusion phase for seven to ten days during which they ate a small range of rarely eaten foods. Foods were then introduced, one by one, to see which ones caused symptoms. Any foods provoking reactions during the reintroduction phase were identified as culprit foods and avoided thereafter. Culprit foods varied from one individual to the next. Forty-four subjects finished the trial. Of these, 36% felt that after food exclusions they were much better and 39% felt they were better. Objective measurements provided support for these findings – decreased pain and number of painful joints, reduced duration of morning stiffness, shorter time to walk 20 yards, better grip strength and improved erythrocyte sedimentation rate (ESR), haemoglobin, fibrinogen and platelet levels. Improvement on dietary therapy was found to be independent of weight loss (Darlington & Ramsey 1993).

To confirm which foods produce symptoms, ideally a blind food challenge with capsules of the 'culprit' foods should be carried out. At a later date, a blind challenge with three of their culprit foods carried out on 15 RA patients produced deterioration in pain, number of painful joints, morning stiffness, grip strength

Table 7.1 Foods most likely to cause intolerance in rheumatoid patients (reproduced from Darlington & Ramsey 1993 with permission of Oxford University Press).

Food	Symptomatic patients affected by food (%)
Corn	57
Wheat	54
Bacon/pork	39
Oranges	39
Milk	37
Oats	37
Rye	34
Eggs	32
Beef	32
Coffee	32
Malt	27
Cheese	24
Grapefruit	24
Tomato	22
Peanuts	20
Sugar (cane)	20
Butter	17
Lamb	17
Lemons	17
Soya	17

and walking time (Darlington & Ramsey 1993). Foods found by Darlington and Ramsey to be most likely to cause problems in RA patients are shown in Table 7.1.

It can be seen from the table that wheat is one of the foods most likely to cause an adverse reaction and RA has frequently been demonstrated to occur concurrently with coeliac disease, where (wheat) gluten is the offending substance (Cordain et al. 2000). Multiple studies of arthritic patients have demonstrated elevated antibody (IgG) levels to gliadin peptides, breakdown products of gluten (O'Farrelly et al. 1988; Cordain et al. 2000). Of those with raised IgG, 86% were also positive for IgA rheumatoid factor (RF) and they had lower villous surface to volume ratio than patients without antibodies or age-matched controls (O'Farrelly et al. 1988). While gluten-free diets have been shown to be effective in reducing arthritic symptoms in coeliac patients (Cordain et al. 2000), no large clinical trials have looked exclusively at a gluten-free diet for arthritis.

A small exclusion study was carried out by Gianfranceschi and colleagues (1996) where food exclusion was tailored to each individual. Twelve RA patients entered a crossover study to evaluate the effects of different normocaloric diets, one of which excluded foods to which the individual had been shown to react on the basis of a dynamometric challenge test (DRIA test). On the exclusion diets, patients had 42% (95% CI 58%, 25%; $p < 0.005$) less joint pain and 40% (95% CI 66%, 3%; $p < 0.005$) reduction in morning stiffness than when on a 'well balanced' diet. The authors comment that for the relief of RA symptoms, the diet cannot be a standard one but should be selected according to individual food sensitivities.

It is clear that food exclusion diets based on eliminating the same foods for all patients will have a low success rate, as culprit foods will vary from one individual to another. By contrast, elimination diets that were effectively personally tailored were successful for 30–40% of subjects with RA (Darlington & Ramsey 1993; Gianfranceschi et al. 1996). For a detailed description of the principles and practice of this type of elimination diet, see Radcliffe (2002) and Darlington and Gamlin (1996). The diet used in Dr Gail Darlington's RA clinic and later applied in Dr Dorothy Pattison's RA clinic is given in Appendix 4 (personal communications, Dr Gail Darlington & Dr Dorothy Pattison 2005).

The difficulties and risks of elimination and reintroduction suggest that elimination and reintroduction of foods should be carried out under the supervision of an appropriate health professional, preferably with the input of a dietitian. Where possible, patients should be given blind challenge tests with the alleged culprit foods at a later date to confirm or refute the initial findings. This will ensure that as wide a diet as possible is maintained and reduce the risk of nutrient deficiency.

According to Rennie and colleagues (2003), it is estimated that probably fewer than 5% of RA patients do have an actual immune sensitivity to specific foods, which is similar to the level found in the general population. As this does not accord with the results reported by Darlington and colleagues, we must ask whether the food sensitivities that appear to be related to RA symptoms are immune sensitivities or whether they result from some other mechanism. We shall address this question in section 7.6.

7.3 Vegan and vegetarian diets

Vegetarian, and to a lesser extent, vegan diets are types of food exclusion with which people are reasonably familiar. These diets can be classified by degree of strictness as follows (Thomas 2001):

- Vegan: no meat, poultry, fish, shellfish, eggs or dairy products
- Lactovegetarian: no meat, poultry, fish, shellfish or eggs but dairy products eaten
- Lacto-ovo-vegetarian: no meat, poultry, fish or shellfish but dairy products and eggs eaten
- Piscatarian vegetarian: no red meat or poultry but fish eaten
- Demi-vegetarian: no red meat but poultry and fish eaten

Studies based largely on vegan or lactovegetarian diets have shown some evidence of success in the RA population. Studies published up to 1997 were systematically reviewed by Muller and colleagues (2001). Of these studies, only four were controlled and investigated the effects of fasting and subsequent vegetarian diets for three months or more (Lindberg 1973; Sköldstam et al. 1979; Sköldstam 1986 and Kjelsden-Kragh et al. 1991). When the results of these four studies were pooled, a statistically and clinically significant beneficial long-term effect was found.

The early study by Sköldstam and colleagues (1979) showed the benefit of a 7–10 day fast on RA disease symptoms in 16 patients but there was a rapid deterioration when patients were switched to a lactovegetarian diet. In the subsequent study, the period of fasting was followed by three months on a vegan diet (Sköldstam 1986). While 11 of 20 patients had undergone subjective improvement during this period, there was no improvement in objective variables such as ESR and C-reactive protein (CRP) and 19 patients had lost weight, a downside to such dietary regimens.

Kjeldsen-Kragh and colleagues (1991) carried out a 13-month placebo-controlled, prospective, randomised, single blind trial in 53 participants with RA, who were allocated to one of two dietary regimens. Patients in the experimental diet group (n = 27) were based at a health farm for the initial four weeks where they fasted for the first seven to ten days (herbal tea, parsley, garlic, vegetable broth, skinned potatoes, carrot juice, beet and celery were allowed). After this, a basic diet of the same foods as were eaten during the fast was followed with a new food item added every two days. Foods were omitted for seven days if pain, discomfort or stiffness occurred. This subsequent diet was vegan, and gluten-free. Refined sugar, citrus fruits, strong spices, salts, preservatives, alcohol, tea and coffee were also avoided. The diet was followed for three and a half months, after which time dairy products and foods containing gluten were reintroduced individually, followed by a lactovegetarian diet for 12 months. Patients in the control group (n = 23), though they were sent to a convalescent home for the initial four weeks, followed a normal omnivorous diet for the entire study.

Clinical examinations were carried out at baseline, one, four, seven, 10 and 13 months, with regular 24 hour dietary recalls at and between these assessments. Almost all disease variables (objective signs) decreased significantly after one month of treatment in the experimental group. Patients were divided into responders and non-responders, based on clinical criteria. Twelve of 27 subjects (44%) in the experimental group and two out of 26 (8%) in the control group were responders to the dietary regimens. When stool samples from the patients in the trial were analysed (Peltonen et al. 1994), it was found that those patients who had improved markedly had had a change in their faecal flora that was not seen in those who had improved only slightly (see section 7.7.4). After one year, 22 patients from the experimental group and 23 from the control group were re-examined. All of the diet responders but only half of the diet non-responders were still following the same diet as that consumed in the study.

In a subsequent study by the same group (see section 7.7.4), of 43 RA patients randomised to an uncooked vegan diet or a normal omnivorous diet, 28% of those on the vegan diet showed a marked improvement, again corresponding to a significant change in faecal flora (Peltonen et al. 1997). In a later review of these studies, Kjeldsen-Kragh (1999) concluded that:

'Fasting, followed by a vegetarian diet has a favourable influence on disease activity in some patients with RA.'

Hafstrom et al. (2001) studied 66 patients with active RA, randomised to receive either a gluten-free vegan diet (38 patients) or a 'well balanced non-vegan diet' (28 patients) for one year. At nine months, nine patients of the 22 remaining in the vegan group (41%) and one patient of the 25 remaining in the non-vegan group (4%) fulfilled the set improvement criteria. Corresponding figures for the intention-to-treat populations were 24% and 4%. The IgG antibody levels against gliadin and β-lactoglobulin decreased but only in the responder subgroup of those on the vegan diet (Hafstrom et al. 2001).

A vegan diet and the early phases of the Kjeldsen-Kragh diet are quite strict and readily lead to weight loss and micronutrient deficiencies. It would therefore be inadvisable for RA patients to carry out these diets without professional support. That said, 25–45% of those capable of sticking to such a regime appear to have a decrease in symptoms. As observed by Kjelsden-Kragh (1999):

'Provided that detrimental effects on nutritional status can be prevented, dietary treatment may prove to be a valuable supplement to the ordinary therapeutic armamentarium for RA.'

7.4 The Mediterranean diet

Fruit and vegetables with their antioxidant components have a central position in the Mediterranean diet, which is widely believed to be a healthy diet. A typical interpretation of the traditional Greek Mediterranean diet is shown in Figure 7.1 (Trichopoulou & Vasilopoulou 2000). Such a diet is rich in antioxidants, n-3 fatty acids and olive oil, which have been shown to be of importance in RA (see Chapters 3, 8 and 9). Thus it was thought that such a Mediterranean diet might suppress disease activity in patients with RA.

RA patients (n = 56) followed either a modified Cretan Mediterranean diet or an ordinary Western (control) diet for 12 weeks (Sköldstam et al. 2003). The diet group were advised to eat large amounts of fruits and vegetables, pulses, cereals, fish (especially fish with a high n-3 fatty acid content), nuts and seeds [with high α-linolenic acid (ALA) content]. Meat (such as pork, beef, lamb or mutton), cured meat, sausage etc. was replaced by poultry, fish or vegetarian dishes and olive oil and canola oil were used for food preparation, baking and in salad dressing. Margarine was based on canola oil. No recommendation was given for alcohol but patients were advised to drink green or black tea.

Clinical examinations were performed at baseline, three, six and 12 weeks while plasma levels of antioxidants and urinary malondialdehyde (MDA), a marker of oxidative stress, were also assessed (Hagfors et al. 2003). In the second half of the 12-week trial, patient-assessed improvements were seen in inflammation, physical functioning and vitality in those on the Mediterranean diet compared to those on the control diet. Though significantly higher intakes of antioxidant-rich foods were recorded, there was no change in urine MDA or plasma levels of antioxidants. However, the plasma levels of vitamin C, retinol and uric acid were inversely correlated with RA disease activity variables (Hagfors et al. 2003). These results indicate that the Mediterranean diet may improve physical functioning and decrease inflammation in RA. However, additional studies are required to confirm these findings.

Part of the benefit of the Mediterranean diet may relate to its higher content of n-3 fatty acids, higher n-3 to n-6 ratio (Hagfors et al. 2005), and content of olive

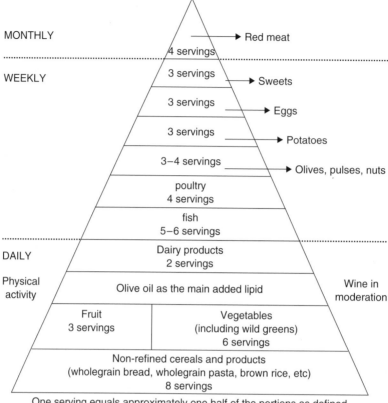

MONTHLY   → Red meat
4 servings

WEEKLY   3 servings   → Sweets

3 servings   → Eggs

3 servings   → Potatoes

3–4 servings   → Olives, pulses, nuts

poultry
4 servings

fish
5–6 servings

DAILY   Dairy products
2 servings

Physical
activity   Olive oil as the main added lipid   Wine in
moderation

Fruit   Vegetables
3 servings   (including wild greens)
6 servings

Non-refined cereals and products
(wholegrain bread, wholegrain pasta, brown rice, etc)
8 servings

One serving equals approximately one half of the portions as defined
in the Greek market regulations

Also remember to:
- drink plenty of water
- avoid salt and replace it with herbs (e.g. oregano, basil, thyme, etc)

Figure 7.1   The traditional Mediterranean diet pyramid depicting dietary guidelines for adults in Greece (reproduced with permission from Trichopoulou & Vasilopoulou 2000).

oil. It has recently been discovered that fresh extra virgin olive oil contains an anti-inflammatory component named oleocanthal (Beauchamp et al. 2005). Concentrations of oleocanthal will vary depending on the variety of the olives, and their age at pressing. A neat oil that strongly stings the throat when sipped will have the best concentration. A 50 g daily dose (4 tablespoonfuls) of such olive oil is equivalent to about 10% of the ibuprofen dose recommended for adult pain relief. Though this is a small dose, it may have additive effects if taken daily with other aspects of the Mediterranean diet.

7.5   Elemental diets

An elemental diet is a routine treatment used to induce remission in active Crohn's disease which, like RA, is an inflammatory condition. Thus it was thought it might be effective in RA. It is considered to be hypoallergenic because it provides food broken down into its simplest form: amino acids, glucose, medium chain triglycerides, vitamins, minerals and trace elements. Though it provides all the calories, vitamins and minerals required, because it is a powdered food, mixed with water, it is a deeply unpopular diet and difficult to sustain. However, it has been used in a number of studies in RA patients.

van de Laar and van der Korst (1992) examined the influence of food allergy or intolerance in 94 patients with seropositive RA over a 12-week period using double-blind, randomised methodology. Patients were monitored while eating their normal diets for four weeks followed by four weeks on one of two dietary regimens:

- An allergen-free elemental diet, free from additives, preservatives and common allergenic components. Participants were also allowed to consume three apples per day, tea, allergen-free chewing gum and sugar
- An elemental diet containing milk allergens and azo dyes, but free from other allergenic substances

After four weeks following either diet, participants returned to their normal dietary intake. Clinical and laboratory parameters of disease activity were scored every two weeks. Improvements were seen in all patients during the four week dietary intervention, based on several disease parameters. When the normal diet was re-established, clinical and subjective parameters reversed. While no significant differences were found between the two groups, it was noted that some individuals seemed to show a marked symptomatic improvement.

The individuals who showed marked improvement were followed up in a subsequent study (van de Laar et al. 1992). The six patients were reintroduced to the non-allergenic elemental diet until symptoms reduced (clinical remission). Then three times per week, double-blind food challenges were given with either an incriminating food (a food causing a positive skin reaction in subjects) or placebo. These challenges showed intolerance for specific foodstuffs in four out of the six patients. Biopsy specimens were taken from the synovial fluid and proximal small intestine in three of these patients before the non-allergenic diet and during the diet, if disease activity had been reduced. Clinical reduction in inflammatory joint parameters was obtained with the allergen-free diet and a reduction in inflammation was also seen histologically, which was, however, only moderate. In two patients, both with raised serum IgE concentrations and specific IgE antibodies to certain foods, a marked reduction of mast cells in the synovial membrane and proximal small intestine was seen. These patients clearly demonstrated an underlying immunological reaction to these foods. It was concluded that food intolerance may exist in a minority of seropositive RA patients, probably in around 5%.

Holst-Jensen et al. (1998) conducted a single-blind randomised study of 30 patients with RA, allocated to either an elemental peptide diet or normal diet for four weeks. Patients were followed for a total of six months. Several outcome measures were assessed such as morning stiffness, pain intensity and patient's global assessment of health. While the diet group saw a statistically significant improvement in level of pain (p = 0.02), Health Assessment Questionnaire score (p = 0.03), and a significant reduction in body mass index (BMI) (p = 0.001), a clear remission was only achieved in one patient. Two further studies in this area (see below) also concluded that elemental feeding is advantageous only to some RA patients.

Haugen and colleagues (1994) carried out a controlled, double-blind pilot study of an elemental diet in treatment of RA. Seventeen patients were included, ten receiving an elemental diet and seven receiving a control soup for three weeks. During the fourth week the patients' normal diets were resumed. A significant improvement was seen in the number of tender joints in the experimental group. Three patients in the experimental group and two in the control group improved in all measured disease variables showing a response in a subset of patients.

Kavanagh et al. (1995) studied 47 patients with RA in a controlled, randomised, double-blind trial to receive one of two diets for four weeks:

- Experimental diet: Elemental 028 (clinically used elemental diet) plus some chicken, fish, rice, carrots, runner beans and bananas to increase patient tolerance
- Elemental 028 taken as a drink substitute, twice a day, plus normal food

After four weeks, foods were reintroduced to the experimental diet one at a time with a period of 48 hours between each introduction. If symptoms worsened, the food was eliminated. Several variables were recorded including morning stiffness and CRP concentration. There was a high default rate with only 38% of participants completing the 24-week study. The elemental diet was successful in achieving initial improvements in grip strength (p = 0.008) and Ritchie score (p = 0.006) although at 24-weeks, after food reintroduction, the difference between the groups disappeared.

Though all of these studies show that an elemental diet can improve RA symptoms in a subset of individuals and may induce remission, improvements in symptoms are only seen while on the diet, re-emerging when the normal diet is recommenced. Given the nature of the elemental diet, the lack of pleasure in consuming it and the difficulty in sustaining it, it is hard to see an argument for its use in RA except perhaps on a temporary basis as a diet of last resort.

7.6   Summary of dietary findings

In summary, controlled studies involving exclusion of foods such as red meat, dairy products, cereals and wheat gluten have reported inconsistent results (Rennie et al. 2003). This is likely to be because only a subgroup of patients (the diet responders) can benefit from dietary modification, and because the foods to which patients are intolerant differ from one individual to the next. In general, it can be said that:

- RA patients can benefit from symptom relief during fasting (though there is a risk of malnutrition), but symptoms recur on reintroduction of food.

- A fast followed by a vegan or lactovegetarian diet can have a longer term benefit on symptoms of RA for up to 45% of those capable of following such a regime.
- There is some evidence that a Mediterranean diet may be of benefit to those with RA.
- An elemental diet is unlikely to be an appropriate option.
- A subgroup of RA patients (30–40%) will benefit from an elimination diet followed by a reintroduction phase to identify 'culprit foods' that they must then avoid.
- A subgroup of patients can remain well, off all medication and controlled by diet alone, for follow-up periods of up to 12 years.

It may therefore be worth trying an elimination diet or a lactovegetarian or vegan diet, possibly following a short fast, for a patient who is not underweight and who has sufficient professional support. If improvement is not seen within a period of three weeks (Darlington & Gamlin 1996), the diet should be abandoned. Although, unlike RA, OA is not primarily an inflammatory condition, OA patients with noticeable joint inflammation, more generalised joint involvement, a family history of RA or other symptoms typical of food intolerance such as headaches, irritable bowel syndrome (IBS), asthma or eczema, may wish to try an elimination diet or other dietary therapy as outlined above (Darlington & Gamlin 1996).

7.7 Possible mechanisms by which exclusion, elemental, vegan and vegetarian diets may exert their effects on RA

A number of mechanisms for dietary effects in RA have been suggested. These are shown schematically in Figure 7.2 and described below.

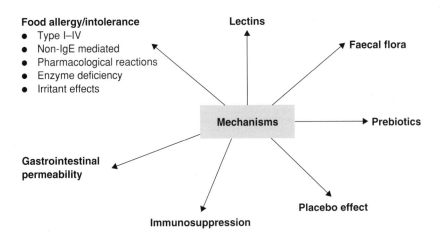

Figure 7.2 Mechanisms by which exclusion, elemental, vegan and vegetarian diets may exert their effects on RA.

7.7.1   Food allergy or intolerance

Only a single layer of epithelial cells separates the individual from enormous amounts of antigens of both bacterial and dietary origin (Kjeldsen-Kragh 1999) though the function of the gut-associated lymphoid tissue (GALT) is to protect the individual from harmful allergens that may pass through the epithelial layer of the intestine (Schley & Field 2002). However, there is evidence from reputable researchers that food allergy or intolerance may have a role in some people with RA, estimates varying between 5 and 32% (Hunter 1991; Darlington & Ramsey 1993; Kjeldsen-Kragh 1999; Haugen et al. 1999). Thus, foods truly can exacerbate arthritis in some patients (Kjeldsen-Kragh 1999; Hunter 1991).

True allergic responses to food are typified by the well recognised peanut or shellfish allergy. Four types of food allergy are recognised:

- *Type I*: An immediate reaction after exposure to a foreign protein. Symptoms include rhinitis, asthma, flushing, lip mouth and throat swelling, breathing difficulties and anaphylaxis. This allergic reaction is IgE-mediated.
- *Type II*: Immediate effects are seen as with type I reactions but this response is confined to cell membranes only.
- *Type III*: Immune-complex reactions which may occur hours after exposure to the antigen. Reactions normally occur in the skin and bronchi.
- *Type IV*: Cell-mediated reactions that occur 24–48 hours after exposure.

With a few exceptions, sensitivities to foods in patients with RA are not acute, allergic (Type I) reactions, nor have abnormal IgE levels or positive skin tests to food extracts been shown in patients with RA undergoing dietary therapy (Darlington & Ramsey 1993; Darlington 2002). Furthermore, immune complexes are not raised in food-sensitive patients, nor do they fall when patients respond to dietary therapy (Darlington 2002). When Kjeldsen-Kragh (1999) measured IgE, IgG, IgM and IgA antibodies against food antigens, no association between the food items to which subjects believed they had adverse reactions and the antibody activity to antigens in these foods was found, indicating that systemic immune reactions against food antigens are not of pathogenic importance in most patients (Kjeldsen-Kragh 1999).

However, some studies of RA patients have demonstrated elevated antibody (IgG) levels, notably for gliadin peptides (from gluten) in association with raised IgA RF (O'Farrelly et al. 1988; Cordain et al. 2000; Darlington 2002). Furthermore, IgG antibody levels against gliadin and β-lactoglobulin decreased in the responder subgroup of those on a vegan diet (Hafstrom et al. 2001). IgG antibodies generally give a more delayed response following antigen exposure and have been implicated in some cases of food sensitivity (Atkinson et al. 2004). Testing for IgG antibodies is simple, commercially available and has shown some value as a basis for food elimination in IBS, though not as yet in RA (Atkinson et al. 2004). Clinical immunologists, however, point out that IgG antibodies are present in healthy individuals and so this mechanism is controversial. Further studies are needed to investigate its relevance to RA.

Food intolerance is believed to be a non-immunologically mediated process and again four types of food intolerance are recognised:

- Non-IgE-mediated: this may be difficult to differentiate from food allergy though with food intolerance, no immunological response is involved.
- Pharmacological: taking large amounts of foods with pharmacologically active constituents can trigger reactions. Pork, tomato, spinach, shellfish, strawberries, chocolate, fish, citrus fruits, 'old' tuna, coffee and alcohol are all examples of foods that may contain or cause the release of vasoactive amines, such as histamine, serotonin, octopamine and phenylephrine. High levels of vasoactive amines may cause disease aggravation in RA patients (Haugen et al. 1999).
- Enzyme deficiency: malabsorption may result if one or more enzyme is absent or deficient, for example lactase deficiency leads to lactose intolerance.
- Irritant effects: some foods may cause irritation to the gastrointestinal tract.

There is no doubt that a subset of RA patients who are not food allergic can benefit from dietary therapy. While for convenience we may describe such patients as food intolerant, this does not necessarily imply that one of the above mechanisms is relevant: one or a number of the mechanisms described below or some completely different explanation may be responsible for dietary alteration of disease symptoms.

7.7.2   Alteration of gastrointestinal permeability

The gastrointestinal tract may play an important role in the pathogenesis of RA (Cordain et al. 2000). A mucosal immune system, gut-associated lymphoid tissue (GALT), protects the intestine, being strategically placed where external pathogens and allergens can gain access to the body (Schley & Field 2002). Despite this protection, increased gut permeability, a result of the gut inflammation that exists in up to 67% of RA patients (Cordain et al. 2000), possibly exacerbated by NSAID and DMARD treatment, can allow the passage of antigens. Thus luminal bacteria and polypeptides may be chronically absorbed in quantities sufficient to produce immunological responses leading to overt expression of RA (Darlington & Ramsey 1993). A strong relationship between gut inflammation and joint inflammation has been recognised for decades in clinical practice (Cordain et al. 2000).

Gut permeability can be increased by strong coffee or tea, highly spiced food, raw pineapple or papaya and excessive amounts of alcohol (Darlington & Gamlin 1996), but also by disease, acetic acid, cereal grains and lectins derived from legumes (Cordain et al. 2000). Omission of such substances from the diet could reduce gastrointestinal permeability, thereby reducing symptoms.

7.7.3   Effect of lectins

It may be possible to reduce peripheral antigenic stimulation by the exclusion of lectins, dietary elements found in legumes and cereals (see section 2.4.5; Darlington

& Ramsey 1993; Cordain et al. 2000). Lectins are carbohydrate-binding gly-coproteins of non-immune origin that may act as immunogens, allergens and gut irritants and may directly interact with bacteria of the digestive tract (Pusztai 1993; Darlington 2002). Foods in the legume or cereals group, such as beans, wheat, peanuts, peas and lentils, contain lectins and indeed foods commonly associated with food allergy such as peanuts and wheat are particularly rich in lectins (Darlington & Ramsey 1993). According to Darlington (2002), with increased consumption of raw and unprocessed foods by 'health conscious' people, we are probably now exposed to greater amounts of dietary lectins than at any time for many decades.

Most lectins are resistant to breakdown by gut proteolytic enzymes and some, such as the phytohaemagglutanin (PHA) from kidney bean (*Phaseolus vulgaris*), survive almost quantitatively (Pusztai 1993). Even less resistant lectins are only about 80% broken down on passage through the gut (Pusztai 1993). Most lectin-containing foods are cooked before they are eaten. Although cooking destroys most lectins, this takes a long time at fairly high temperatures and some lectins may simply be resistant to cooking (Cordain et al. 2000; Freed 1999). Wheat, rye, barley, oats, maize and particularly kidney beans, have all shown residual lectin activity despite cooking (Cordain et al. 2000).

It has been suggested that lectins may have a role in the pathogenesis of food intolerance in RA (Darlington & Ramsey 1993). They have been used to produce experimentally induced RA in rabbits (Brauer et al. 1983). Lectins bind specifically to glycosylated membrane receptors on gut epithelial cells and can be endocytosed, generating an immune response (Pusztai 1993). Not only do lectins interact with enterocytes and lymphocytes, they trigger mast cells directly, and by binding to the lining of the gut wall, increase its permeability (Darlington & Ramsey 1993). Translocation of dietary and gut-derived antigens to peripheral tissues such as liver, spleen, kidney and blood can then occur (Cordain et al. 2000).

Animal experiments have shown that legume and cereal lectins are also capable of altering gut microflora (Pusztai 1993). Some lectins, notably PHA and soya bean agglutinin (SBA), act as growth signals for the gut, resulting in accelerated cell turnover and increasing the number of juvenile cells on the small intestinal villi. These juvenile cells have an increased number of mannose receptors, allowing the attachment of more *E. coli* to the gut wall resulting in *E. coli* overgrowth. (On the other hand, by competitively blocking adhesion sites for bacteria, some lectins can selectively *inhibit* bacterial binding to the gut, reducing pathogenic infections.)

The increased intestinal permeability noted above that results from lectin-binding facilitates the translocation of gut pathogens to the periphery (for references, see Cordain et al. 2000). This may be a particular problem in the case of gut patho-gens such as *E. coli* and *Lactobacillus lactis* that contain the Q(K/R)RAA shared epitope (see section 2.4.2), potentially triggering cross-reactivity with the con-served amino acid sequence in individuals susceptible to RA by virtue of carrying the MHC class II HLA-DR4 and HLA-DR1 alleles (Cordain et al. 2000).

In vitro, lectins do have antidotes: they have specific chemical reactivity with saccharides so their action can be blocked by simple sugars (Cordain et al. 2002). Table 7.2 shows these sugar specificities, e.g. wheat lectin, rice and barley lectins

Table 7.2 Examples of foods containing lectins and their *in vitro* sugar specificities (adapted from Cordain et al. 2002).

Plant name	Sugar specificity
Peanut, groundnut	Galactose
Jack bean	Mannose, Glucose
Horse gram	N-acetylglucosamine
Hyacinth bean	Not available
Soya bean	Galactose, N-acetylglucosamine
Barley	N-acetylglucosamine
Lentil	Mannose, Glucose
Winged bean	Fucose
Rice	N-acetylglucosamine
Mung bean	Not available
Scarlet runner bean	N-acetylglucosamine
Lima bean	N-acetylglucosamine
Kidney bean	N-acetylglucosamine
Garden pea, split pea	Mannose, Glucose
Castor bean	Galactose, N-acetylglucosamine
Potato	Diacetylchitobiose
Wheat	N-acetylglucosamine
Horse bean, broad bean	Mannose, Glucosamine

can be blocked by N-acetylglucosamine. Therefore, if wheat or wheat lectin (wheatgerm agglutinin) is a suspected trigger food for RA symptoms, oral N-acetylglucosamine oligomers may be an effective treatment.

Despite the above considerations, which have mostly been determined from animal work, vegan and vegetarian diets that have shown success in a subset of RA patients must be rich sources of lectins, calling into question the importance of lectins as triggers for RA. Furthermore, exposure to lectins is likely to have occurred during the evolutionary development of our digestive system (Pusztai 1993). Nonetheless, it would be sensible for anyone with a tendency for inflammatory joint disease to ensure that foods rich in lectins are always thoroughly cooked and to be on the lookout for an adverse reaction to kidney beans (*Phaseolus vulgaris*), a particularly rich source of phytohaemagglutinin (Freed 1999).

7.7.4 Alteration to gut flora: pre- and probiotic dietary components

As previously explained (see section 2.4.6), intestinal flora differ between RA patients and normal controls (Peltonen et al. 1997; Toivanen 2001, 2003). For instance, the majority of RA patients were found to have an abnormally abundant faecal flora of atypical *Clostridium perfringens* (Darlington & Ramsey 1993; Kjelsden-Kragh 1999). This same bacterium was associated with the development of symptoms of arthritis in pigs following feeding with a fish-powder diet, demonstrating that diet can affect gut flora and lead to the development of arthritis (Darlington & Ramsey 1993; Kjeldsen-Kragh 1999).

If abnormal gut flora or a disorder of bacterial fermentation in the colon were a causal factor in the appearance of RA symptoms, then dietary manipulation that altered intestinal microflora could well be beneficial. Though the mechanism by which dietary change may alter gut flora to reduce arthritic symptoms is unclear, such a change might reduce the antigenic challenge of the gut, thereby influencing the degree of joint inflammation (Kjeldsen-Kragh 1999). Some examples follow.

Patients with active RA have antibodies to *Proteus mirabilis* in their serum (Ebringer et al. 1985; Kjeldsen-Kragh 1999). In a group of RA patients, a change to a vegetarian diet caused a significant decrease in IgG antibody activity to *Proteus mirabilis*, which was significantly more pronounced in those who improved on the diet than in the non-responders or omnivores (for references, see Kjeldsen-Kragh 1999). This decline correlated significantly with a reduction in a composite index of disease activity.

When RA patients changed from an omnivorous to a vegetarian diet, a significant alteration in the bacterial composition of the faeces was observed (as estimated by cellular fatty acid profile) that correlated with changes in disease activity (Peltonen et al. 1994). Faecal flora from patients experiencing the largest improvement in symptoms on the vegetarian diet (high improvement index defined as $\geq 20\%$ improvement in five or six of six disease activity parameters) was significantly different from those on the same diet with a low improvement index (Peltonen et al. 1994). Similar methodology was applied in a later study where 43 patients were randomised either to a vegan diet (an uncooked diet rich in *Lactobacilli*) or to a continuation of their normal omnivorous diets (Peltonen et al. 1997). A significant ($p = 0.001$) diet-induced change in faecal flora was observed in the test group but not in the control group. Furthermore, after one month of the vegan dietary regimen, in the test group, those with a high improvement index (28%) had significantly ($p = 0.001$) different faecal flora from those with a low improvement index. It therefore appears that changes in faecal flora brought about by a vegetarian or vegan diet in a percentage of individuals are associated with improvement in RA activity (Peltonen et al. 1997).

A diet with significant pre- or probiotic components may alter intestinal flora, thereby influencing RA disease activity. A prebiotic is a fermentable fibre that passes into the colon to become a selective substrate for a number of beneficial colonic bacteria (Schley & Field 2002) while a probiotic (e.g. live yoghurt) contains active bacterial components associated with beneficial effects such as certain lactobacilli or bifidobacteria.

Prebiotic dietary components may favour the growth of beneficial bacterial strains (Gibson & Roberfroid 1995) and may therefore have a role to play in RA disease modification. There is strong evidence that consumption of prebiotic fibres such as inulin and oligofructose (FOS) increases the proportion of beneficial lactic acid bacteria in the human colon (Schley & Field 2002). Furthermore, there are convincing preliminary data to suggest that the consumption of prebiotic fibres can modulate immune parameters in GALT, secondary lymphoid tissues and peripheral circulation (Schley & Field 2002). Changes in the intestinal microflora provoked by prebiotic components may mediate immune changes by:

(1) The direct contact of lactic acid bacteria or bacterial products with immune cells in the intestine
(2) The production of short-chain fatty acids from fibre fermentation that have immunomodulatory and anti-inflammatory properties
(3) Changes in mucin production that might result in reduced bacterial translocation across the gut barrier (Gibson & Roberfroid 1995; Schley & Field 2002)

There is some evidence that probiotics in the diet may be beneficial in inflammatory arthritis. Treatment of rats with *Lactobacillus rhamnosus GG* (LGG), either live or heat killed, had a significant ($p < 0.001$) preventive and therapeutic effect on experimentally induced arthritis (Baharav et al. 2004). The best anti-inflammatory effect on clinically active arthritis in these rats was found with commercial yoghurts containing LGG, or to a lesser extent, *Lactobacillus bulgaricus*. The fact that the anti-inflammatory effect did not depend on the viability of the micro-organism indicates that a heat-stable bacterial wall, cell membrane or intracellular component is responsible for the effect, or alternatively that systemic immuno-modulation by bacterial or milk-derived factors occurs (Baharav et al. 2004). A human study had a rather less successful outcome. Probiotic treatment with capsules of LGG *vs.* placebo was instigated in a group of 21 patients with RA over a 12-month period. At the end of this time, the LGG group showed a reduction in the number of tender and swollen joints and improved subjective wellbeing but there were no statistically significant differences in disease activity between the LGG and control groups as assessed by clinical parameters, biochemical variables and a health assessment questionnaire (Hatakka et al. 2003). The authors believe that more studies are warranted on the effects of probiotic bacteria in RA.

In summary, the beneficial effect of dietary treatment seen in some RA patients may result from alterations in colonic microflora caused by the dietary change that affect gut permeability, fermentation and immunity thereby reducing joint inflammation (Schley & Field 2002). The potential of pre- and probiotic dietary components in the amelioration of RA has not yet been fully explored.

7.7.5 Weight reduction and associated immunosuppression

Although most of the dietary information in this chapter is relevant primarily to patients with RA, weight reduction can definitely benefit patients with OA, in particular decreasing the risk of development of OA of the knees, hips and hands (Darlington 2002). The relevant mechanisms – reduced mechanical load on weightbearing joints and lower production of inflammatory mediators by adipose tissue – are discussed in section 3.6.

In many dietary studies, RA patients lost weight in the experimental group (Kjeldsen-Kragh 1999; Darlington & Ramsey 1993; Kavanagh et al. 1995; Holst-Jensen et al. 1998; Darlington, Ramsey & Mansfield 1986). As dietary energy re-striction is associated with immunosuppression (Kjeldsen-Kragh 1999; Darlington & Ramsey 1993), the clinical improvements seen in these studies could be secondary to malnutrition (Kjeldsen-Kragh 1999) partly explaining why symptoms recommence on return to the normal diet, as weight increases. However, weight reduction over time did not differ significantly between diet responders and non-responders (Kjeldsen-Kragh 1999). Many RA patients lose weight during periods of disease activity without having associated benefit (Darlington & Ramsey 1993). It is therefore unlikely that weight reduction associated with dietary change is the main factor in improvement of symptoms in diet responders.

7.7.6   Placebo effect

Though the placebo effect may have contributed to the clinical responses noted in some studies it is insufficient to explain all of the significant improvements seen in studies of food exclusion or dietary modification, such as vegan or elemental diets (Darlington & Ramsey 1993; Darlington et al. 1986). The effects of the placebo response generally fade over time. In a study of one-year duration (Kjeldsen-Kragh 1999), clear objective signs of decreased disease activity in the diet responders were still apparent at the end of the study, suggesting that the effect was not simply due to a placebo response.

7.8   Risks of undertaking dietary modifications

Although a subgroup of RA patients will benefit from an elimination diet followed by a reintroduction phase to identify 'culprit foods' that must then be avoided, such a strategy should only be tried under supervision of a dietitian or a GP, as inappropriate or excessive exclusion may lead to macronutrient deficiency or weight loss, micronutrient deficiency, and ultimately, malnutrition. Supervision is essential to ensure a balanced diet is achieved while trying to elucidate possible problems with food.

As explained in section 7.7.3, lectins present in pulses and grains may potentially cause adverse effects. While thorough cooking of such foods – which reduces lectin activity – may suffice, exclusion of lectins would include the removal of staple carbohydrate foods, including rice and bread. As it is important for the diet to contain carbohydrate foods, alternatives should be sought – wheat-free carbohydrate foods might be tried – to ensure that the diet is well balanced.

Vegetarian diets are far less extreme and are acceptable to many people in the normal population and might therefore be tried by RA sufferers. However, these diets, and in particular the stricter vegan diet, are not risk-free. Vegetarians and vegans are at increased risk of some micronutrient deficiencies, in particular of vitamin D, vitamin B_{12}, riboflavin, iron, calcium, iodine, selenium and zinc, where the richest or most bioavailable sources are from animal products. The risk of deficiency will depend on how strict the diet is, with the vegan diet being the strictest (Thomas 2001). Table 7.3 shows where vitamin D, vitamin B_{12}, riboflavin and calcium may be found in a vegan or vegetarian diet: for example, vitamin B_{12} is found in textured vegetable protein.

Table 7.3 Vegan and vegetarian sources of certain micronutrients commonly associated with foods of animal origin (Thomas 2001).

Micronutrients	Vegetarian and vegan sources
Vitamin D	Fortified: soya milk, breakfast cereals, soya cheese, soya yoghurts and vegan margarines
Vitamin B_{12}	Fortified: yeast extract, vegetable stock, soya milk, textured soya protein and breakfast cereals
Riboflavin	Yeast extract, wheat germ, almonds, soya beans, tempeh, pumpkin seeds, mushrooms, avocado and fortified breakfast cereal
Calcium	Soya cheese, tofu, kidney beans, haricot beans, almonds, brazil nuts, hazel nuts, green leafy vegetables, dried figs, white/brown/wholemeal bread and fortified soya milk

To prevent or decrease the risk of malnutrition, it would be wise to advise RA patients wishing to try a dietary strategy to follow a vegetarian diet, preferably a piscatarian vegetarian diet in which fish, including oily fish, is eaten. Oily fish is likely to be beneficial in inflammatory arthritis (see Chapter 9). If other more extreme diets are to be undertaken, advice and support should be sought from a dietitian.

References

Atkinson W, Sheldon TA, Shaath N, Whorwell PJ (2004) Food elimination based on IgG antibodies in irritable bowel syndrome: a randomised controlled trial. Gut 53(10), 1459–64.

Baharav E, Mor F, Halpern M, Weinberger A (2004) *Lactobacillus* GG bacteria ameliorate arthritis in Lewis rats. *Journal of Nutrition* 134(8), 1964–69.

Beauchamp GK, Keast RS, Morel D, Lin J, Pika J, Han Q, Lee CH, Smith AB, Breslin PA (2005) Phytochemistry: ibuprofen-like activity in extra virgin olive oil. *Nature* 1, 437(7055), 45–46.

Brauer R, Thoss K, Henzgen S, Waldman G (1985) Lectin-induced arthritis of rabbit as a model of rheumatoid arthritis. In: *Lectins, vol IV* (TC Bog-Hansen and E van Driessche, eds). Berlin, Walter de Gruyter & Company, pp. 29–38.

Cordain L, Toohey L, Smith MJ, Hickey MS (2000) Modulation of immune function by dietary lectins in rheumatoid arthritis. *British Journal of Nutrition* 83(3), 207–17.

Danao-Camara TC, Shintani TT (1999) The dietary treatment of inflammatory arthritis: case reports and review of the literature. *Hawaii Medical Journal* 58(5), 126–31.

Darlington LG, Ramsey NW, Mansfield JR (1986) Placebo-controlled, blind study of dietary manipulation therapy in rheumatoid arthritis. *The Lancet* 1(8475), 236–8.

Darlington LG, Ramsey NW (1993) Clinical Review – Review of dietary therapy for rheumatoid arthritis. *British Journal of Rheumatology* 32, 507–14.

Darlington G, Gamlin L (1996) Diet and arthritis. A comprehensive guide to controlling arthritis through diet. London, Vermilion.

Darlington LG (2002) Joints and arthritic disease. In: *Food Allergy and Intolerance*, 2nd edition (J Brostoff, SJ Challacombe, eds). London, WB Saunders, pp 747–60.

Ebringer A, Ptaszynska T, Corbett M, Wilson C, Macafee Y, Avakian H, Baron P, James DC (1985) Antibodies to proteus in rheumatoid arthritis. *The Lancet* 10, 2(8450), 305–7.

Freed DL (1999) Do dietary lectins cause disease? *British Medical Journal* 17, 318(7190), 1023–24.

Gibson GR, Roberfroid MB (1995) Dietary modulation of the human colonic microbiota: introducing the concept of prebiotics. *Journal of Nutrition* 125(6), 1401–12.

Gianfranceschi P, Fasani G, Speciani AF (1996) Rheumatoid arthritis and the drop in tolerance to foods. *Annals of the New York Academy of Sciences* 78, 379–81.

Hafstrom I, Ringertz B, Spangberg A, Von Zweigbergk L, Brannemark S, Nylander I, Ronnelid J, Laasonen L, Klareskog L (2001) A vegan diet free of gluten improves the signs and symptoms of rheumatoid arthritis: the effects on arthritis correlate with a reduction in antibodies to food allergens. *Rheumatology* 40(10), 1175–79.

Hagfors L, Leanderson P, Sköldstam L, Andersson J, Johansson G (2003) Antioxidant intake, plasma antioxidants and oxidative stress in a randomized, controlled, parallel, Mediterranean dietary intervention study on patients with rheumatoid arthritis. *Nutrition Journal* 2, 5.

Hagfors L, Nilsson I, Sköldstam L, Johansson G (2005) Fat intake and composition of fatty acids in serum phospholipids in a randomized, controlled, Mediterranean dietary intervention study on patients with rheumatoid arthritis. *Nutrition and Metabolism* (London) 10, 2(1), 26 (Epub ahead of print).

Hatakka K, Martio J, Korpela M, Herranen M, Poussa T, Laasanen T, Saxelin M, Vapaatalo H, Moilanen E, Korpela R (2003) Effects of probiotic therapy on the activity and activation of mild rheumatoid arthritis – a pilot study. *Scandinavian Journal of Rheumatology* 32(4), 211–15.

Haugen MA, Kjeldsen-Kragh J, Forre O (1994) A pilot study of the effect of an elemental diet in the management of rheumatoid arthritis. *Clinical and Experimental Rheumatology* 12(3), 275–79.

Haugen M, Fraser D, Forre O (1999) Diet therapy for the patient with rheumatoid arthritis? *Rheumatology* (Oxford) 38(11), 1039–44.

Holst-Jensen SE, Pfeiffer-Jensen M, Monsrud M, Tarp U, Buus A, Hessov I, Thorling E, Stengaard-Pedersen K (1998) Treatment of rheumatoid arthritis with a peptide diet: a randomized, controlled trial. *Scandinavian Journal of Rheumatology* 27(5), 329–36.

Hunter JO (1991) Food allergy – or enterometabolic disorder? *The Lancet* 338, 495–96.

Kavanagh R, Workman E, Nash P, Smith M, Hazleman BL, Hunter JO (1995) The effects of elemental diet and subsequent food reintroduction on rheumatoid arthritis. *British Journal of Rheumatology* 34, 270–73.

Kjeldsen-Kragh J, Haugen M, Borchgrevink CF (1991) Controlled trial of fasting and one-year vegetarian diet in rheumatoid arthritis. *The Lancet* 338, 899–902.

Kjeldsen-Kragh J (1999) Rheumatoid arthritis treated with vegetarian diets. *American Journal of Clinical Nutrition* 70(suppl), 594S–600S.

Kroker G, Stroud R, Marshall R, Bullock T, Carroll FM, Greenberg M, Randolph T, Rea W, Smiley R (1984) Fasting and RA: a multicenter study. *Clinical Ecology* 2, 137–144.

Lindberg E (1973) Konnen Ernahrungfaktoren die chronische Polyarthritis beeinflussen? (Can nutritional factors modify chronic polyarthritis?) *Zeitschrift fur Physiotherapie* 25, 119–29.

Martin RH (1998) The role of nutrition and diet in rheumatoid arthritis. *Proceedings of the Nutrition Society* 57(2), 231–4.

Muller H, de Toledo FW, Resch KL (2001) Fasting followed by vegetarian diet in patients with rheumatoid arthritis: a systematic review. *Scandinavian Journal of Rheumatology* 30(1), 1–10.

O'Farrelly C, Marten D, Melcher D, McDougall B, Price R, Goldstein AJ, Sherwood R, Fernandes L (1988) Association between villous atrophy in rheumatoid arthritis and a rheumatoid factor and gliadin-specific IgG. *The Lancet* 8, 2(8615), 819–22.

Panush RS, Carter RL, Katz P, Kowsari B, Longley S, Finnie S (1983) Diet therapy for rheumatoid arthritis. *Arthritis and Rheumatism* 26(4), 462–71.

Panush RS (1991) Does food cause or cure arthritis? *Rheumatic Disease Clinics of North America* 17, 259–72.

Peltonen R, Kjeldsen-Kragh J, Haugen M, Tuominen J, Toivanen P, Forre O, Eerola E (1994) Changes of faecal flora in rheumatoid arthritis during fasting and one-year vegetarian diet. *British Journal of Rheumatology* 33(7), 638–43.

Peltonen R, Nenonen M, Helve T, Hanninen O, Toivanen P, Eerola E (1997) Faecal microbial flora and disease activity in rheumatoid arthritis during a vegan diet. *British Journal of Rheumatology* 36(1), 64–68.

Pusztai A (1993) Dietary lectins are metabolic signals for the gut and modulate immune and hormone functions. *European Journal of Clinical Nutrition* 47(10), 691–99.

Radcliffe MJ (2002) Elimination diets as a diagnostic tool. In: *Food Allergy and Intolerance*, 2nd edition (J Brostoff, SJ Challacombe, eds). London, WB Saunders, pp. 817–29.

Rennie KL, Hughes J, Lang R, Jebb SA (2003) Nutritional management of rheumatoid arthritis: a review of the evidence. *Journal of Human Nutrition and Dietetics* 16(2), 97–109.

Schley PD, Field CJ (2002) The immune-enhancing effects of dietary fibres and prebiotics. *British Journal of Nutrition* 87(suppl 2), S221–30.

Sköldstam L, Larsson L, Lindstrom FD (1979) Effect of fasting and lactovegetarian diet on rheumatoid arthritis. *Scandinavian Journal of Rheumatology* 8(4), 249–55.

Sköldstam L (1986) Fasting and vegan diet in rheumatoid arthritis. *Scandinavian Journal of Rheumatology* 15(2), 219–21.

Sköldstam L, Magnusson K-E (1991) Fasting, intestinal permeability and rheumatoid arthritis. *Rheumatic Disease Clinics of North America* 17, 363–71.

Sköldstam L, Hagfors L, Johansson G (2003) An experimental study of a Mediterranean diet intervention for patients with rheumatoid arthritis. *Annals of the Rheumatic Diseases* 62(3), 208.

Thomas B (2001) *Manual of Dietetic Practice*, 3rd edition. Oxford, Blackwell Science.

Toivanen P (2001) From reactive arthritis to rheumatoid arthritis. *Journal of Autoimmunity* 16, 369–71.

Toivanen P (2003) Normal intestinal microbiota in the aetiopathogenesis of rheumatoid arthritis. *Annals of the Rheumatic Diseases* 62(9), 807–11.

Trichopoulou A, Vasilopoulou E (2000) Mediterranean diet and longevity *British Journal of Nutrition* 84, Suppl 2, S205–9.

van de Laar MAFJ, van der Korst JK (1992) Food intolerance in rheumatoid arthritis I. A double-blind, controlled trial of the clinical effects of elimination of milk allergens and azo dyes. *Annals of the Rheumatic Diseases* 51, 298–302.

van de Laar MAFJ, Aalbers M, Bruins FG, Van Dinther-Janssen ACHM, van der Korst JK, Meijer CJLM (1992) Food intolerance in rheumatoid arthritis II. Clinical and histological aspects. *Annals of the Rheumatic Diseases* 51, 303–6.

8 Role of micronutrients in the amelioration of rheumatoid arthritis and osteoarthritis

8.1 Introduction

As micronutrients have many important roles within the body, poor dietary intake or status of certain micronutrients may predispose to incidence or progression of arthritic disease. Some micronutrients work as antioxidants, either directly or as components of antioxidant enzymes. Many, such as vitamin C, selenium, zinc, copper and iron, have additional roles unrelated to their functions in antioxidant systems. Others such as vitamin D and boron are not seen as antioxidants, but the former appears to influence risk of RA and progression of OA. Brief mention will also be made in this chapter of potassium and magnesium, though they are not, strictly speaking, micronutrients.

8.2 Antioxidants in the body

Reactive oxygen and nitrogen species (ROS and RNS) are produced by inflamed tissue, within joints, and by hypoxic reperfusion mechanisms (Blake et al. 1989; Adam 1995; McAlindon et al. 1996a). They characterise RA, and to a lesser extent, OA (McAlindon et al. 1996a; see section 2.4.7). Because of its ability to scavenge or limit the production of species such as superoxide, hydrogen peroxide, peroxynitrite, and some metal ions, the antioxidant defence system of the body plays an important part in ameliorating inflammation and slowing disease progression. A wide variety of antioxidants exist in different body compartments, as shown in Table 8.1.

Catalase, superoxide dismutase (SOD) and glutathione peroxidase (GPx) are intracellular antioxidant enzymes that are dependent on iron (catalase), copper, zinc and manganese (SOD) and selenium (mainly GPx) for their function. Extracellularly, for the most part, these antioxidant enzymes are scarce and thus antioxidant protection is supplied by small molecule antioxidants, the most important of which are glutathione (GSH), ascorbate (vitamin C), α-tocopherol (vitamin E) and uric acid. Vitamins C and E and glutathione are present in the cell (or cell membrane, in the case of vitamin E) as well as the plasma. Antioxidant properties have also been ascribed to β-carotene, a precursor of vitamin A, although to a lesser extent. Important plasma antioxidants include transferrin, lactoferrin and ferritin that transport or store iron, and caeruloplasmin that binds copper, keeping them from catalysing oxidation reactions such as the Fenton reaction that can produce the dangerous hydroxyl radical from hydrogen peroxide (Halliwell & Gutteridge

Table 8.1 Types of antioxidants (modified from Bender & Bender 1997).

	In plasma	Intracellular
Hydrophilic	Vitamin C	Vitamin C in cytosol or mitochondria
	Uric acid	GSH in cytosol or mitochondria
	GPx 2, 3 & selenoprotein P	GPx 1 in cytosol
	Transferrin, lactoferrin & ferritin	Thioredoxin reductase (selenoenzyme)
	Caeruloplasmin	Catalase in peroxisomes
	Bilirubin	CuZnSOD in cytosol
	Glutathione	MnSOD in mitochondria
	Albumin (as radical scavenger)	Ubiquinol in mitochondria
	Plant flavonoids	
Hydrophobic	Vitamin E	Vitamin E in membrane or mitochondria
	Carotenoids	GPx 4 in membranes
	Lutein	
	Zeaxanthin	
	Ubiquinol	
	Cryptoxanthin	
	Lycopene	

Abb: GSH (glutathione), SOD (superoxide dismutase) and GPx (glutathione peroxidase)

1999a). The concentrations of many of these antioxidant micronutrients depend upon the nutritional intake of the individual.

Antioxidants also have an important role in attenuating the formation of, or removing (e.g. GPx), pro-inflammatory eicosanoids resulting from the interaction of arachidonic acid (AA) with reactive oxygen species (ROS) (Adam 1995; Rayman 2000) (see Chapter 9).

8.3   Vitamins A, C and E and β-carotene and their role in RA and OA

Most studies of the effect of antioxidants on RA and OA have involved the use of the dietary antioxidants, β-carotene and vitamins C and E. These have been carried out by a number of groups and are outlined below.

8.3.1   Description and functions of vitamins A, C and E and β-carotene

Vitamin A is a term generally applied to retinol and retinoic acid that is usually taken to mean intake of preformed vitamin A plus provitamin A carotenoids, which can be cleaved in the body to give retinol. There are around 50 carotenoids (e.g. α-, β- and γ- carotenoids and cryptoxanthin) which are potential sources of vitamin A (Bender & Bender 1997). Though vitamin A has limited antioxidant properties, β-carotene is a more potent antioxidant. Of the dietary carotenoids, β-carotene is the most common and the most frequently studied in rheumatic diseases.

Vitamin C has two main functions that are relevant to arthritis: it acts as an antioxidant and it is necessary for collagen synthesis. It is the most important water-soluble antioxidant in intracellular and extracellular compartments, scavenging the superoxide, hydroxyl, thiyl and peroxyl radicals. It is needed for connective tissue synthesis and repair, being required for glycosaminoglycan synthesis and by the enzyme lysyl-hydroxylase for the hydroxylation of specific prolyl and lysyl residues in procollagen that stabilise the mature collagen fibril (Darlington & Stone 2001). Ascorbate significantly increases sulphated proteoglycan content of chondrocytes partly by reducing the activity of the desulphating aryl sulphatases (Schwartz & Adamy 1977). Vitamin C is used up in conditions of oxidative stress despite the regeneration of its reduced form from GSH and NADPH (Darlington & Stone 2001) and so low vitamin C status is common in those with rheumatic diseases.

Vitamin E has eight forms α-, β-, γ- and δ-tocopherols and tocotrienols, the most biologically active of which is considered to be α-tocopherol. α-tocopherol is the most common form of vitamin E in the UK diet whereas γ-tocopherol is the commonest in the US diet where soya products represent a greater proportion of the food intake. Vitamin E is the most important lipophilic antioxidant, scavenging peroxyl radicals and terminating the free radical lipid peroxidation chain reaction. It also inhibits arachidonic acid (AA) release from phospholipids and reduces eicosanoid formation resulting in a mild anti-inflammatory effect (Adam 1995). Though it is consumed in these processes, it can be regenerated by GSH (with the help of GPx) and ascorbic acid (vitamin C).

8.3.2   Studies of vitamins A, C and E and β-carotene in RA and OA

A number of studies show that low antioxidant status is a risk factor for RA. A nested case control study within a Finnish cohort of 1419 adult men and women investigated antioxidant status in relation to RA (Heliövaara et al. 1994). During a follow-up period of 20 years, 14 individuals, initially free of arthritis, developed RA. Two matched controls were selected for each case. Serum α-tocopherol, β-carotene and selenium concentrations were measured in the stored serum samples. Elevated risk of RA was observed in association with low levels of each nutrient. A significantly higher risk of RA (RR 8.34; 95% CI 1.0, 71.0; p-trend 0.03) was observed in the lowest tertile of antioxidant index compared with the highest tertile.

In a prospective cohort study, Comstock and colleagues (1997) investigated 21 out of 50 patients who developed RA from a group of 20 305 healthy individuals, 2–15 years after blood donation in 1974. Each case was matched to four controls. The stored serum samples from cases and controls were examined blind for β-carotene, retinol and α-tocopherol. Individuals with RA were found to have had lower serum concentrations of α-tocopherol, retinol and β-carotene at baseline than their matched controls: only β-carotene was significantly lower. Both these studies suggest an association between low antioxidant status and RA risk.

Knekt et al. (2000) also carried out a prospective investigation of α-tocopherol status and RA risk. This nested case control study within a Finnish cohort of 18 709 men and women, free of arthritis at the baseline examination in 1973–1978, identified 122 people with RA, 34 of whom were negative for rheumatoid factor. Each case was matched with three controls. After the first 10 years of follow up, the relative risk for the highest compared to the lowest tertile of serum α-tocopherol in both rheumatoid factor positive and negative subjects was 0.44 (95% CI 0.19, 0.99), showing a significant reduction in risk at higher α-tocopherol status.

Paredes et al. (2002) investigated status of vitamins A, E, lipid profile and inflammatory markers in 30 patients with RA and 30 controls. Patients were found to have significantly higher levels of inflammatory markers than controls and lower plasma vitamin A status. Vitamin E status was similar in both groups. The conclusion drawn was that chronic inflammation affects antioxidant vitamin levels in RA patients.

Vitamin E has been the subject of several supplementation trials that indicate differing influences on clinical outcome in OA and RA. Scherak and Kolarz (1991) supplemented 38 RA patients and 44 OA patients daily with 1200 mg d-α-tocopherol or diclofenac (an NSAID) for three weeks in a double-blind manner. They found no significant correlation between vitamin E and clinical improvement in OA, but in RA, there was a significant inverse correlation between the increase in plasma vitamin E and pain score (r = −0.503; p = 0.033). Similar findings were obtained by Edmonds and colleagues (1997) who carried out a randomised, placebo-controlled, double-blind trial in which 42 RA patients took either 1200 mg d-α-tocopherol or placebo alongside antirheumatic drugs (NSAIDs, analgesics and DMARDs) for 12 weeks. In this study, pain parameters were also found to be significantly decreased in the vitamin E treatment group though clinical indices of inflammation or oxidative modification were not affected. A further randomised, double-blind study in 85 hospitalised patients with chronic RA, which compared vitamin E (3 × 400 mg RRR-α-tocopherol acetate/d) with diclofenac-sodium, showed benefits in other disease parameters as well as pain (Wittenborg et al. 1998). After three weeks of treatment, both groups showed significant improvement in all clinically assessed parameters i.e. morning stiffness, Ritchie Index, grip strength and pain: both physicians and patients considered α-tocopherol treatment to be as effective as diclofenac (Wittenborg et al. 1998).

In agreement with the findings of Scherak and Kolarz (1991), two other studies found no effect of vitamin E treatment on OA. Wluka and colleagues (2002) found no beneficial effect of vitamin E in the management of OA, neither on cartilage volume loss nor on symptoms, in a group of 136 participants with knee OA. This was a well designed, randomised, placebo-controlled study of two years duration examining the effect of supplementation with 500 IU of vitamin E. Brand et al. (2001) also used 500 IU supplements of vitamin E in their shorter six month randomised, double-blind, placebo-controlled study of 77 patients with OA. As with the previous study, no benefit in the management of knee OA was found. However, in contrast to these results, McAlindon and Felson (1997) describe a

German study of 56 OA patients in which improvements in pain at rest, pain on movement and a reduction in analgesic use resulted from taking 400 mg α-tocopherol/d compared with placebo for six weeks.

Some studies of RA and OA have also included vitamin C in their investigations. McAlindon and colleagues (1996a) conducted a prospective observational study of the effect of dietary antioxidant nutrients (vitamin C, E and β-carotene) on OA of the knee as part of the Framingham Osteoarthritis Cohort Study. Participants' knees were evaluated by radiography between 1983–85 and again between 1992–93. Dietary intake of vitamin E, C and β-carotene was assessed by a Food Frequency Questionnaire (FFQ) administered between 1988–89. Of 640 patients assessed, incident and progressive OA had occurred in 81 and 68 patients' knees respectively. No significant association was found between any antioxidant nutrient and OA incidence. However, a threefold reduction in risk of OA progression, which related predominantly to a reduced risk of cartilage loss, was found for both the middle tertile (adjusted OR 0.3; 95% CI 0.1, 0.8) and the highest tertile (adjusted OR 0.3; 95% CI 0.1, 0.6) of vitamin C intake. Those with high vitamin C intake also had a reduced risk of developing knee pain (adjusted OR 0.3; 95% CI 0.1, 0.8). A reduced risk of OA progression was also seen for β-carotene (adjusted OR 0.4; 95% CI 0.2, 0.9) and vitamin E intake, though the latter was seen in the male subgroup only. The use of a FFQ for estimating dietary intake is known to be a rather inaccurate measure and this must be borne in mind when assessing the significance of the findings of this study, though it must be acknowledged that the vitamin C effects were large. In contrast to these findings, no effect of dietary antioxidants vitamin C or β-carotene was seen in the 136 OA patient study of Wluka and colleagues (2002) described above.

Cerhan et al. (2003) conducted a prospective cohort study of 29 368 women from 1986 to 1997, identifying 152 cases of RA. After controlling for other risk factors, greater intakes (highest *vs.* lowest tertile) of both supplemental vitamin C (RR 0.7; 95% CI 0.48, 1.9; p-trend 0.08) and vitamin E (RR 0.72; 95% CI 0.47, 1.12; p-trend 0.06) were inversely associated with RA. No association was identified, however, with total carotenoid levels, nor with α- or β-carotene, lycopene or lutein/zeaxanthin, but there was a significant association with β-cryptoxanthin, the main source of which is citrus fruits. There was also some suggestion that the intake of fruit and cruciferous vegetables might be protective against the development of RA (Cerhan et al. 2003).

The benefit of increased levels of antioxidant nutrients was explored in RA subjects following a Mediterranean diet. Statistically significant, though weak, inverse correlations with some disease activity variables were seen for retinol, vitamin C and uric acid (Hagfors et al. 2003).

8.3.3 Conclusions and recommendations from these studies

Taking an overall view of these studies of dietary intake and supplementation, it appears that while vitamin E generally has no effect in OA, it may exert a significant analgesic effect in RA. This is in keeping with previous findings of the ability of α-tocopherol to influence complex neuropathic pain syndromes (Edmonds et al. 1997). Edmonds and colleagues (1997) have postulated that the analgesic effect may be due to an interaction between α-tocopherol and nitric oxide. In the light of these effects, vitamin E status should be adequately maintained, at the very least by advising adequate intake by dietary means. Alternatively a short period (up to 12 weeks) of vitamin E supplementation (though the level of 1200 mg/d used in some of the studies quoted above is very high) could be recommended to RA patients to see if a reduction in pain is noticed or if a concomitant reduction in NSAID dose might be achieved (Abate et al. 2000). In either case, a sufficient intake of vitamin C is required to ensure the regeneration of vitamin E at the membrane water interface.

With respect specifically to vitamin C, the threefold reduced risk of OA progression and development of knee pain seen at medium and high dietary intakes of vitamin C in the Framingham Osteoarthritis Cohort Study is hard to ignore, though these effects were not reproduced in the study of Wluka and colleagues (2002). Those suffering from OA should therefore be advised to ensure that their dietary intake of vitamin C is at least up to the RNI/RDA. In the latest UK National Diet and Nutrition Survey of people aged 65 and over, 33% of free living participants and 45% of those in institutions had an intake of vitamin C below the RNI. This finding was supported by the data on vitamin C status, which showed that 4% of the free living and 40% of those in institutions had unacceptably low plasma levels (Bates et al. 1999). If considering advising vitamin C supplementation for those who find it difficult to consume enough fruit or vegetables, note that vitamin C absorption alters with intake: at intakes below 180 mg/d, 70% is absorbed, but when intakes exceed 1 g/d, absorption reduces to 15%. According to Bender (2002), in healthy individuals, an intake of 100 mg/d is likely to saturate tissues, but this may not be the case in subjects under considerable oxidative stress and more may be needed to optimise non-haem iron absorption (Bender 2002). However, even in this case, daily supplement levels above 500 mg are probably just a waste of money. Furthermore, several authors (e.g. Fisher & Naughton 2004) have noted that at high doses, vitamin C may become a pro-oxidant, particularly if being co-supplemented with iron.

There does not seem to be a strong case for specifically increasing the intake of β-carotene, but given the elevated risk of RA associated with low serum levels of β-carotene, it would be sensible to ensure a good dietary intake of carotenoid-rich vegetables. Indeed the dietary intake of all antioxidant nutrients needs to meet at least recommended intake levels in RA patients, in the light of their chronic inflammatory challenge and resultant low antioxidant status.

8.4   Selenium in RA and OA

8.4.1   Functions of selenium relevant to RA and OA

Selenium, a metalloid, is an important nutrient for human health (Rayman 2000). It is best known in the context of the selenoproteins that have selenocysteine at the active centre, many of which function as enzymes: 25 selenoproteins are known to be encoded in the human genome. Of most importance to those with rheumatic diseases are selenoproteins that function as antioxidant enzymes, most notably the family of glutathione peroxidases (GPxs), but also perhaps the less well known family of thioredoxin reductases (TRRs) and selenoprotein P (SelP), though the latter is not usually considered as an enzyme (Rayman 2000). These all have anti-inflammatory potential, for instance:

(1) GPx dampens the propagation of ROS by reducing lipid hydroperoxides, unstable compounds that could break down to give further reactive free radicals and cytotoxic species, to harmless alcohols.
(2) GPx metabolises hydroperoxide intermediates produced in eicosanoid synthesis by the lipoxygenase and cyclo-oxygenase pathways thereby preventing the production of inflammatory prostaglandins and leukotrienes (Rayman 2002).
(3) GPx, and particularly SeP, can scavenge peroxynitrite ($ONOO^-$), a highly damaging ROS/RNS product of the reaction between nitric oxide (NO) and superoxide (O_2^-) (Rayman et al. 2003), both of which are produced in the oxidatively stressed joint (Darlington & Stone 2001).

Peroxynitrite breaks down under the acidic conditions found in inflammation and ischaemia to give the hydroxyl radical, which has been found in the synovial fluid of arthritic subjects and which is known to break down hyaluronic acid and disrupt proteoglycans (Darlington & Stone 2001). The involvement of peroxynitrite in RA can be inferred from the finding of nitrotyrosine, a product of attack on protein, in the serum and synovial fluid of RA patients but not controls (Darlington & Stone 2001).

Selenium has further non-antioxidant effects that may well be helpful in arthritic conditions. Firstly, it may reduce the ability of matrix metalloproteinases (MMPs) to cause cartilage breakdown by inducing tissue inhibitors of MMPs (TIMPs) (Yoon et al. 2001). Secondly, it may inhibit neovascularisation, which is central to the development and perpetuation of rheumatoid synovitis. Vascular endothelial growth factor (VEGF), the main mediator of angiogenesis, is found in the synovial fluid and serum of patients with RA, and its expression is correlated with disease severity (Clavel et al. 2003). Following VEGF stimulation, vascular endothelial cells secrete MMPs that break down the surrounding tissue matrix allowing the penetration of the new blood vessel sprout (Jiang et al. 1999). After the first events of angiogenesis, the enzymatic activity of MMPs can be held in check by the coexpression of their inhibitors i.e. TIMPs (Kolb et al. 1999). Selenium has been shown to reduce the formation of new microvessels by inhibiting the expression of VEGF and reducing the activity of MMPs in another context (Jiang et al. 1999), possibly by upregulating TIMPs (Yoon et al. 2001). At levels of intake of around 200 µg/d, monomethylated selenium metabolites are formed in sufficient quantity to inhibit neo-angiogenesis and have been shown to do so (Jiang et al. 1999, 2000).

Table 8.2 Selenium (μg/l) in plasma or serum from RA patients in different parts of the world (reproduced from Tarp 1994 with permission of the Danish Medical Bulletin).

Authors	Country	RA patients	Controls
Aaseth et al.	Norway	94 ± 25 (23)	129 ± 9 (10)
Sullivan et al.	Nebraska, USA	120 ± 30 (10)	120 ± 10 (37)
Mötönen et al.	Finland	75 ± 9 (10)	90 (range 71–119;20)
Tarp et al.	Denmark	70 ± 13 (87)	80 ± 11 (288)
Tarp et al.	Denmark	69 ± 19 (40)	80 ± 11 (288)
Schmidt et al.	Germany	70 ± 13 (50)	82 ± 9 (10)
Peretz et al.	Belgium	77 ± 20 (45)	84 ± 15 (45)
Tarp et al.	Denmark	64 (range 57–74(6))	86 (range 72–111(6))
Borglund et al.	Sweden	66 ± 9 (7)	77 ± 2 (5)
Arnaud et al.	France	47 ± 21 (21)	71 ± 22 (21)
Morisi et al.	Italy	85 ± 13 (18)	90 (4201)
Tarp et al.	Denmark	71 ± 15 (28)	80 ± 11 (288)
Jacobsson et al.	Sweden	77 ± 16 (38)	85 ± 13 (57)
O'Dell et al.	Nebraska, USA	148 ± 42 (101)	160 ± 25 (20)
Tarp et al.	Denmark	61 ± 17 (9)	89 ± 12 (8)

8.4.2 Selenium status in OA and RA patients

Low concentrations of selenium have been measured in plasma or serum of RA patients from different parts of the world when compared to controls (Tarp 1994, 1995; see Table 8.2).

Tarp has calculated that the mean reduction in concentration in studies quoted in the table is 10%. Similarly, a decrease in erythrocyte or whole blood selenium content has been found in most studies that have determined selenium in these matrices (Tarp 1995). The suggestion that selenium concentration drops in response to inflammation or as a result of the acute phase response is supported by a number of studies that showed an association between selenium concentration and clinical indices and biochemical parameters of inflammation (Tarp 1995; Maehira et al. 2002). Furthermore, in a longitudinal study on 28 RA patients, selenium concentrations were found to be low in periods of disease activity and normal in periods of low activity (Tarp et al. 1989). The finding of Meltzer and colleagues (1989) that RA patients and healthy Norwegians had an identical intake of selenium per kg body mass demonstrates that factors other than intake account for the differences in status observed.

There appears to be only one study that has evaluated selenium status in OA patients (Jordan et al. 2005). The Johnston County Osteoarthritis Project, a population-based epidemiological study of black and white people in North Carolina, measured selenium status by neutron activation analysis in 940 newly enrolled participants of mean age 59.6 years. A preliminary account of the study has been given in abstract form. Radiographic knee OA was defined as Kellgren–Lawrence grade 2–4. Adjusted least squares means for selenium were lower in those with any knee OA, bilateral knee OA and severe knee OA ($p \le 0.05$) as compared with those with normal X-rays. For every increase of 0.1 μg/g selenium, the odds of knee OA, bilateral knee OA and severe knee OA were decreased by 15–20%. For those in the highest compared to the lowest tertile of toenail selenium, the odds (95% CI) of knee OA were 0.62 (0.37–1.02), for bilateral knee OA 0.79 (0.31–0.97) and severe knee OA 0.56 (0.34–0.94). Gender interactions were significant for severity of knee OA with strong effects in women. Race interactions were seen for any knee OA and laterality knee OA with strong effects in African Americans. This calls into question whether low selenium may be a potentially modifiable risk factor for OA and suggests the need for intervention studies.

8.4.3   Prospective and intervention studies with selenium

While some studies have found that higher selenium status is associated with lower RA risk, others have not. For instance, Tarp and colleagues (1989) found no association between an initial low selenium concentration and the course of RA.

Heliövaara et al. (1994) carried out a nested case control study in a Finnish cohort of 1419 adults. Fourteen individuals developed RA in this cohort over a 20 year period. Each case was matched to two controls. A non-significant increased risk of developing RA was found in the lowest tertile of serum selenium (RR 1.63; 95% CI 0.57, 4.69; p-trend = 0.11).

Knekt et al. (2000) carried out a nested case control study within a Finnish prospective study cohort of 18 709 men and women with no arthritis at the outset. One hundred and twenty two people with RA (88 positive for RF, 34 negative for RF) were identified in 1989. Each case was matched with three controls. The adjusted relative risk between the highest and lowest tertiles of serum selenium was 0.16 (95% CI 0.04, 0.69; p-trend = 0.02) for RF-negative arthritis, showing a significant risk reduction with higher selenium status. There was no association for RF-positive RA (Knekt et al. 2000).

Intervention studies with selenium in RA are tabulated in Table 8.3. Three double-blind, randomised, placebo-controlled studies showed significant improvements in measurable parameters of disease activity. In the first, Peretz et al. (1992) studied 15 women suffering from recent onset RA (< 5 years). In addition to their conventional treatments, they received either 200 μg/d of selenium-enriched yeast or matched placebo for a period of 90 days. Significant improvements were seen in pain (p < 0.01), number of involved joints (p < 0.05) and delayed hypersensitivity skin reaction (p < 0.05), showing improved cellular immunity.

Interestingly, the second study, that of Aaseth and colleagues (1998), required an eight-month period with a dose of 600 μg selenium as selenium-enriched yeast for a significant beneficial effect to be established: no significant improvement was seen at four months. The authors suggest that the lack of response following treatment with lower doses (as in earlier studies) or a shorter treatment period, indicate that the apparent clinical efficacy cannot simply relate to an antioxidant effect, as it requires the accumulation of an unphysiologically high amount of selenium (Aaseth et al. 1998). An alternative explanation may be that selenium metabolism in polymorphonuclear leucocytes is impaired, as suggested by Tarp (1995), who found that selenium supplementation was unable to raise the level of

Table 8.3 Intervention studies with selenium in RA (modified from Tarp 1995).

Study	No. of patients	Daily Se dose	Treatment period	Result
Tarp et al. 1985	40	256 µg Se-yeast	6 mth	Non-significant
Petersson et al. 1991*	20	Not given	6 mth	Non-significant
Jäntti et al. 1991	28	150 µg	8 wk	Non-significant
Peretz et al. 1992	15	200 µg Se-yeast	3 mth	Sig. reduction in pain ($p < 0.01$) and joint involvement ($p < 0.05$) in recent onset RA
Heinle et al. 1997[†]	70	200 µg Na_2SeO_3	3 mth	Sig. decrease in RA symptoms, inflammation, NSAID and cortisone use
Aaseth et al. 1998§	47	600 µg Se-yeast	8 mth	Sig. improvement in pain, grip strength and morning stiffness
Peretz et al. 2001	55	200 µg Se-yeast	3 mth	Non-significant except for arm movements and health perception

* Plus vitamins A, C and E
† Both active and placebo tablets contained a low dose of vitamin E
§ Both supplementation and placebo groups received additional fish oil supplementation

selenium in polymorphonuclear leucocytes in RA patients, though it increased significantly in the controls. No serious toxic effects were seen at this 600 µg/d dose. {Certain immune system and anti-cancer effects of selenium also require relatively high amounts of selenium (Rayman 2005)}.

The third study that showed significant effects of selenium treatment included fish oil in the supplements given to both active treatment and placebo groups (Heinle et al. 1997). A decrease in inflammatory parameters as well as in the number of tender and swollen joints was found on supplementation with 200 µg/d sodium selenite for three months. It is possible that the presence of the fish oil potentiated the effect of selenium. As selenium affects the production of eicosanoids (see section 8.4.1), a synergistic effect between selenium and fish oil (see Chapter 9) can perfectly well be envisaged.

It is notable that a second double-blind placebo-controlled study by Peretz and colleagues (2001) failed to replicate the clinical benefit of selenium found in their earlier study (1992). In the second study, 55 RA patients also received either 200 µg/d of selenium as selenium-enriched yeast or a placebo for a period of 90 days. Significant improvements were seen in a number of clinical disease parameters in both selenium and placebo groups. The only benefits exclusive to the selenium treatment were significant improvements in arm movements and quality of life. This study differed from the earlier study by including patients whose disease was more severe and of longer standing. If the effect of selenium is partly antiangiogenic as explained above, it may be more successful in early disease and may also require a longer time than three months for the effect to be established in patients with more severe disease and a longer disease history.

Table 8.4 Selenium intake data for a number of countries (Rayman 2004).

Country	Selenium intake (µg/person/d)	Reference
Australia	57–87	Fardy et al. 1989
Austria	48	Simma & Pfannhauser 1998 (cited by Combs 2001)
Belgium	28–61	Robberecht et al. 1994
Czech Republic	10–25 (estimate)	Kvícala et al. 1996
Canada	98–224	Gissel-Nielsen 1998 (cited by Combs 2001)
China	7–4990	Combs 2001
Croatia	27	Klapec et al. 1998 (cited by Combs 2001)
Denmark	38–47	Danish Government Food Agency 1995
France	29–43	Lamand et al. 1994
Germany	35	Alfthan & Neve 1996
Japan	104–199	Miyazaki et al. 2001
Netherlands	39–54	van Dokkum 1995
	67	Kumpulainen 1993
New Zealand	55–80	Vannoort et al. 2000
Poland	30–40 (calculated)	Wasowicz et al. 2003
Serbia	30	Djujic et al. 1995
Slovakia	38	Kadrabová et al. 1998
Sweden	31	Swedish National Food Administration 1989
	38	Kumpulainen 1993
Switzerland	70	Kumpulainen 1993
UK	29–39	MAFF 1997
USA	106	Food and Nutrition Board 2000
Venezuela	200–350	Combs & Combs 1986 (cited by Combs 2001)

8.4.4 Recommendations for selenium intake

Marginal selenium deficiency exists in a number of countries or areas within countries. Levels of selenium intake recommended by authorities in different countries average out at around 53 µg/d for women and 60 µg/d for men (Rayman 2004). For example, recommended dietary intake levels of selenium in the UK (Reference Nutrient Intake, RNI) are 75 µg/d for men and 60 µg/d for women while in the North America (RDA), 55 µg/d is recommended for both men and women (see Appendix 3 which gives RNIs/RDAs for various nutrients) though this is likely to be revised upwards as a result of more recent work (Xia et al. 2005). A compilation of selenium intake data across the world is shown in Table 8.4 (Rayman 2004).

While the intake of selenium in New Zealand, formerly low, appears to have increased in the last decade as a result of importation of Australian wheat (Thomson & Robinson 1996; Vannoort et al. 2000), that in a number of European countries has declined owing to reduced importation of selenium rich, North American wheat for breadmaking (Rayman 1997; Adams et al. 2002). For instance, selenium intake in the UK has fallen in the last 25 years or so from around 60 µg/d to 29–39 µg/d (Rayman 2002), the latter being approximately half of the UK RNI. Comparison of the values in Table 8.4 with recommended levels shows that

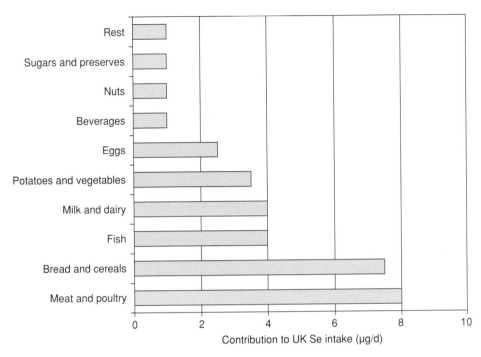

Figure 8.1 Contribution to UK daily selenium intake from different food groups (MAFF Joint Food Safety and Standards Group 1997).

recommended daily intakes are not now achieved in the majority of European countries together with parts of China. Selenium status is therefore an important issue for the general population in a number of countries where it is found in good concentrations only in a small number of foods such as Brazil nuts, organ meats and fish. Figure 8.1 shows the main food sources of selenium in the UK.

On the evidence presented above, RA patients appear to have lower selenium status than healthy individuals and a greater requirement for antioxidants owing to the oxidative stress and inflammation associated with their condition and recent evidence suggests the same is true for OA patients. Taking into consideration the fact that in many countries, RDA/RNI levels of selenium intake cannot be provided by the normal diet, supplementation should be considered (Adam 1995). In order to optimise the antioxidant effects of the selenoenzymes, a daily supplement of 50–100 µg would be realistic. However, Adam (1995) has suggested that an intake of 300 µg/d is necessary to improve the status of RA patients and this dose is only half of the 600 µg/d found to be effective in the study of Aaseth and colleagues (1998). If selenium is indeed acting through an effect on angiogenesis, a daily dose of around 200 µg is probably necessary to provide a sufficient level of the active metabolite, methyl selenol, and this may have to be continued for up to a year if benefit is to be seen.

However, when considering selenium supplementation, it must be remembered that selenium is a toxic nutrient. Several expert panels have recommended that it is prudent to restrict adult intake from all sources to an upper limit of 400–450 μg/d (Rayman 2000). The UK Food Standards Agency (FSA) expert group on vitamins and mineral has recommended that a maximum of 450 μg of selenium should be consumed per day to leave a sufficient margin of safety. On the assumption that:

> '. . . a maximum intake of 100 μg per day will be obtained from food, a margin of 350 μg per day selenium is available for supplementation or other additional intake.' (UK Expert Group on Vitamins and Minerals 2003)

In studies in the UK and Denmark, each on 500 people, no adverse effects were found in elderly people consuming 300 μg/d selenium, as selenium-enriched yeast over periods up to five years (Rayman 2004), nor was any evidence of selenium toxicity found in people living in South Dakota whose natural dietary intakes over their lifetimes were as high as 724 μg/d (Longnecker et al. 1991). However, some sensitive individuals have experienced adverse effects at 600 μg/d (Whanger 1996) so this level of supplementation cannot be recommended on the basis of sparse evidence of benefit.

8.5   Copper, zinc and RA and OA

8.5.1   Functions of copper and zinc relevant to RA and OA

Zinc and copper are key components of important metalloenzymes. Zinc in particular has a very wide range of functions including: regulation of synthesis; regulation of hormone action; digestion and degradation of connective tissue e.g. collagen by the zinc collagenases and proteoglycans by stromelysin; and the better known function in the cytosolic antioxidant enzyme, superoxide dismutase (CuZnSOD), where zinc holds the structure together (Frausto da Silva & Williams 2001a). Copper, as the cuproenzyme lysyl oxidase, has a key role in building the extracellular matrix by cross-linking proteins such as collagen and elastin. The synthetic and degradative functions of copper and zinc respectively are key to connective tissue management. These need to be kept in balance and vitamin D has a role here (Frausto da Silva & Williams 2001b). In the context of arthritis, the fact that copper deficiency can impair collagen formation (Frausto da Silva & Williams 2001c) is an important, though scarce mentioned, consideration, while its ability to scavenge superoxide as CuZnSOD in the inflamed joint, forming the less toxic H_2O_2 product, is well recognised (Aaseth et al. 1998). Dietary deficiency of either copper or zinc will markedly decrease tissue concentration of CuZnSOD resulting in peroxidative damage (Fang et al. 2002; Adam 1995).

8.5.2   Copper and zinc status in OA and RA patients

Zinc and copper intakes, estimated from a three day food diary, were reported to be low in RA patients in a US study (Kremer & Bigaouette 1996) but comparable to those of the normal diet in a Finnish study (Honkanen et al. 1991a) where intakes were recorded over seven days. A five day dietary survey of 48 RA patients in New Zealand suggested that only 10% achieved the recommended dietary intake of zinc (Stone et al. 1997). Low serum zinc has certainly been reported in RA patients (Helliwell et al. 1984; Peretz et al. 1993; Naveh et al. 1997), but it is argued that it is more likely to be a consequence of inflammation and disease activity than of reduced dietary intake (Honkanen et al. 1991b; Peretz et al. 1993). In inflammatory rheumatic diseases, zinc concentration decreases in plasma owing to the redistribution of the element within body compartments under the influence of the acute phase response (Shenkin 1995): increased concentrations are seen in mononuclear leukocytes, urine and synovial fluid (Peretz et al. 1993; Adam 1995). Patients may not be deficient in zinc but simply be in a state of element redistribution. Conversely, copper levels increase with the acute phase response and are normally elevated as a result of inflammation (Shenkin 1995).

SOD activity was significantly lower in 23 RA patients in Indiana than in 47 age matched controls (DiSilvestro et al. 1992). Similarly, in a comparison of 97 RA patients with 97 matched controls in Korea, a significantly lower plasma activity of SOD was found in the RA patients (Bae et al. 2003). Such data suggest that there might be some benefit in increasing the activity of this enzyme that can remove superoxide.

8.5.3   Intervention studies with copper and zinc

In the light of the above considerations, studies have looked at the effects of zinc supplementation on clinical outcomes of RA. These have been contradictory. High dose zinc has been shown to improve symptoms in one study (Simkin 1977) but not in others (Peretz et al. 1993; Adam 1995). Peretz et al. (1993) studied nine controls and 18 RA patients aged 24–64 years treated with NSAIDs who were randomly assigned, via a double-blind design, to receive either placebo or zinc supplementation (45 mg zinc/d) for two months. Clinical and biological assessments were undertaken at baseline, 30 and 60 days. The study concluded that zinc supplementation did not produce any beneficial effect measurable with the selected indicators of inflammatory status and disease activity (Peretz et al. 1993). No significant side effects were noted, even though the supplement provided three times the USA RDA. However, two cases did report a worsening of disease. Naveh and colleagues (1997) studied zinc absorption in 13 patients with low RA activity, 16 patients with high RA activity, and 8 controls, after ingestion of 50 mg 'elemental' zinc. Initially, plasma zinc was significantly lower in the RA groups than in the controls. After supplementation, plasma zinc rose in the control group from 111 ± 7 µg/dl to a peak of 200 ± 24 µg/dl over two hours but showed no significant increase in the RA groups. Twenty-four-hour urinary zinc excretions before and after zinc ingestion were significantly lower for the RA groups than for the control group. These results suggest zinc malabsorption and therefore zinc deficiency in the RA patients (Naveh et al. 1997). This malabsorption may suggest why no benefits were seen after zinc supplementation in the Peretz et al. (1993) study.

In a US prospective cohort study of 29,000 women aged 55–69 years at base-line, 152 cases of RA were identified over 11 years (Cerhan et al. 2003). Greater use of supplemental zinc (RR 0.39; 95% CI 0.17, 0.88; p trend, 0.03) was inversely associated with RA while any use of supplemental copper (RR 0.54; 95% CI 0.42, 1.01) and manganese (RR 0.50; 95% CI 0.23, 1.07) showed suggestive inverse associations with RA. However, these associations do not prove causality.

Early uncontrolled work on copper supplementation in RA reported beneficial effects (Aaseth et al. 1998). A later study by DiSilvestro and colleagues (1992) administered 2 mg of copper/d for four weeks to 23 RA subjects and 47 matched controls. Before supplementation, erythrocyte CuZnSOD activity was significantly lower in RA patients than in controls but increased in 18 out of 23 RA patients following supplementation, suggesting *marginal copper status in RA patients* (DiSilvestro et al. 1992).

Intra-articular injections of CuZnSOD have been shown to reduce joint inflammation and provide benefit in both RA and OA suggesting the need for adequate intakes of both of these micronutrients (Aaseth et al. 1998; Darlington & Stone 2001).

8.5.4   Recommendations for intake of copper and zinc in RA and OA

The important effects relating to the need for concerted synthesis and degradation of connective tissue outlined above, in addition to the role of both zinc and copper in SOD, suggest the need for adequate intakes of both of these micronutrients. It is therefore of some concern that in the latest UK National Diet and Nutrition Survey of people aged 65 and over, the intake of copper fell below the RNI in 82% of free living participants and in 90% of those in institutions, while the corresponding figures for zinc were 62% and 54% (Bates et al. 1999). Intake figures were better in the adult survey though even then, median intake was below the RNI in women of all ages (70–82% of RNI) (Henderson et al. 2003). We believe that the dietary intake of copper and zinc should reach the RDA/RNI level for these nutrients. Given the potential of copper to catalyse redox reactions producing the hydroxyl radical (Fenton reaction), supplementation with copper above RDA/RNI levels is to be avoided, while doses of zinc more than twice the RDA/RNI may impair copper absorption (Berger 2002).

8.6   Iron in RA and OA

8.6.1   Functions of iron relevant to RA and OA

The primary function of iron is in the facilitation of oxygen utilisation and storage in the muscles. It also serves as an important stimulator of cell proliferation and immunoglobulin formation (Adam 1995). Iron has both pro- and antioxidant functions. As part of the enzyme catalyse, it behaves as an antioxidant, converting hydrogen peroxide to water and oxygen. However, as a component of endoperoxide synthetase it is proinflammatory, determining the extent of eicosanoid biosynthesis (Adam 1995). It appears that iron may have a relatively specific influence on synovitis as opposed to inflammation generally (Morris et al. 1995). In addition, ferrous iron can catalyse the formation of the damaging hydroxyl radical in the Fenton reaction (Adam 1995; Halliwell & Gutteridge 1999a). Iron status therefore needs to be balanced between these functions.

In active RA, the inflamed synovium is subject to recurrent traumatic micro-bleeding and iron is deposited as ferritin in the synovium (Blake et al. 1990). The ischaemia reperfusion cycles that occur within the inflamed joint (see section 2.4.7) lead to the production of superoxide ($O_2^{\cdot-}$) from the enzyme xanthine oxidase (Blake et al. 1990). Superoxide can mobilise iron from ferritin. Free iron (or haem) has the capacity to form the highly toxic and destructive hydroxyl radical from $O_2^{\cdot-}$ and hydrogen peroxide by the Fenton reaction (Blake et al. 1990; Adam 1995). This causes tissue damage within the joint (Blake et al. 1990). Thus within this context, a high iron status is contraindicated in OA and RA patients.

8.6.2 Iron status in OA and RA patients

Anaemia is a common co-morbidity in individuals with RA, mild anaemia being present in between 33% and 60% of patients, depending on the study (Wilson et al. 2004). Anaemia in RA is multifactorial in nature (Fitzsimons & Sturrock 2002). While in many cases it is iron deficiency anaemia resulting from gastrointestinal bleeding provoked by the use of NSAIDs, around 60% or so of the time it is a manifestation of the anaemia of chronic disease associated with RA (Punnonen et al. 2000; Fitzsimons & Sturrock 2002). Thus low levels of plasma iron are often seen in RA despite packed iron stores (Adam 1995). The mechanism of the anaemia of chronic disease in RA is not fully understood but is thought to relate to the increased production of inflammatory cytokines, especially IL-1 and TNF-α. The drop in plasma iron correlates closely with the activity of the inflammatory process (Halliwell & Gutteridge 1999b). Excess levels of cytokines are responsible for a decrease in erythropoietin response in the bone marrow, leading to inadequate erythropoiesis even in the presence of adequate iron stores (Fitzsimons & Brock 2001; Fitzsimons & Sturrock 2002; Wilson et al. 2004). Other possible causes of anaemia and haematological manifestations of RA have been reviewed (ARC for Research 1995; Bowman 2002).

It is important to distinguish those patients whose anaemia might benefit from simple iron therapy from those with anaemia of chronic disease where the underlying disorder is the source of the problem. In the latter case, treatment with epoietin (a synthetic version of endogenous erythropoietin, which stimulates the production of red blood cells) can improve haemoglobin levels (Wilson et al. 2004). In order to distinguish between these two causes of anaemia, haematological tests can be used (Table 8.5).

Table 8.5 Biochemical tests to identify the cause of anaemia (modified from ARC for Research 1995).

Investigation	Normal values	Comments
Haemoglobin g/dl	12.0–16.0 (women) 13.5–18.0 (men)	Commonly around 10 g/dl in anaemia of chronic disease
Mean corpuscular volume (MCV) fl	75–95	Above 70 fl in anaemia of chronic disease
Mean corpuscular haemoglobin concentration (MCHC) g/dl	32–36	Reduced in iron deficiency
Serum iron μmol/l	13–32	Reduced in iron deficiency and anaemia of chronic disease
Total iron binding capacity (TIBC) μmol/l	45–70	Reduced in active RA. In iron deficiency this is normally greater than 55 μmol/l
% Transferrin saturation	< 50% (women) < 40% (men)	Low in iron deficiency anaemia and anaemia of chronic disease
Serum ferritin μg/l	25–400	An acute phase reactant therefore may be elevated in active RA. More than 60 μg/l in anaemia of chronic disease; less than 60 μg/l in iron deficiency
Serum soluble transferrin receptor (sTfR)	average 5.0 ± 1.0 mg/l, but commercial assays give disparate values	Considerably elevated in iron deficiency anaemia but remains normal in the anaemia of inflammation

The anaemia of chronic disease can be recognised from these tests by the following characteristics (Fitzsimons & Brock 2001):

- Decreased concentration of serum iron, transferrin and total iron-binding capacity
- Normal or raised ferritin – ferritin levels rise and fall with inflammation in the acute phase response and can therefore be independent of reticuloendothelial (RE) iron stores
- Increased erythrocyte sedimentation rate (ESR)
- Red cells which are often normochromic normocytic but may show hypochromic, microcytic indices, similar to the effects of iron deficiency, especially in RA patients
- Normal or only slightly raised soluble transferrin receptor (sTfR) in serum as opposed to an increased concentration in response to iron deficiency anaemia as the expression is upregulated. This test has high sensitivity and specificity for distinguishing iron deficiency anaemia from anaemia of chronic disease in anaemic RA patients but is less generally available and rather expensive

8.6.3 Effect of resolution of anaemia on RA symptoms and quality of life

The impact of resolution of anaemia on symptoms and quality of life (QOL) has been reviewed by Wilson and colleagues (2004). In 12 studies reviewed, resolution of anaemia, generally by treatment with epoietin (for anaemia of chronic disease), was associated with improvements, some of which were significant, in numbers of swollen joints, pain score, grip strength, energy levels and QOL.

8.6.4 Recommendations for iron intake

While an adequate intake of dietary iron is important, high iron levels, as discussed previously, may lead to the generation of reactive oxygen and nitrogen species (including the hydroxyl radical via the Fenton reaction), lipid peroxidation and oxidative stress (Fisher & Naughton 2004). Iron supplementation may therefore be detrimental, worsening inflammation, and should not be given unless there is evidence from the tests outlined above of a true deficiency. In fact there is some evidence that mild iron deficiency may actually be beneficial, suppressing joint inflammation (Blake et al. 1990).

8.7 Vitamin D in OA and RA

8.7.1 Role of vitamin D in relation to OA and RA

Changes in periarticular bone are a well recognised part of the natural history of OA. Patients with osteoarthritis of the knee who have bone scan abnormalities adjacent to the knee have a higher rate of disease progression than those without such changes (McAlindon & Felson 1997). Normal bone metabolism is dependent on the presence of vitamin D, which may come from the diet (vitamin D_2 in foods of plant origin, vitamin D_3 in foods of animal origin) or from the action of sunlight (UVB) on the skin (vitamin D_3). Vitamin D is converted into the active hormone, calcitriol (1,25-dihydroxyvitamin D), by hydroxylation reactions in the liver and kidneys (see Figure 8.2). If vitamin D concentration is low, there will be adverse effects on calcium metabolism and bone formation resulting in a reduced ability of bone to respond optimally to pathophysiological processes in OA (McAlindon & Felson 1997). This may lead to disease progression.

Vitamin D has further functions relevant to arthritis. Articular cartilage, particularly from OA, seems to be sensitive to the effects of vitamin D: it appears to stimulate the synthesis of proteoglycan by articular chondrocytes (McAlindon & Felson 1997). Furthermore, vitamin D hormone, 1,25-dihydroxyvitamin D, modulates T-cell immunity and can act as an immunosupressant in conditions involving hyperactive T-cell immunity such as RA (DeLuca & Cantorna 2001). Though the mechanism is unclear, it appears to involve a change in cytokine expression patterns (DeLuca & Cantorna 2001).

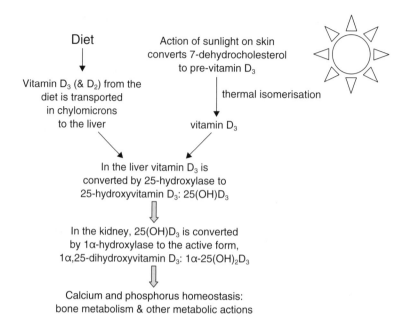

Figure 8.2   Vitamin D metabolism (adapted from Zittermann 2003).

8.7.2   Studies looking at the relationship between vitamin D and arthritis

The extent of disease activity was found to be associated with vitamin D hormone levels: serum 1,25-dihydroxyvitamin D concentrations were reduced in patients with a high compared to a low disease activity (for references see Zittermann 2003).

The association of supplemental and dietary vitamin D and RA risk was invest-igated in a prospective cohort of 29 368 women, aged 55–59 (the Iowa Women's Health study), with no history of RA at baseline (Merlino et al. 2004; see section 3.9 and Table 3.2). Total intake and supplemental vitamin D were significantly inversely associated with RA risk in these older women.

Supplementation with 1,25-dihydroxyvitamin D in autoimmune animal models of RA, one of which was collagen-induced arthritis, markedly suppressed disease activity (DeLuca and Cantorna 2001). However, human trials of vitamin D in RA have not shown such a clear outcome. Of five small intervention studies described by Zittermann (2003), three showed a significant improvement in pain and disease activity. Those that showed benefit used high doses: 250 μg/d vitamin D (10 000 IU) or 50 μg/d 25-hydroxyvitamin D, or 2 μg/d 1α,25-dihydroxyvitamin D (calcitriol) (Zittermann 2003).

With regard to OA, the effect of vitamin D was investigated within the Framingham OA Cohort study (McAlindon et al. 1996b). Two measures of vit-amin D status were assessed – dietary intake and serum 25-hydroxyvitamin D. No

Table 8.6 Association of serum 25-hydroxyvitamin D concentration and development or progression of radiographic OA over 8 years (reproduced with permission from Felson et al. 2000).

Serum 25-Hydroxy-vitamin D concentration	Odds ratio (95% CI)		
	Development of knee osteoarthritis*	Progression of knee osteoarthritis*	Severe narrowing of the hip joint space†
Lowest third	0.9 (0.5–1.9)	2.9 (1.0–8.3)	3.3 (1.1–9.9)
Middle third	0.9 (0.5–1.8)	2.8 (1.0–7.9)	3.2 (1.1–9.7)
Highest third	1.0 (referent)	1.0 (referent)	1.0 (referent)

* Based on data for progressive and incident knee osteoarthritis on radiography from the Framingham study. No association was found for incident disease
† Based on data from the Study of Osteoporotic Fractures Research Group. A woman could have no or mild narrowing at baseline. A weaker association was found for other definitions of hip osteoarthritis

effects were seen on disease incidence (Table 8.6). However, a three to fourfold increase in risk of progression of OA was seen in the middle and low tertiles of vitamin D intake (OR lowest *vs.* highest tertile, 4.0, 95% CI, 1.4, 11.6) and serum concentration (OR 2.9, 95% CI 1.0, 8.3).

From their findings, McAlindon and colleagues (1996b) concluded that:

'... *persons with either relatively low dietary intake of vitamin D or serum 25(OH)D levels less than approximately 74.88 nmol/l (30 ng/ml) have a substantially increased risk for progression of osteoarthritis of the knee.*'

The association between serum vitamin D and progression of knee OA found in the Framingham study is shown in Table 8.6 (Felson et al. 2000). Further evidence for the effect of vitamin D on OA was found by the Study of Osteoporotic Fractures Research Group, which showed that high serum concentration of vitamin D protected against both incident and progressive (see Table 8.6) hip OA (Lane et al. 1999). Vitamin D intakes below 9.7 μg/d appear to enhance OA progression (Zittermann 2003).

8.7.3 Vitamin D intake and status

Circulating levels of 25-hydroxyvitamin D are regarded as the best indicator of vitamin D status and concentrations below 40–50 nmol/l are thought to reflect vitamin D insufficiency (Zittermann 2003). Subjects living close to the equator or with good outdoor skin exposure have mean 25-hydroxyvitamin D serum levels of 107 nmol/l and upper levels of around 160 nmol/l (Zittermann 2003). There is therefore a case for adequate concentrations of 25-hydroxyvitamin D being between 100 and 200 nmol/l, at which level no disturbances in vitamin D-dependent body functions occur (Peacock 1995). There is a marked seasonal variation in 25-hydroxyvitamin D concentrations, even in healthy people. UVB radiation from the sun that can produce vitamin D in the skin is negligible from October to April at

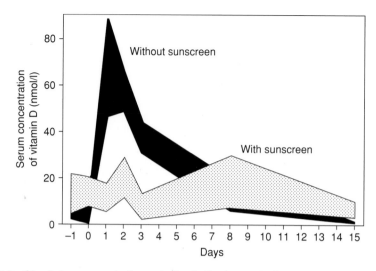

Figure 8.3 Circulating concentrations of vitamin D after a single exposure to one minimal erythemal dose of simulated sunlight with either a sunscreen of SPF 8 or a topical placebo cream (reproduced with permission from Holick 2004).

the latitude of 52° N, and from November to February at 42° N (Zittermann 2003). Low vitamin D status is widespread at northern latitudes in the general population. Though it is thought that summer exposure, if adequate, should provide sufficient stores for the winter months, this is frequently not the case. People with dark skins produce no more than 5–19% of the vitamin D produced in light-skinned people (Holick 2004). Furthermore, the fear of skin cancer has greatly increased the use of sunscreens: even use of a relatively low factor sunscreen (SPF 8) reduces the production of pre-vitamin D_3 by more than 95% (Figure 8.3) (Holick 2004). Intake from diet is therefore more important in northern latitudes, particularly for those who are institutionalised or housebound.

Vitamin D status in different European population groups during summer and winter has been tabulated by Zittermann (2003). This shows that with the exception of Norway, where vitamin D-rich fatty fish consumption is relatively high, vitamin D status in Europe in winter is insufficient as defined above. Low dietary intakes of vitamin D and calcium have been reported in RA patients (Morgan et al. 1997; Martin 1998) while epidemiological data indicate that more than 60% of rheumatic patients have 25-hydroxyvitamin D concentrations below 50 nmol/l and 16% have levels clearly in the deficiency range (< 12.5 nmol/l) (Zittermann 2003).

No UK recommendations (RNIs) exist for adults under 65, but findings from the National Diet and Nutrition Survey of adults aged 19–64 found median daily intake in the UK, at 3.1 µg for men and 2.3 µg for women to be well below currently accepted adequate intake values of 5–10 µg/d (Henderson et al. 2003). Overall, 14% of men and 15% of women had a plasma concentration of 25-hydroxyvitamin D lower than 25 nmol/l. Adequate levels of intake rise to 15 µg/d

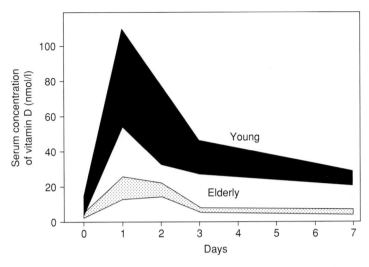

Figure 8.4 Circulating concentrations of vitamin D in response to a whole-body exposure to one minimal erythemal dose of simulated sunlight in healthy young and elderly subjects (reproduced with permission from Holick 2004).

for elderly subjects with insufficient vitamin D skin synthesis (Zittermann 2003). Intakes in Germany and the Netherlands are almost as low and are just adequate (around 5 μg/d) in Finland where more fatty fish is consumed (Zittermann 2003). In the UK, the 1994–1995 National Diet and Nutrition Survey of people aged 65 and over showed that the RNI for vitamin D (10 μg/d) was not met by 97% of the free living nor by 99% of those in institutions, 37% of whom have plasma concentrations of 25-hydroxyvitamin D less than 25 nmol/l (Bates et al. 1999). The reasons for particular problems in this population group, which are likely to be replicated in other northern European countries, are:

- The low levels of UVB irradiation at these latitudes
- The significant age-related decline in the ability of vitamin D to be synthesised in the skin after exposure to UVB light (see Figure 8.4)
- The reduced outdoor activity that is common in the elderly

A further difficulty in achieving adequate vitamin D status is the low vitamin D content of most foods (see section 8.7.4). The recognition of this problem has led to the mandatory fortification of some foods with vitamin D in a number of countries. Staple foods such as milk and margarine are fortified in the USA and Canada. In the UK, vitamin D is required by law to be added to margarine and is also added to most reduced fat and low fat spreads. Data from the Food and Agriculture Organization (FAO) published in 1995 showed that at that time margarine was also fortified by mandate in Australia, Columbia, Ecuador, Pakistan and Sweden and within the last 10 years, other countries may well have followed suit. The majority of countries in Europe and the rest of the world do not have

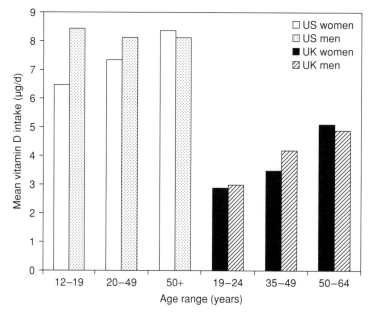

Figure 8.5 Average daily intake levels of vitamin D in the US and UK according to age and gender (data from Calvo et al. 2005; Henderson et al. 2003).

mandatory fortification (Calvo et al. 2005). Optional fortification of foods such as margarine, fat spreads, vegetable oil, and some breakfast cereals is allowed in most countries and contributes considerably to vitamin D intake. Though Japan and Norway have little or no fortification of foods, both countries have relatively good vitamin D intakes owing to their high fish consumption: Japanese women, 7.1 μg/d; Norwegian women 5.9 μg/d, Norwegian men 6.8 μg/d (compared with US men 8.12 μg/d, US women 7.33 μg/d; UK men 4.2 μg/d, UK women 3.7 μg/d) (Calvo et al. 2005). Average daily intake levels of vitamin D according to age and gender in the US and the UK are shown in Figure 8.5 (Calvo et al. 2005; Henderson et al. 2003). The higher intake in the US is a result of a greater level of food fortification, notably in milk, and to a greater use of supplements. Supplements contributed 30% and 40% to total vitamin D intake in men and women respectively in the US, whereas the corresponding figures were 12% and 24% in the UK (Calvo et al. 2005; Henderson et al. 2003). Current sources of vitamin D in the US and UK diets are shown in Figure 8.6 (Calvo et al. 2005; Henderson et al. 2003).

8.7.4   Recommendations for vitamin D intake

Given the immunosuppressant properties of vitamin D, its importance to calcium metabolism, bone formation, proteoglycan synthesis, modulation of cytokine expression and reduction of OA progression, it is clearly a crucial nutrient for arthritic patients. Patients should therefore be advised to increase their consumption of vitamin D.

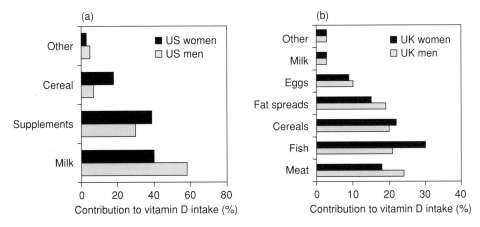

Figure 8.6 Dietary sources of vitamin D (a) in the US (data from Calvo et al. 2005) and (b) in the UK (data from Henderson et al. 2003).

Current dietary recommendations, as shown in Appendix 3, are believed by a number of workers to be far below the optimal level required to maintain adequate circulating 25-hydroxyvitamin D, which may be as much as 100 μg/d (Zittermann et al. 2003). In the context of RA, oral doses of 50 μg/d or greater of vitamin D or 25-hydroxyvitamin D were able to improve outcome (for references see Zittermann 2003).

Achieving the levels used in the supplementation studies from foods would be extremely difficult, as only a few foods are good sources of vitamin D, as can be seen from Table 8.7, which gives the vitamin D content of foods in the US diet (Mahan & Escott-Stump 2004). Vitamin D is found naturally in some animal products, notably oily fish, meat and egg yolk, resulting in higher intakes of vitamin D in meat and fish eaters than in vegetarians and vegans, as seen in the EPIC-Oxford study (Davey et al. 2003; see Figure 8.7).

Unless patients have a good intake of oily fish or spend time in the sun, they should be advised to take supplements of vitamin D, up to a level of 25 μg/d in OA patients, particularly if over 65 years, institutionalised, housebound, dark-skinned living at latitudes > 50°, or if they wear enveloping clothing. As plasma vitamin D concentrations are significantly lower in winter, most notably from January to March in the UK (Henderson et al. 2003), this is the most important time to consider supplementing intake. Cod liver oil is a commonly used supplement in arthritic patients and supplies around 5 μg/g of vitamin D. However, it also contains about 1600 μg/g vitamin A, and such a dose is therefore contraindicated in pregnancy owing to teratogenic effects which may occur at intakes greater than 1800 μg/d (remembering that diet also contributes to vitamin A intake). Apart from pregnancy, there is a risk of toxicity from a chronic intake of vitamin A of 15 mg (15 000 μg ≡ 50 000 IU)/d or more.

In trying to ameliorate arthritic symptoms or slow progression of OA, a balance must be struck between an effective intake and one that avoids toxicity. Being a fat

Table 8.7 Vitamin D content of foods available in North America (adapted from Mahan & Escott-Stump 2004).

Food item	Vitamin D (IU/100 g)	Vitamin D (µg/100 g)	Portion Size (g)	Vitamin D (µg/portion)
Breakfast cereals				
All-Bran	140	3.5	50	1.8
Frosted Flakes	140	3.5	50	1.8
Corn Flakes	140	3.5	50	1.8
Special K	140	3.5	50	1.8
Raisin Bran	152	3.8	50	1.9
Just Right with fruit and nuts	108	2.7	50	1.4
Apple Jacks	140	3.5	50	1.8
Honey and Nut Crunch	140	3.5	50	1.8
Natural raisin bran	152	3.8	50	1.9
Dairy and egg products				
Milk (cow, fortified, skimmed, semi-skimmed and whole)*	40	1.0	200	2.0
Goat milk (whole)	12	0.3	200	0.6
Cheddar cheese	12	0.3	40	0.1
Whipping cream	52	1.3	30	0.4
Egg (whole)	52	1.3	70	0.9
Fats				
Butter	56	1.4	10	0.1
Margarine (fortified)	60	1.5	10	0.2
Fish				
Salmon (canned, pink)	624	15.6	150	23
Sardines (canned in tomato sauce)	480	12.0	150	18
Tuna (canned in oil)	236	5.9	150	8.9
Meat				
Beef (liver)	16	0.4	150	0.6
Beef (sausage)	44	1.1	150	1.7
Vegetables				
Mushrooms (Shitake, dried)	1660	41.5	—	—
Mushrooms (Shitake, fresh)	100	2.5	401.0	

* Fortified in the US

soluble vitamin, vitamin D can accumulate in the body to toxic levels. Excess may lead to hypercalcaemia and hypercalciuria, resulting in the deposition of calcium in soft tissues, demineralisation of bones and irreversible renal and cardiovascular toxicity (UK Expert Group on Vitamins and Minerals 2003). No adverse effect on calcium levels was observed in a five-month supplementation study of vitamin D_3 at 100 µg/d in 63 adults aged 23–56. However, one study did report development of hypercalcaemia (serum calcium > 2.75 mmol/l) in two subjects in a six-month supplementation study with 50 µg/d vitamin D in females above the age of 60 and males above the age of 65 (UK Expert Group on Vitamins and Minerals 2003). According to the UK Expert Group on Vitamins and Minerals (2003), long-term

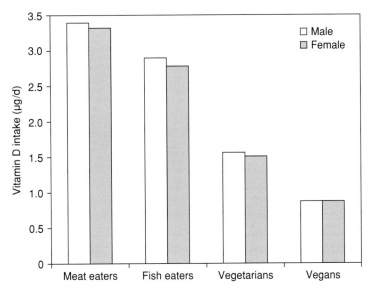

Figure 8.7 Mean daily intake of vitamin D by diet group and gender (data from Davey et al. 2003).

intakes of 25 μg/d appear to be well tolerated and may be necessary to prevent deficiency in some groups. Higher intakes should only be taken under medical guidance and for limited periods.

8.8 Boron and arthritis

Boron is not yet accepted as an essential nutrient for humans but it is known to interact with the metabolism of calcium, vitamin D and magnesium, all of which are important in bone metabolism (Devirian & Volpe 2003). Boron appears to normalise the disturbed energy substrate utilisation caused by vitamin D deficiency and may benefit bone mineral density when dietary intake of calcium, magnesium and vitamin D are low (Devirian & Volpe 2003). In other words, it appears to be a conditionally essential nutrient with regard to bone health.

High levels of dietary boron (20 μg/g) postponed the onset and lessened the severity of arthritis in rats (Bai & Hunt 1995) and there is some rather poor quality evidence for a benefit of boron in human arthritis (Devirian & Volpe 2003). Possible mechanisms that have been suggested for this beneficial effect are the purported ability of boron to control the inflammatory process and affect steroid hormones by its interaction with hydroxyl groups (Bai & Hunt 1995; Devirian & Volpe 2003). Controlled, adequately sized studies are required in humans.

There is no dietary requirement for boron but good dietary sources are apples, grapes, tomatoes, celery, almonds and bananas (Nielsen 1988). Drinking water is another source, probably because of detergent residues, though content varies with location.

8.9   Magnesium and arthritis

Magnesium, the second most abundant cation in cellular systems, is a nutrient that has many biological functions including structural, control and regulatory (Tam et al. 2003). It plays an important role in the immune system and affects cytokine secretion. Increased levels of pro-inflammatory cytokines such as IL-6 and TNF-α have been detected in animals deprived of magnesium for three weeks (Tam et al. 2003). Magnesium is required for the function of integrins, cell-surface receptors that are important in cartilage development and chondrogenesis (see Goggs et al. 2005). Though there are no relevant human studies showing benefit of magnesium in arthritis, advice to increase intake is probably warranted, as according to the latest UK National Diet and Nutrition Surveys of adults and the elderly, many individuals fail to achieve recommended intakes of magnesium (Henderson et al. 2003; Finch et al. 1998). Women in all age groups and men aged 19–24 fail to reach the RNI. Of those aged 65 or over, 22% of free living and 31% of those in institutions did not even achieve the LRNI (Lower Reference Nutrient Intake) which, by definition, is only adequate for 2.5% of the population (Finch et al. 1998).

8.10   Potassium and arthritis

Potassium may have a role in RA according to Weber (2003) who notes that low cell potassium is always seen in RA. Weber (2003) also reports that he has seen RA 'dramatically relieved, perhaps cured' with potassium. Potassium is another nutrient of which intakes are notably low in the UK. For instance, 30% of the free living and 37% of those in institutions aged 65 or above fail to meet the LRNI. No controlled studies have been conducted but this is an interesting area that may warrant further study.

8.11   Recommendations for achieving optimal micronutrient status in OA and RA

People rarely consume products as single nutrients. Foods are a complex mixture of known nutritional factors and other beneficial components, many of which may not yet be recognised. Fruits and vegetables fall into this category: they are rich sources of many antioxidant micronutrients, flavonoids, isothiocyanates, fibre, prebiotics and many other valuable compounds that have not yet been put in bottles. Therefore by eating dietary sources of nutrients, additional benefits may accrue. Rich dietary sources of some micronutrients are listed in Table 8.8.

Consumption of fortified foods is a helpful way of increasing the intake of some nutrients in countries that allow or encourage fortification practices. Flour, margarines/spreads and breakfast cereals are staple foods that are commonly fortified, as is milk in North America. Fortification of margarine with vitamins A and D is mandatory in a number of countries: 600–1500 μg of vitamin A and 5–13.3 μg of vitamin D are added per 100 g margarine, depending on the country (FAO 1995). Nutrients fortified in foods may be more bioavailable than when taken as

Table 8.8 Rich food sources of specific nutrients of relevance to RA/OA (data from Bender & Bender 1997; Thomas 2001).

Vitamin C	Vitamin D	Vitamin E	Selenium	Copper	Zinc	Magnesium	Potassium	Calcium	Boron
Berries and currants (i.e. blackcurrants)	Oily fish	Vegetable oils	Brazil nuts	Crab, prawns, lobster, mussels	Red meat	Green leafy vegetables	Fruit: such as bananas, apricots, citrus fruit, rhubarb, blackcurrants, dried fruit, fruit juice	Milk	Apples
Citrus fruit	Dairy products	Margarine	Kidney	Liver	Liver	Meat	Vegetables: such as mushrooms, beetroot, tomatoes	Dairy products	Grapes
Fruit juice	Eggs	Wholegrain cereals	Liver	Kidney	Kidney	Wholegrain cereals and pulses	Potatoes	Fish containing soft bones	Tomatoes
Vegetables (especially green leafy vegetables)	Margarine and butter	Nuts and seeds	Fish	Plain chocolate	Fish and shellfish	Some hard drinking water	Pulses	Green leafy vegetables	Celery
Potatoes (and sweet potato)	Meat	Fried foods	Shellfish	Beans and lentils	Milk and milk products	Milk and milk products	Chocolate, cocoa	Food containing white flour	Almonds
Potato chips	Cereal products	Meat, fish, eggs	Lentils and pulses	Brazil nuts	Pulses	Chocolate	Coffee	Pulses	Bananas
									Drinking water

supplements, as illustrated by the following example. Leonard and colleagues (2004) compared bioavailability of a 400 IU vitamin E supplement with vitamin E-enriched breakfast cereal in five subjects. They found that bioavailability was greater in the fortified food and that supplemental vitamin E, being a fat-soluble vitamin, if accompanied by a low fat meal, was poorly absorbed. This example illustrates the usefulness of fortified foods in the achievement of adequate vitamin, mineral and trace element status.

Where adequate amounts of a micronutrient cannot be obtained from foods, the UK RNI or US RDA (see Appendix 3) can normally be used as a reasonable guide to dose, as levels set should be adequate for 97.5% of the population and well below toxic intakes. There can be occasional problems of bioavailability where the intake of one nutrient may have antagonistic effects on others. Copper, zinc and iron use the same transporters, therefore an increase in one may affect the absorption of the others (Adam 1995). In practice, this appears to be more of a problem for copper in competition with zinc than for zinc in competition with iron. Furthermore, antioxidants do not work singularly but synergistically (Darlington & Stone 2001), requiring one another for removal of reaction products or their own regeneration. These considerations suggest that supplementation of single nutrients is usually inadvisable.

In general, if supplementation is required to achieve adequate nutritional status, it would be preferable to supplement with a good quality multivitamin and mineral supplement containing all the nutrients mentioned in this chapter at RDA/RNI level. This is more likely to maintain micronutrient homeostasis. That said, on the basis of the studies presented here, there is clearly a case for supplementing certain nutrients, notably vitamin D but also vitamin E (in RA) and selenium (in RA), at a higher level, at least for an experimental period, to see if any improvement is experienced. Vegetarians and vegans need to take particular care to have adequate intakes of vitamin D and selenium.

Supplements may provide well over the RNI/RDA. While this is unlikely to matter very much in the case of water soluble nutrients such as vitamin C where excess is excreted in the urine, fat soluble vitamins may build up slowly over time to toxic levels. For example, vitamin A consumed in supplement form at 1000 µg RE (retinol equivalents) per day, may lead to liver damage within ten years. Similarly, vitamin D at high levels may become toxic over prolonged periods. Selenium is also toxic at elevated doses, as explained in section 8.4.4. It is important that both the RNI/RDA and the potential toxic dosage are known. Signs of toxicity should be monitored in those taking potentially toxic supplements at levels above the RNI/RDA.

References

Aaseth J, Haugen M, Forre O (1998) Rheumatoid arthritis and metal compounds – perspectives on the role of oxygen radical detoxification. *Analyst* **123**, 3–6.

Abate A, Yang G, Dennery P, Oberle S, Schroder H (2000) Synergistic inhibition of cyclo-oxygenase-2 expression by vitamin E and aspirin. *Free Radical Biology and Medicine* **29**, 1135–42.

Adam O (1995) Review – Anti-inflammatory diet in rheumatic diseases. *European Journal of Clinical Nutrition* **49**, 703–17.

Adams ML, Lombi E, Zhao F-J, McGrath S (2002) Evidence of low selenium concentrations in UK bread-making wheat grain. *Journal of the Science of Food and Agriculture* **82**, 1160–65.

ARC (Arthritis and Rheumatism Council) for Research (1995) *Collected Reports on the Rheumatic Diseases*, pp. 3–10, 20–43, 49–51, 168–77, 186–97, 218–21, 229–35, 245–55.

Bae S-C, Kim S-J, Sung M-K (2003) Inadequate antioxidant nutrient intake and altered plasma antioxidant status of rheumatoid arthritis patients. *Journal of the American College of Nutrition* **22**(4), 311–15.

Bai Y, Hunt CD (1995) Dietary boron alleviates adjuvant-induced arthritis (AIA) in rats. *Journal of the Federation of American Societies for Experimental Biology* (FASEB), **A576**.

Bates CJ, Prentice A, Cole TJ, van der Pols JC, Doyle W, Finch S, Smithers G, Clarke PC (1999) Micronutrients: highlights and research challenges from the 1994–95 National Diet and Nutrition Survey of people aged 65 years and over. *British Journal of Nutrition* **82**, 7–15.

Bender DA (2002) *Introduction to Nutrition and Metabolism*, 3rd edition. London, Taylor and Francis, pp. 402–5.

Bender DA, Bender AE (1997) *Nutrition: a Reference Handbook*. Oxford, Oxford University Press, pp. 228, 257, 272, 372, 432, 436.

Berger A (2002) What does zinc do? *British Medical Journal* **325**, 1062–63.

Blake DR, Merry P, Stevens C, Dabbagh A, Sahinoglu T, Allen R, Morris C (1990) Iron free radicals and arthritis. *Proceedings of the Nutrition Society* **49**, 239–45.

Blake DR, Merry P, Unsworth J, Kidd BL, Outhwaite JM, Ballard R, Morris CJ, Gray L, Lunec J (1989) Hypoxic-reperfusion injury in the inflamed human joint. *The Lancet* **1**, 289–93.

Bowman SJ (2002) Hematological manifestations of rheumatoid arthritis. *Scandinavian Journal of Rheumatology* **31**(5), 251–59.

Brand C, Snaddon J, Bailey M, Cicuttini F (2001) Vitamin E is ineffective for symptomatic relief of knee osteoarthritis; a six-month double-blind, randomised, placebo-controlled study. *Annals of the Rheumatic Diseases* **60**(10), 946–49.

Calvo MS, Whiting SJ, Barton CN (2005) Vitamin D intake: a global perspective of current status. *Journal of Nutrition* **135**(2), 310–16.

Cerhan JR, Saag KG, Merlino LA, Mikuls TR, Criswell LA (2003) Antioxidant micronutrients and risk of rheumatoid arthritis in a cohort of older women. *American Journal of Epidemiology* **157**(4), 345.

Clavel G, Bessis N, Boissier MC (2003) Recent data on the role for angiogenesis in rheumatoid arthritis. *Joint Bone Spine* **70**(5), 321–26.

Comstock GW, Burke AE, Hoffman SC, Helzlsouer KJ, Bendich A, Masi AT, Norkus EP, Malamet RT, Gershwin (1997) Serum concentrations of alpha tocopherol, beta carotene and retinol preceding the diagnosis of rheumatoid arthritis and systemic lupus erythematosus. *Annals of the Rheumatic Diseases* **56**(5), 323–25.

Darlington LG, Stone TW (2001) Review article – Antioxidants and fatty acids in the amelioration of rheumatoid arthritis and related disorders. *British Journal of Nutrition* **85**, 251–69.

Davey GK, Spencer EA, Appleby PN, Allen NE, Knox KH, Key TJ (2003) EPIC-Oxford: lifestyle characteristics and nutrient intakes in a cohort of 33 883 meat-eaters and 31 546 non-meat-eaters in the UK. *Public Health Nutrition* **6**, 259–69.

DeLuca HF, Cantorna MT (2001) Vitamin D: its role and uses in immunology. *Journal of the Federation of American Societies for Experimental Biology* **15**, 2579–85.

Devirian TA, Volpe SL (2003) The physiological effects of boron. *Critical Reviews in Food Science and Nutrition* **43**, 219–31.

DiSilvestro, RA, Marten J, Skehan M (1992) Effects of copper supplementation on ceruloplasmin and copper-zinc superoxide dismutase in free living rheumatoid arthritis patients. *Journal of the American College of Nutrition* **11**, 177–80.

Edmonds SE, Winyard PG, Guo R, Kidd B, Merry P, Langrish-Smith A, Hansen C, Ramm S, Blake DR (1997) Durative analgesic activity of repeated oral doses of Vitamin E in the treatment of rheumatoid arthritis. Results of a prospective placebo-controlled double-blind trial. *Annals of the Rheumatic Diseases* **56**, 649–55.

Fang YZ, Yang S, Wu G. (2002) Free radicals, antioxidants, and nutrition. *Nutrition* **18**, 872–79.

FAO (1995) *Food and Nutrition paper 60. Food fortification: technology and quality control.* Annex 7. www.fao.org/docrep/w2840e/w2840e0e.htm

Felson DT, Lawrence RC, Dieppe PA, Hirsch R, Helmick CG, Jordan JM, Kington RS, Lane NE, Nevitt MC, Zhang Y, Sowers M, McAlindon T, Spector TD, Poole AR, Yanovski SZ, Ateshian G, Sharma L, Buckwalter JA, Brandt KD, Fries JF (2000) Osteoarthritis: new insights. Part 1: the disease and its risk factors. *Annals of Internal Medicine* 133, 635–46.

Finch S, Doyle W, Lowe C, Bates CJ, Prentice A, Smithers G, Clarke PC (1998) *National Diet and Nutrition Survey: People aged 65 years and over, 1994–1995. Report of the diet and nutrition survey.* London, The Stationery Office, (computer file) 2nd edition. Colchester, Essex, UK Data Archive (distributor), November 2001, SN, 4036.

Fisher AEO, Naughton DP (2004) Iron supplements: the quick fix with long-term consequences. *Nutrition Journal* 3, 2.

Fitzsimons EJ, Brock JH (2001) The anaemia of chronic disease. *British Medical Journal* 322, 811–12.

Fitzsimons EJ, Sturrock RD (2002) The chronic anaemia of rheumatoid arthritis: iron banking or blocking? *The Lancet* 360, 1713–14.

Frausto da Silva JJR, Williams RJP (2001a) *The Biological Chemistry of the Elements: The Inorganic Chemistry of Life*, 2nd edition. Oxford, Oxford University Press, pp. 426–28.

Frausto da Silva JJR, Williams RJP (2001b) ibid., p. 301.

Frausto da Silva JJR, Williams RJP (2001c) ibid., pp. 424–25, 538–543.

Goggs R, Vaughan-Thomas A, Clegg P, Carter S, Innes J, Mobasheri A (2005) Nutraceutical therapies for degenerative joint diseases: a critical review. *Critical Reviews in Food Science and Nutrition* 45, 145–64.

Hagfors L, Leanderson P, Skoldstam L, Andersson J, Johansson G (2003) Antioxidant intake, plasma antioxidant and oxidative stress in a randomised, controlled, parallel, Mediterranean dietary intervention study on patients with rheumatoid arthritis. *Nutrition Journal* 2, 5.

Halliwell B, Gutteridge J (1999a) *Free Radicals in Biology and Medicine*, 3rd edition. Oxford, Oxford University Press, pp. 53–55.

Halliwell B, Gutteridge J (1999b) ibid., p. 336.

Heinle K, Adam A, Gradl M, Wiseman M, Adam O (1997) Selenium concentration in erythrocytes of patients with rheumatoid arthritis. Clinical and laboratory chemistry infection markers during administration of selenium (Article in German) *Medizinische Klinik* (Munich) 92, Suppl 3, 29–31.

Heliövaara M, Knekt P, Aho K, Aaran R-K, Alfthan G, Aromaa A (1994) Serum antioxidants and risk of rheumatoid arthritis. *Annals of the Rheumatic Diseases* 53, 51–53.

Helliwell M, Coombes EJ, Moody BJ, Batstone GF, Robertson J (1984) Nutritional status in patients with rheumatoid arthritis. *Annals of the Rheumatic Diseases* 43, 386–90.

Henderson L, Irving K, Gregory J, Bates C, Prentice A, Perks J, Swan G, Farron M (2003) *Food Standards Agency The National Diet and Nutrition Survey: adults aged 19 to 64 years.* www.statistics.gov.uk/downloads/theme_health/NDNS_v3.pdf

Holick MF (2004) Vitamin D. In: *Nutrition and Bone Health* (MF Holick, B Dawson-Hughes, eds), Totowa, NJ, Humana Press, pp. 403–40.

Honkanen VE, Lamberg-Allardt CH, Vesterinen MK, Lehto JH, Westermarck TW, Metsa-Ketela TK, Mussalo-Rauhamaa MH, Konttinen YT (1991a) Plasma zinc and copper concentrations in rheumatoid arthritis: influence of dietary factors and disease activity. *American Journal of Clinical Nutrition* 54, 1082–86.

Honkanen V, Konttinen YT, Sorsa T, Hukkanen M, Kemppinen P, Santavirta S, Saari H, Westermarck T (1991b) Serum zinc, copper and selenium in rheumatoid arthritis. *J Trace Elem Electrolytes Health Dis.* 5, 261–3.

Jäntti J, Vapaatalo H, Seppälä E, Ruutsalo H-M, Isomäki H (1991) Treatment of rheumatoid arthritis with fish oil, selenium, vitamins A and E and placebo. *Scandinavian Journal of Rheumatology* 20, 225 (abstract only).

Jiang C, Jiang W, Ip C, Ganther H, Lu J (1999) Selenium-induced inhibition of angiogenesis in mammary cancer at chemopreventive levels of intake. *Molecular Carcinogenesis* 26(4), 213–25.

Jiang C, Ganther H, Lu J (2000) Monomethyl selenium-specific inhibition of MMP-2 and VEGF expression: implications for angiogenic switch regulation. *Molecular Carcinogenesis* **29**(4), 236–50.

Jordan J, Fang F, Arab L, Morris J, Renner J, Helmick C, Hochberg M (2005) Low selenium levels are associated with increased risk for osteoarthritis of the knee. *Abstract no. 1189, American College of Rheumatology/Association of Rheumatology Health Professionals Annual Scientific Meeting*, November 12–17, San Diego, California.

Knekt P, Heliövaara M, Aho K, Alfthan G, Marniemi J, Aromaa A (2000) Serum selenium, serum alpha-tocopherol, and the risk of rheumatoid arthritis. *Epidemiology* **1**(4), 402–5.

Kremer JM, Bigaouette J (1996) Nutrient intake of patients with rheumatoid arthritis is deficient in pyridoxine, zinc, copper and magnesium. *Journal of Rheumatology* **23**(6), 990–94.

Kolb C, Mauch S, Krawinkel U, Sedlacek R (1999) Matrix metalloproteinase-19 in capillary endothelial cells: expression in acutely, but not in chronically, inflamed synovium. *Experimental Cell Research* **10**, 250(1), 122–30.

Lane NE, Gore LR, Cummings SR, Hochberg MC, Scott JC, Williams EN, Nevitt MC (1999) Serum vitamin D levels and incident changes of radiographic hip osteoarthritis: a longitudinal study. Study of Osteoporotic Fractures Research Group. *Arthritis and Rheumatism* **42**(5), 854–60.

Leonard SW, Good CK, Gugger ET, Traber MG (2004) Vitamin E bioavailability from fortified breakfast cereals is greater than that from encapsulated supplements. *American Journal of Clinical Nutrition* **79**, 86–92.

Longnecker MP, Taylor PR, Levander OA, Howe M, Veillon C, McAdam PA, Patterson KY, Holden JM, Stampfer MJ, Morris JS et al. (1991) Selenium in diet, blood, and toenails in relation to human health in a seleniferous area. *American Journal of Clinical Nutrition* **53**, 1288–94.

Maehira F, Luyo G, Miyagi I, Oshiro M, Yamane N, Kuba M, Nakazato Y (2002) Alterations of serum selenium concentrations in the acute phase of pathological conditions. *Clinica Chimica Acta* **316**, 137–46.

MAFF Joint Food Safety and Standards Group (1997) *Food Surveillance Information Sheet* **126**, October 1997.

Mahan LK, Escott-Stump (2004) *Krause's Food, Nutrition and Diet Therapy*, 11th edition. Philadelphia, WB Saunders, pp. 1144–58.

Martin RH (1998) The role of nutrition and diet in rheumatoid arthritis. *Proceedings of the Nutrition Society* **57**, 231–34.

McAlindon T, Felson DT (1997) Nutrition: risk factors for osteoarthritis. *Annals of the Rheumatic Diseases* **56**, 397–402.

McAlindon TE, Jacques P, Zhang Y, Hannan MT, Aliabadi P, Weissman B, Rush D, Levy D, Felson DT (1996a) Do antioxidant micronutrients protect against the development and progression of knee osteoarthritis? *Arthritis and Rheumatism* **39**(4), 648–56.

McAlindon TE, Felson DT, Zhang Y, Hannan MT, Aliabadi P, Weissman B, Rush D, Wilson PW, Jacques P (1996b) Relation of dietary intake and serum levels of vitamin D to progression of osteoarthritis of the knee among participants in the Framingham Study. *Annals of Internal Medicine* **125**, 353–59.

Meltzer H, Bibow K, Ronneberg R, Haugen M, Holm H (1989) The intake of selenium and other nutrients in a group of Norwegian rheumatics. In: *Selenium in Biology and Medicine* (ed. A Wendel). Springer, Berlin, pp. 238–41.

Merlino LA, Curtis J, Mikulus TR, Cerhan JR, Criswell LA, Saag KG (2004) Vitamin D intake is inversely associated with rheumatoid arthritis: results from the Iowa Women's Health Study. *Arthritis and Rheumatism* **50**, 72–77.

Morgan SL, Anderson AM, Hood SM, Matthews PA, Lee JY, Alarcón GS (1997) Nutrient intake patterns, body mass index and vitamin levels in patients with rheumatoid arthritis. *Arthritis Care and Research* **10**, 9–17.

Morris CJ, Earl JR, Trenam CW, Blake DR (1995) Reactive oxygen species and iron – a dangerous partnership in inflammation. *International Journal of Biochemistry and Cell Biology* **27**, 109–22.

Naveh Y, Schapira D, Ravel Y, Geller E, Scharf Y (1997) Zinc metabolism in rheumatoid arthritis: plasma and urinary zinc and relationship to disease activity. *Journal of Rheumatology* **24**, 643–66.

Nielsen FH (1988) Nutritional significance of the ultratrace elements. *Nutrition Reviews* **46**, 337–41.

Paredes S, Girona J, Hurt-Camejo E, Vallve JC, Olive S, Heras M, Benito P, Masana L (2002) Antioxidant vitamins and lipid peroxidation in patients with rheumatoid arthritis: association with inflammatory markers. *Journal of Rheumatology* **29**, 2271–77.

Peacock M (1995) Nutritional aspects of hip fractures. *Challenges of Modern Medicine* **7**, 213–22.

Peretz A, Neve J, Duchateau J, Famaey JP (1992) Adjuvant treatment of recent onset rheumatoid arthritis by selenium supplementation: preliminary observations. *British Journal of Rheumatology* **31**, 281–86.

Peretz A, Neve J, Jeghers O, Pelen F (1993) Zinc distribution in blood components, inflammatory status and clinical indexes of disease activity during zinc supplementation in inflammatory rheumatic diseases. *American Journal of Clinical Nutrition* **57**(5), 690–94.

Peretz A, Siderova V, Neve J (2001) Selenium supplementation in rheumatoid arthritis investigated in a double-blind, placebo-controlled trial. *Scandinavian Journal of Rheumatology* **30**(4), 208–12.

Petersson I, Majberger E, Palm S, Larsen A (1991) Treatment of rheumatoid arthritis with selenium and vitamin E. *Scandinavian Journal of Rheumatology* **20**, 218.

Punnonen K, Kaipiainen-Seppanen O, Riittinen L, Tuomisto T, Hongisto T, Penttila L (2000) Evaluation of iron status in anemic patients with rheumatoid arthritis using an automated immunoturbidimetric assay for transferrin receptor. *Clinical Chemistry and Laboratory Medicine* **38**(12), 1297–300.

Rayman MP (1997) Dietary selenium: time to act. *British Medical Journal* **314**, 387–88.

Rayman MP (2000) The importance of selenium to human health. *The Lancet* **356**, 233–241.

Rayman MP (2002) The argument for increasing selenium intake. *Proceedings of the Nutrition Society* **61**, 203–15.

Rayman MP, Bode P, Redman CWG (2003) Low selenium status is associated with the occurrence of the pregnancy disease preeclampsia in UK women. *American Journal of Obstetrics and Gynecology* **189**, 1343–49.

Rayman MP (2004) The use of high-selenium yeast to raise selenium status: how does it measure up? *British Journal of Nutrition* **92**, 557–73.

Rayman MP (2005) Selenium in cancer prevention: a review of the evidence and mechanism of action. *Proceedings of the Nutrition Society* **64**, 527–42.

Simkin PA (1977) Zinc sulphate in rheumatoid arthritis. *Progress in Clinical and Biological Research* **14**, 343–56.

Scherak O, Kolarz MD (1991) Vitamin E and rheumatoid arthritis. *Arthritis and Rheumatism* **34**(9), 1205–6.

Schwartz E, Adamy L (1977) Effect of ascorbic acid on arylsulfatase activities and sulfated proteoglycan metabolism in chondrocyte cultures. *Journal of Clinical Investigation* **60**, 96–106.

Shenkin A (1995) Trace elements and inflammatory response: implications for nutritional support. *Nutrition.* Jan–Feb; **11**(1 Suppl), 100–5.

Stone J, Doube A, Dudson D, Wallace J (1997) Inadequate calcium, folic acid, vitamin E, zinc and selenium intake in rheumatoid arthritis patients: results of a dietary survey. *Seminars in Arthritis and Rheumatism* **27**(3), 180–85.

Tam M, Gomez S, Gonzalez-Gross M, Marcos A (2003) Possible roles of magnesium on the immune system. *European Journal of Clinical Nutrition* **57**(10), 1193–97.

Tarp U, Overvad K, Thorling EB, Graudal H, Hansen JC (1985) Selenium treatment in rheumatoid arthritis. *Scandinavian Journal of Rheumatology* **14**(4), 364–68.

Tarp U, Graudal H, Overvad K, Thorling E, Hansen J (1989) Selenium in rheumatoid arthritis. A historical prospective approach. *Journal of Trace Elements and Electrolytes in Health and Disease* B, 93–95.

Tarp U (1994) Selenium and the selenium-dependent glutathione peroxidase in rheumatoid arthritis. *Danish Medical Bulletin* **41**, 264–74.

Tarp U (1995) Selenium in rheumatoid arthritis. A review. *Analyst* **120**, 877–81.

Thomas B (2001) *Manual of Dietetic Practice*, 3rd edition. Oxford, Blackwell Science.

Thomson CD, Robinson MF (1996) The changing selenium status of New Zealand residents. *European Journal of Clinical Nutrition* **50**(2), 107–14.

UK Expert Group on Vitamins and Minerals (2003) Annex 4. *Current Usage of Vitamin and Mineral Supplements in the UK*. Food Standards Agency, May 2003. ISBN 1-904026-11-7. www.food.gov.uk/multimedia/pdfs/vitmin2003.pdf

Vannoort R, Cressey P, Silvers K (2000) 1997/1998 *New Zealand Total Diet Survey*. Part 2: Elements. Wellington, Ministry of Health.

Weber CE (2003) Potassium for rheumatoid arthritis. *British Medical Journal* **318**(7190), 1023–24.

Whanger P, Vendeland S, Park Y-C, Xia Y (1996) Metabolism of sub-toxic levels of selenium in animals and humans. *Annals of Clinical and Laboratory Science* **26**, 99–113.

Wilson A, Yu HT, Goodnough LT, Nissenson AR (2004) Prevalence and outcomes of anaemia in rheumatoid arthritis: a systematic review of the literature. *American Journal of Medicine* **116** (suppl 7A), 50S–57S.

Wittenborg A, Petersen G, Lorkowski G, Brabant T (1998) Effectiveness of vitamin E in comparison with diclofenac sodium in treatment of patients with chronic polyarthritis (Article in German) *Zeitschrift fur Rheumatologie* **57**(4), 215–21.

Wluka AE, Ttuckey S, Brand C, Cicuttini FM (2002) Supplementary vitamin E does not affect the loss of cartilage volume in knee osteoarthritis: a 2 year double-blind randomised placebo-controlled study. *Journal of Rheumatology* **29**(12), 2585–91.

Xia Y, Hill KE, Byrne DW, Xu J, Burk RF (2005) Effectiveness of selenium supplements in a low-selenium area of China. *American Journal of Clinical Nutrition* **81**, 829–34.

Yoon SO, Kim MM, Chung AS (2001) Inhibitory effect of selenite on invasion of HT1080 tumor cells. *Journal of Biological Chemistry* **276**, 20085–92.

Zittermann A (2003) Vitamin D in preventative medicine: are we ignoring the evidence? *British Journal of Nutrition* **89**(5), 552–72.

9 Polyunsaturated fatty acids in the treatment of arthritis

9.1 Essential fatty acids and their nomenclature

Fatty acids are the building blocks of fats (triacylgerols), phospholipids and glycolipids, the latter two occurring in biological membranes. Though dietary fat had long been recognised as an important source of energy for mammals, in the late 1920s researchers demonstrated a dietary requirement for particular fatty acids (MacLean et al. 2004). While mammalian cells can introduce double bonds into the fatty acid chain, they cannot do so at positions 3 and 6 to produce α-linolenic acid (ALA) and linoleic acid (LA), known as the essential fatty acids. No other fatty acids in foods are considered essential because they can all be synthesised from the short-chain fatty acids (MacLean et al. 2004).

Fatty acids are often referred to using the number of carbons in the acyl chain, followed by a colon, followed by the number of double bonds in the chain: the position of the double bond, counting from the methyl end of the chain, is also given. Thus α-linolenic acid (ALA) is known as 18:3n-3 {or 18:3(ω-3)} and linoleic acid (LA) as 18:2n-6 {or 18:2(ω-6)}, as illustrated in Figure 9.1. ALA is the parent compound of the n-3 series of fatty acids and LA the parent of the n-6 series. Similarly, oleic acid, though not an essential fatty acid, is the parent of the n-9 series. ALA and LA are known as polyunsaturated fatty acids (PUFAs), as they have more than one double bond. Having 18 carbon atoms, they are short-chain PUFAs but they can be converted to longer 20- and 22-carbon PUFAs, the so-called long-chain PUFAs (LC PUFAs), of which eicosapentaenoic acid (EPA, 20:5n-3), docosahexaenoic acid (DHA, 22:6n-3), dihomo-γ-linolenic acid (DGLA, 20:3n-6) and arachidonic acid (AA, 20:4n-6), are examples (Figure 9.1).

9.2 Role of fatty acids: relevance to arthritis

Fatty acids have a number of functions in the body (Adam 1995):

- As a source of energy which can be stored
- As structural components of phospholipids in biological membranes
- As functional components of phospholipids in membranes, regulating membrane fluidity and membrane-bound enzyme function
- For lipid transport
- For cell signalling
- As precursors of important biological mediators

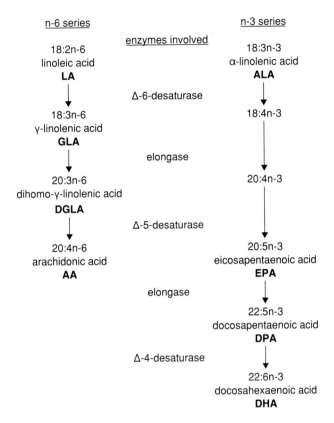

Figure 9.1 Desaturation and chain elongation of essential fatty acids.

The relevance of essential fatty acids to arthritis is largely connected with this last function, namely that they are the precursors of important biological mediators. N-3 fatty acids, in particular, are important immunomodulatory nutrients, which influence both cytokine production and lipid-derived metabolites (hormone-like substances known as eicosanoids) to create anti-inflammatory responses. The way in which n-3 PUFAs modify the inflammatory process and how they interact with the other group of essential fatty acids, the n-6 PUFAs, is relevant to an understanding of their role in arthritis.

9.3 Metabolism of polyunsaturated fatty acids

9.3.1 Conversion to long-chain PUFAs

Following ingestion, LA (n-6) and ALA (n-3) are metabolised in the liver by a complex set of synthetic pathways that share several enzymes, as shown in Figure 9.1 (MacLean et al. 2004). They undergo stepwise chain elongation and desaturation, competing for the same enzymes. The conversion from parent fatty acids LA and ALA to the long-chain PUFAs – DGLA, AA, EPA and DHA – where it occurs, occurs only slowly in humans, indicating that metabolism is inefficient (Adam 1995; MacLean et al. 2004). Thus the amount of DGLA, for example, is less than 1% of total fatty acid in plasma lipids, not only because of slow conversion but also because the amount of this precursor is negligible in a typical Western diet (Adam 1995). The diet (meat and meat products) is the source of AA, as no appreciable amounts of this fatty acid are formed from ingested LA (Adam 1995; Adam et al. 2003; Mantzioris et al. 1995). As regards conversion from ALA, less than 1% of plasma ALA was utilised for long-chain PUFA synthesis in human subjects eating either beef- or fish-based diets (Pawlosky et al. 2003). Nonetheless, prolonged intake of ALA results in appreciable levels of EPA (Adam 1995; Mantzioris et al. 1995), though dietary EPA is approximately sevenfold more efficient than dietary ALA in elevating tissue EPA (James et al. 2003). Furthermore, conversion from EPA to DHA is severely restricted, resulting in a conversion rate of ALA to DHA of only a few per cent, particularly with an n-6-PUFA-rich diet (Gerster 1998). Oily fish is the predominant source of EPA and DHA in the Western diet.

9.3.2   Formation of eicosanoids from PUFA precursors

Eicosanoids are hormone-like agents formed from 20-carbon (Greek: *eikosi* = 20) fatty acid precursors by the action of cyclo-oxygenase (Cox-1, Cox-2) or lipoxygenase (5-, 12-, 15-Lox) enzymes. They exert their effects locally, either in the cells that synthesise them or in adjacent cells (MacLean 2004). The eicosanoid family includes subgroups of substances, including the prostaglandins, leukotrienes and thromboxanes. Unesterified (free) AA (20:4n-6) is the precursor of a group of eicosanoids that includes series-2 prostaglandins and series-4 leukotrienes, while EPA (20:5n-3) gives rise to a group of eicosanoids that includes the series-3 prostaglandins and series-5 leukotrienes (Figure 9.2).

With a typical Western diet, formation of eicosanoids from EPA is both limited and slow, while from DGLA (20:3n-6), it is negligible (Adam 1995; Broadhurst et al. 2002). Though the production of eicosanoids from endogenously formed AA is low, meat and meat products are a ready source of exogenous AA, which, following release from membrane phospholipids by phospholipases (Adam 1995; Adam

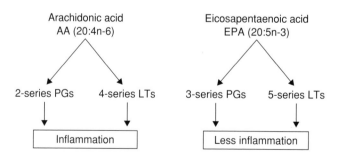

Figure 9.2   Eicosanoid precursors, AA and EPA (after P. Calder, personal communication, 2003).

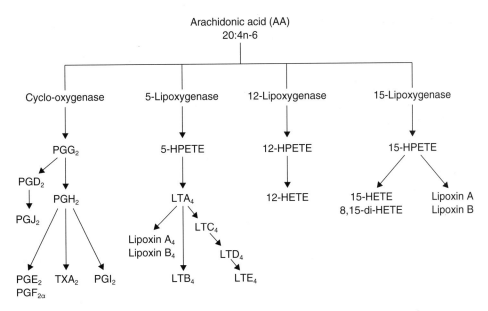

Figure 9.3 Synthesis of eicosanoids from arachidonic acid (AA) leading to prostaglandins (PG), leukotrienes (LT), hydroxy fatty acids (HETE) and lipoxins (Adam 1995; Calder & Field 2002).

et al. 2003), acts as the substrate for the production of series-2 prostaglandins, series-4 leukotrienes, hydroxy fatty acids and lipoxins (Figure 9.3). Because the membranes of most cells contain much larger amounts of AA compared to the amounts of DGLA and EPA, the series-2 prostaglandins and series-4 leukotrienes are those most commonly produced (Calder & Zurier 2001).

9.4   Inflammatory potential of eicosanoids

AA and EPA are metabolised to eicosanoid products that differ considerably in inflammatory potential. The eicosanoid products of AA, the series-2 prostaglandins and series-4 leukotrienes {e.g. prostaglandin E_2 (PGE_2) and leukotriene B_4 (LTB_4)} are pro-inflammatory. It is exogenous AA that is related to increased eicosanoid formation, the amount produced correlating with inflammatory severity in RA. By contrast, the EPA-derived prostaglandins attenuate these pro-inflammatory effects and are associated with anti-inflammatory responses (MacLean et al. 2004). Table 9.1 shows the eicosanoids formed and their relative inflammatory potential (see also Figure 9.2).

9.5   Eicosanoids in arthritis

A strong inflammatory reaction is present both in RA and late-stage OA patients (Curtis et al. 2004a). Cellular activation induces Cox-2, leading to a markedly elevated production of prostaglandins, while the infiltrating leucocytes and

Table 9.1 Eicosanoids produced from n-3 and n-6 fatty acids and their inflammatory potential (Calder & Zurier 2001; MacLean et al. 2004).

Family	Substrate fatty acid	Eicosanoids produced	Inflammatory potential
n-6	Dihomo-γ-linolenic acid DGLA (20:3n-6)	Series 1-Prostaglandins (e.g. PGE_1, PGD_1, PGF_{1a}) Thromboxane A_1 15-OH-DGLA	Less inflammatory
n-6	Arachidonic acid AA (20:4n-6)	Series 2-Prostaglandins (i.e. PGE_2, PGD_2, PGF_{2a}, PGH_2, PGI_2) Series 4-Leukotrienes (i.e. LTB_4–E_4) Thromboxane A_2 5-eicosatetraenoic acid (5-HETE)	Pro-inflammatory
n-3	Eicosapentaenoic acid EPA (20:5n-3)	Series 3-Prostaglandins (e.g. PGE_3, PGH_3, PGI_3) Series 5-Leukotrienes (i.e. LTB_5–E_5) Thromboxane A_3	Less inflammatory

synoviocytes present in RA are important sources of eicosanoids, particularly under the influence of TNF-a and other pro-inflammatory cytokines (Calder & Zurier 2001). PGE_2, LTB_4, 5-HETE (a product of AA metabolism by 5-Lox) and platelet-derived activating factor (another phospholipid-derived inflammatory mediator) are found in the synovium of patients with active RA while expression of both Cox-1 and Cox-2 are increased (Calder & Zurier 2001).

Eicosanoids derived from AA produced in arthritic joints are associated with the following undesirable effects (Calder & Zurier 2001).

PGE_2:
- Is pro-inflammatory
- Increases vascular permeability
- Increases vasodilation
- Increases blood flow
- Increases local pyrexia
- Potentiates pain caused by other agents
- Promotes the production of matrix metalloproteinases (see 9.7.5)
- Stimulates bone resorption

LTB_4:
- Increases vascular permeability
- Enhances local blood flow
- Is a potent chemotactic agent for leucocytes
- Induces release of lysosomal enzymes

- Enhances the generation of reactive oxygen species
- Enhances production of pro-inflammatory cytokines, TNF-a, IL-1 and IL-6

5-HETE:
- is an agonist for the LTB_4 receptor

Platelet activating factor:
- promotes production of TNF-a and increases vascular permeability

9.6   Rationale for the use of specific PUFAs in the treatment of arthritis

Certain PUFAs, notably EPA and ALA of the n-3 class and DGLA of the n-6 class, have suppressive effects on the production of a range of lipid and cytokine mediators of inflammation and of the degradative enzymes that occur in joints (James et al. 2003). PUFAs are known to be important cell signalling molecules and many of these effects may operate through their ability to alter gene expression (Simopoulos 1999).

In addition to reduction of symptoms (Caughey et al. 1996), some favourable effects of n-3 PUFAs/GLA/DGLA are listed below and are expanded upon in the following section (Arita et al. 2005; Calder & Zurier 2001; Cleland et al. 2004; Curtis et al. 2004b; James et al. 2003; MacLean et al. 2004):

- Production of less biologically potent eicosanoids than those from AA
- Competitive inhibition of enzymes that metabolise AA to pro-inflammatory eicosanoids
- Production of anti-inflammatory prostaglandins (PGE_1 from DGLA)
- Decreased production of inflammatory cytokines
- Inhibition of the proliferation of lymphocytes
- Inhibition by n-3 PUFAs of the production of cartilage-degrading enzymes
- Attenuation of NF-κB (TNF-α stimulates NF-κB which triggers gene transcription).

9.7   Beneficial effects of GLA, DGLA and n-3 PUFAs

9.7.1   Effects on eicosanoids

Gamma linolenic acid (GLA), DGLA and n-3 PUFAs are able to decrease pro-inflammatory n-6 eicosanoid formation if the intake is sufficiently high compared to that of AA, and (to a lesser extent) LA. They do this by decreasing the amount of AA in membrane phospholipids and competively inhibiting the production of AA-derived eicosanoids from Cox and 5-Lox (James et al. 2003). For example, when healthy subjects were supplemented with fish oil providing 2.1 g EPA + 1.1 g DHA/d for 12 weeks, the amount of AA in plasma phospholipids and mononuclear cells decreased by 20% while that of EPA increased, altering the ratio of AA:EPA from 23:1 to 1.5:1 in plasma phospholipids and from 28:1 to 6:1 in mononuclear cells (Yaqoob et al. 2000).

Table 9.2 Modification of pro-inflammatory and other effects of eicosanoids by altering the dietary content of PUFAs (Belch & Hill 2000; Simopoulos 1999).

Fatty acid ingested	Eicosanoid effect	Properties of eicosanoid affected
EPA/DHA/GLA/DGLA	$\downarrow$ PGE$_2$	Associated with pain, inflammation and vascular permeability
EPA/DHA/GLA/DGLA	$\downarrow$ TXA$_2$	Potent aggregator and vasoconstrictor
EPA/DHA/GLA/DGLA	$\downarrow$ LTB$_4$	Inducer of inflammation, and of leucocyte chemotaxis and adherence, enabling leucocytes to move from the circulatory system into tissues
EPA/DHA	$\uparrow$ LTB$_5$	Weak inducer of inflammation and a chemotactic agent – 10 to 100 times less potent than LTB$_4$
EPA/DHA	$\uparrow$ TXA$_3$	Weak vasoconstrictor and platelet aggregator
EPA/DHA	$\uparrow$ PGI$_3$ $\leftrightarrow$ PGI$_2$	Both are active vasodilators and inhibitors of platelet aggregation
GLA/DGLA	$\uparrow$ PGE$_1$	Inhibitory effect on polymorphonuclear leucocytes and lymphocytes; inhibitor of leukotriene synthesis and ultimately, suppresser of inflammation

DGLA (20:3n-6), formed from dietary GLA (18:3n-6), is a competitive substrate for Cox, producing PGE$_1$ (Calder & Zurier 2001). Although PGE$_1$ can induce the signs of inflammation, its action on polymorphonuclear leucocytes and lymphocytes is mostly inhibitory: thus it reduces leucocyte chemotaxis and the margination and adherance of leucocytes in blood vessels (Belch & Hill 2000). It has a number of anti-inflammatory effects including inhibition of TNF, IL-1 and IL-6 production by macrophages and inhibition of myeloperoxidase and superoxide production by neutrophils (Calder & Zurier 2001). Furthermore, DGLA has an inhibitory effect on LT synthesis (Belch & Hill 2000): 15-Lox metabolises DGLA to 15-hydroxy-DGLA which is an inhibitor of 5- and 12-Lox, thereby decreasing the production of damaging leukotrienes, notably LTB$_4$, and 5-HETE from AA (Calder & Zurier 2001).

The effects of ingestion of EPA/DHA and GLA/DGLA on raising or lowering concentrations of specific eicosanoids together with the properties of the eicosanoid affected are summarised in Table 9.2.

As is apparent from the table, these influences on eicosanoid production will create an anti-inflammatory and anti-aggregatory response, thereby influencing RA expression and reported symptoms. Benefits may also be apparent in late-stage OA where there is a clear inflammatory component. This suggests that there may be positive benefit to be gained from increasing dietary sources of the n-3 fatty acids, EPA and DHA, and/or of the n-6 fatty acids GLA/DGLA, particularly while decreasing dietary sources of AA.

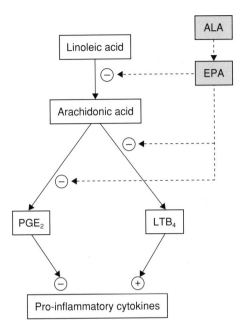

Figure 9.4 Effects of n-3 PUFA on cytokine production (after Calder 1997).

9.7.2 Effects on cytokine production

Overproduction of pro-inflammatory and immunoregulatory cytokines is associated with chronic inflammatory disease (Calder 1997). Both TNF-α and IL-1β are present in rheumatoid synovium and synovial fluid and have been implicated as mediators of the joint pathology of RA, i.e. synovial hyperplasia, leucocyte infiltration, cartilage degradation and expression of adhesion molecules necessary for leucocyte extravasion (movement from the circulatory system into tissues) (Caughey et al. 1996; MacLean et al. 2004). Both cytokines mediate the systemic effects of inflammation, stimulate T- and B-lymphocyte proliferation and promote further cytokine release (Calder 1997).

Eicosanoids are able to modulate the production of cytokines (Calder 1997). Dependent on the nature of the eicosanoid, the effects differ: thus while PGE$_2$, derived from AA, suppresses the production of TNF, IL-1, IL-6 and IL-2, the series-4 leukotrienes, also derived from AA, enhance their production (Figure 9.4, Calder 1997). If the production of *all* AA-derived eicosanoids is suppressed by providing sufficient n-3 PUFA substrates (particularly EPA) to compete for metabolism by Cox and Lox, then production of inflammatory cytokines will be reduced (Figure 9.4, Calder 1997). While ALA may also help suppress n-6 derived eicosanoid products to some extent by competing for a common enzyme, Δ-6-desaturase, in the eicosanoid synthetic pathway (MacLean et al. 2004), it is probably more likely to do so by acting as a precursor of EPA as demonstrated by Caughey and colleagues (1996).

Several human studies in both healthy volunteers and RA patients have shown that supplementation of the diet with n-3 PUFAs (generally > 2.4 g/d EPA + DHA) resulted in reduced *ex vivo* production of a number of cytokines (to include IL-1, IL-6, TNF and/or IL-2 depending on the study) by peripheral blood mononuclear cells (for references, see Calder 1997; Calder & Zurier 2001). Furthermore, EPA and DHA inhibited the cytokine-induced upregulation of adhesion molecules on the surface of endothelial cells in culture and inhibited the production of IL-1β and TNF-α by human monocytes (for references, see Calder & Zurier 2001). Interestingly, although dietary ALA (flaxseed oil) decreased *ex vivo* TNF-α and IL-1β production in monocytes from healthy volunteers, 13.7 g ALA/d for four weeks was only about 30% as effective as 2.7 g/d EPA plus DHA (Calder & Zurier 2001; Caughey et al. 1996). As EPA increased to around 1% of total fatty acid intake, cytokine production reached a minimum (Caughey et al. 1996). However, not all studies report a cytokine-inhibitory effect of fish oil on healthy humans (see 9.7.3) (Calder & Zurier 2001; James et al. 2003).

Beneficial immunological effects have also been seen on supplementation with GLA: monocytes from healthy human volunteers ingesting 2.4 g/d of GLA from GLA-rich oils showed a decreased production of pro-inflammatory cytokines, decreased lymphocyte reactivity and neutrophil chemotaxis (Calder & Zurier 2001).

Sundrarjun and colleagues (2004) investigated the effect of feeding RA patients a low-n-6 PUFA diet supplemented with fish oil on serum pro-inflammatory cytokines and clinical variables. Sixty patients with active RA were randomly assigned to one of three dietary groups:

(1)   A diet low in n-6 PUFAs with a fish oil supplement (fish oil group)
(2)   A diet low in n-6 PUFAs and placebo (placebo group)
(3)   No special intervention (control group)

At week 18, the fish oil group had significant elevations in EPA and DHA and significant reductions in LA, C-reactive protein and soluble TNF-receptor p55, compared with baseline. At week 24, in both the fish oil and placebo groups there were significant reductions in IL-6 and TNF-α, demonstrating a beneficial effect both of a low n-6 diet and of additional fish oil (Sundrarjun et al. 2004).

To summarise, backed by a biochemical rationale, the studies quoted suggest beneficial reductions in levels of inflammatory cytokines from increasing dietary intake of n-3 fatty acids, particularly of EPA, and that the effect may be improved by reducing the intake of n-6 fatty acids (with the exception of GLA). However, as mentioned above, not all studies have reported a cytokine-inhibitory effect of dietary n-3 fatty acids (Calder & Zurier 2001; James et al. 2003).

9.7.3   Effects of fish oils on cytokine production depend on genotype

The lack of consistency in the reported effects of fish oil on cytokine production has been noted above and can be explained by genetic differences that affect the production of TNF-α, a mediator of the joint pathology of RA and of the systemic effects of inflammation (Calder 1997). TNF-α production varies widely between healthy individuals owing to polymorphisms in the promoter regions of TNF-α and lymphotoxin-α (TNF-β) genes that influence the amount of TNF-α produced after an inflammatory stimulus (Grimble et al. 2002). The TNF-α gene has polymorphisms described as *TNF*1* and *TNF*2* while the lymphotoxin-α gene has polymorphisms *TNFB*1* and *TNFB*2* (Grimble et al. 2002). The *TNFB*2/ TNFB*2* genotype (i.e. homozygosity for *TNFB*2*) is that associated with high inherent TNF-α production.

Grimble and colleagues (2002) carried out a study in 111 healthy young men to examine the relationships between polymorphisms in the TNF genes, baseline levels of TNF synthesis and the effects of fish oils. They found that homozygosity for TNFB*2 (i.e. *TNFB*2/TNFB*2*) was 2.5 times more frequent in the highest than the lowest tertile of TNF-α production and that most (86%) individuals with a high inherent level of TNF-α production are sensitive to the anti-inflammatory effects of fish oil. However, in the highest tertile, responsiveness to fish oil appeared unrelated to TNFB genotype. By contrast, individuals with medium or low levels of inherent TNF-α production are more likely to experience anti-inflammatory effects of fish oil if they are heterozygous for the TNFB alleles (i.e. *TNFB*1/ TNFB*2*) (Grimble et al. 2002). In the middle tertile of TNF-α production, the *TNFB*1/TNFB*2* genotype was six times more frequent than other TNFB genotypes among responsive individuals.

The effects are complex but overall they can be summarised as follows (James et al. 2003):

- In the highest tertile of TNF-α production, fish oil inhibits TNF-α production
- In the middle tertile, fish oil has no effect on TNF-α production
- In the lowest tertile, fish oil stimulates TNF-α production

9.7.4   Effects on lymphocyte proliferation

Treatment with EPA/GLA/DGLA causes inhibition of the proliferation of T-lymphocytes, including that of human synovial lymphocytes stimulated by mitogens (Calder & Zurier 2001). This leads to a decreased production of IL-2, demonstrating a decreased Th1 response and immunosuppression (Calder & Zurier 2001).

9.7.5   Effects of n-3 PUFA on cartilage integrity

Loss of proteoglycan (aggrecan) from cartilage is an early event leading to degradation and joint tissue destruction in degenerative joint diseases (Curtis et al. 2002a). In the arthritic joint, exposure of cartilage to pro-inflammatory cytokines upregulates the activity of cartilage degrading enzymes, aggrecanases and matrix metalloproteinases (MMPs) with catabolic effects, and increases the expression levels of mediators of inflammation such as Cox-2, 5-Lox, IL-1 and TNF-α (Curtis et al. 2002b, 2004a; James et al. 2003).

The potential benefit of n-3 PUFA on cartilage pathology was shown using cultures of human osteoarthritic cartilage harvested from patients who had undergone knee replacement surgery. When these cultures were treated with n-3 PUFA (ALA and EPA), the level of cartilage-degrading aggrecanase and collagenase were decreased while the m-RNA expression of the ADAMTS-4 (an aggrecanase), MMP-13 (a collagenase) and MMP-3 (a stromelysin) was abolished (Curtis et al. 2002a, 2002b). Similarly the m-RNA expression of a number of mediators of inflammation, Cox-2, 5-Lox, TNF-α, IL-1α and IL-1β was abolished. By contrast, addition of n-6 PUFA had no effect.

In a small study carried out in Wales, 10–12 weeks prior to knee replacement surgery, 31 OA patients were randomised to receive 2 capsules/d containing 1000 mg cod liver oil or placebo oil (similar to oil content of the UK diet) that contained the same amount of vitamins A and D. Six patients dropped out of the study leaving 14 on cod liver oil and 11 on placebo. A preliminary report of the results of the study stated that in 86% of patients given cod liver oil greatly reduced levels of aggrecanase were found in cartilage and joint tissue taken at surgery compared with 26% of those on placebo (Curtis et al. 2004b). There was a similar reduction in collagenase activity in 73% of patients on cod liver oil but only in 18% of those on placebo. Furthermore, gene expression for aggrecanases was reduced in 93% of cod liver oil patients and there was a reduced level of the inflammatory mediators, IL-1 and TNF (Curtis et al. 2004b).

The results of these studies imply that n-3 PUFA ingestion may impede disease progression by halting or slowing the production of degradative and inflammatory factors in cartilage degeneration in both RA and OA patients. Furthermore, those that have suffered sporting injuries that predispose to early onset of OA should consider taking cod liver oil or otherwise increase their n-3 PUFA intake to abrogate further joint damage.

9.8 Epidemiology of n-3 PUFA and arthritis

Epidemiological evidence supports the hypothesis that consumption of fish prevents the development of RA. Though the Japanese have a higher prevalence of HLA DR alleles that confer susceptibility to RA compared with most other populations, they have a lower rate of the disease. This has been attributed to their higher intake of n-3 fats derived from fish (see James et al. 2003). The prevalence of RA is also lower in the Inuit, who eat large amounts of fish and marine mammals with a high n-3 PUFA content (Horrobin 1987).

Further evidence of preventive effects of fish eating comes from a case control study. Women with RA were reported to have lower baked or grilled fish consumption than healthy controls. Being in the top 10% of n-3 fat intake (> 1.6 g/d) was associated with a 60% decreased risk of RF-positive RA (see James et al. 2003).

9.9 Interventions with GLA and DGLA in arthritic patients

As explained in sections 9.7.1–9.7.3, a diet rich in GLA (18:3n-6) elevates concentrations of its derivative DGLA (20:3n-6), and increases the incorporation of DGLA into cell membranes with beneficial effects (Belch & Hill 2000). Only limited amounts of GLA are available from normal foods, largely owing to the slow and inefficient formation from the parent fatty acid, LA (see 9.3.1). However, certain plant and seed oils including those of *Oenothera biennis* (evening primrose oil – EPO), *Boragio officianalis* (borage/starflower oil) and *Ribes nigrum* (blackcurrant seed oil – BCSO) are concentrated sources (Leventhal et al. 1993, 1994; Adam 1995). Such concentrated sources are needed to achieve the necessary levels of DGLA. Based on studies in healthy volunteers, Calder and Zurier (2001) concluded that immunological effects required an intake of between 1 and 2.4 g GLA/d.

A number of double-blind, placebo-controlled trials of GLA in RA patients have been carried out, though many have had inappropriate study designs according to current knowledge: doses were too low, not continued for sufficiently long to show effect or an inappropriate placebo was used (Belch & Hill 2000). Of five studies that used between 0.36 and 2.8 g/d GLA, for periods of from 12–52 weeks, all reported some measure of clinical improvement – reduction in duration of morning stiffness, number of swollen and painful joints and/or reduced use of non-steroidal anti-inflammatory drugs (NSAIDs) (Calder & Zurier 2001). It appears that only two studies (described below) used 2 g or more of GLA in the daily dose.

Blackcurrant seed oil (BCSO) is rich in both GLA and ALA. A 24-week, randomised, double-blind, placebo-controlled trial in patients with RA was carried out by Leventhal and colleagues (1994). Treatment with 10.5 g/d BCSO (2 g GLA, 1.5 g ALA and 5 g LA/d) for six months resulted in a modest but statistically significant reduction in overall pain and joint tenderness. However, only a small group, 14 participants, completed the study, possibly because they were required to swallow 15 large capsules per day.

Zurier and colleagues (1996) compared 2.8 g/d GLA against a placebo of sunflower seed oil in a six month, single blind study in 56 patients with RA. After the initial six month period, all participants were given GLA for a subsequent six months. A statistically significant reduction in signs and symptoms of RA disease activity was seen in those using GLA compared to those on placebo. Disease activity also improved in the final six-months of the study in both groups.

Thus it seems that in RA patients, GLA at a daily level of intake between 1 g and 2.8 g can improve symptoms, but all researchers are agreed that further well designed studies of adequate power are required that are double-blind, and use an appropriate (inert) placebo (Adam 1995; Belch & Hill 2000; Darlington & Stone 2001).

9.10   Interventions with fish oil in RA patients

There have been around 20 studies of the use of fish oil (EPA, 20:5n-3 + DHA, 22:6n-3) in RA, dating back to the first reported publication in 1985. In most of the studies in which clinical outcomes were measured, fish oil ingestion resulted in an improvement in at least two outcome measures. Dependent on the study, significant improvements have been seen in morning stiffness, tender joints, swollen joints, patient or physician assessment of disease activity, pain, grip strength, NSAID intake and in biochemical parameters, LTB4, IL1, CRP and ESR. Fish oil interventions in RA have been favourably reviewed by a number of authors (Ariza-Ariza 1998; Calder & Zurier 2001; Darlington & Stone 2001; Kremer 2000) but none of these reviews was systematic in nature. There does, however, appear to be a consistent effect of reduction of number of tender joints and amount of morning stiffness in RA patients treated for 12 weeks or more with a minimum daily dose of fish oil containing 3 g EPA/DHA (Kremer 2000). In a randomised, double-blind, placebo-controlled study designed to look specifically at the possibility of discontinuing NSAID use, Kremer and colleagues (1995) reported that some patients taking 130 mg/kg body weight/d (7–10 g/d) of fish oil were able to discontinue NSAIDs without experiencing a disease flare. This is likely due to the long retention of EPA in cell lipids (Adam 1995).

The doses used in fish oil studies have mostly been from 1–7 g (EPA + DHA)/d, averaging 3.3 g/d (Calder & Zurier 2001). One study used more than one dose of EPA plus DHA, that of Kremer and colleagues (1990). Both doses (2.9 and 5.9 g/d) brought about clinical improvement but the improvement reached significance sooner with the higher dose.

In order to assess systematically the results of trials with fish oil in RA, two meta-analyses have been carried out, the first by Fortin and colleagues (1995). Inclusion criteria for this trial included:

(1) Double-blind, placebo-controlled study
(2) Use of at least one of seven predetermined outcome measures
(3) Results reported for both placebo and treatment groups at baseline and follow-up
(4) Randomisation
(5) Parallel or crossover design

Seven published studies were included and three additional trials were found by contacting researchers in the field. The meta-analysis showed that dietary fish oil supplementation for three-months significantly reduced tender joint count {rate difference (95% CI) = −2.9 (−3.8, −2.1), p = 0.001} and morning stiffness {rate difference (95% CI) = −25.9 (−44.3, −7.5), p < 0.01} compared with the various control oils (Fortin et al. 1995). For the other outcome variables – swollen joint count, grip strength, patient and physician global assessment and erythrocyte sedimentation rate (ESR) – improvements did not come close to significance (p > 0.10).

In a later meta-analysis of randomised controlled trials in RA, MacLean and colleagues (2004) evaluated 21 studies chosen according to stringent inclusion criteria for the US Department of Health and Human Services. The outcome measures included in the meta-analysis are shown in Table 9.3, as are the pooled random effect estimates for these four outcomes. Figure 9.5 shows the patient assessment of pain as measured in the nine included studies and the overall estimated effect size (MacLean et al. 2004). Though the effect sizes are all in the direction

Table 9.3 Summary of numbers of studies in meta-analysis and pooled random estimate of effect sizes of n-3 PUFA relative to placebo (data from MacLean et al. 2004).

Outcome measure	No. of studies describing outcome	No. of studies in meta-analysis	Effect size (95% CI)
Patient assessed pain	19	9	−0.19 (−0.43, 0.06)
Swollen joint count	15	6	−0.13 (−0.35, 0.08)
Disease activity – ESR	16	6	−0.32 (−0.83, 0.19)
Patient global assessment	8	5	−0.30 (−0.90, 0.30)
Tender joint count*	10	6	−0.29 (−3.8, −2.1)*

* MacLean et al. (2004) do not assess this outcome measure, saying it was assessed in a previous meta-analysis (Fortin et al. 1995) from which they cite the result shown

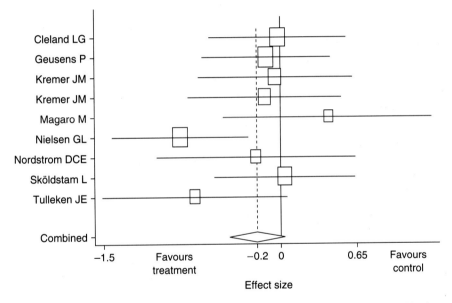

Figure 9.5 Patient-assessment of pain as measured in the nine studies included in the meta-analysis and the overall estimated effect size (MacLean et al. 2004).

of benefit from fish oil treatment, none reaches significance. Though the authors do not themselves assess the effect on tender joint count, they point to the fact that it has already been assessed in a previous meta-analysis and quote the result obtained there (Fortin et al. 1995).

The authors also identified seven studies that assessed the effect of fish oil on NSAID requirement among patients with RA. These were not subjected to meta-analysis but to a qualitative analysis. Among these studies, there was significant reduction in requirement relative to placebo in three, significant reduction relative to baseline requirements in three, and no difference in one (MacLean et al. 2004).

One study that assessed the effect of n-3 PUFA on steroid requirement, demonstrated significant improvement relative to placebo.

Thus in summary, while individual studies have shown significant effects, the two meta-analyses are in agreement that there is no significant effect on swollen joint count, ESR and patient's global assessment. Significant beneficial effects that do not seem to be in dispute relate to number of tender joints, duration of morning stiffness, and requirement for NSAID treatment.

An interesting study that has been published since these meta-analyses were carried out compared the effect of fish oil (3 g/d EPA + DHA) given both alone and with olive oil (6.8 g oleic acid = 9.6 ml), with placebo (soy oil) over a 24-week period (Berbert et al. 2005). Fifty-five patients started the study, of whom 12 withdrew. The investigators were not blinded. Though both fish oil groups improved significantly in a number of clinical parameters, with greater benefits appearing at 24 weeks than at 12 weeks, those who also received olive oil showed accentuated improvement which appeared more rapidly. The authors suggest that the increased effectiveness of fish oil when given with olive oil may relate to the ability of the latter to decrease the expression of intercellular adhesion molecule-1, and to increase the incorporation of n-3 fatty acids in cell membranes. They also suggested that eicosatrienoic acid (ETA, 20:3n-9) synthesised from oleic acid when n-6 fatty acids are restricted, inhibits the synthesis of LTB_4, altering the balance of eicosanoids towards a less inflammatory mixture, as proposed by James and colleagues (2000).

Some explanation for the modest effects observed in most intervention studies may be afforded by the effect of genotype on inflammatory cytokine release in response to fish oil treatment as explained in section 9.7.3. Thus when data are aggregated without consideration of each subject's inherent *ex vivo* TNF-α production or TNF-α or lymphotoxin-α genotype, there may be no overall effect (Grimble et al. 2002). This allows the possibility that only individuals with specific genotypes will benefit from fish oil supplementation, whereas others will either derive no benefit or even experience a worsening in their condition (Yaqoob 2003).

Of interest, the US National Center for Complementary and Alternative Medicine (NCCAM) has planned a study with marine and botanical oils involving 260 RA patients but the initiation of this study appears to have been delayed.

9.11 Interventions with fish oil in RA patients with reduced n-6 PUFA intake

At least two studies have investigated the effect of fish oil on clinical outcomes against a background of a reduced intake of n-6 PUFA on the basis that the latter has a negative effect on tissue concentrations of n-3 fatty acids (James et al. 2000).

In the first, Volker and colleagues (2000) gave RA patients 40 mg/kg body weight/d (2–3 g/d) of n-3 PUFAs for 15 weeks while ensuring that the patients consumed less than 10 g/d of n-6 PUFA. After 15 weeks there were significant improvements in the duration of morning stiffness, pain score, number of swollen joints, patients' and physicians' global assessment of disease activity and overall health assessment.

In a double-blind crossover study with a two-month washout between treatments, the effect of three-months' treatment with fish oil (30 mg/kg body weight/d) or placebo on RA patients already receiving one of two alternative diets was investigated (Adam et al. 2003). Patients had already been on either a normal Western diet or an anti-inflammatory diet that provided less than 90 mg/d AA for eight months. The anti-inflammatory diet was a modified lactovegetarian diet including only plant-derived fats and oils, no egg yolk and reduced fat dairy products. Meat was limited to not more than two servings of 120 g/week. Sixty of the initial 68 patients completed the study. While the anti-inflammatory diet alone reduced the number of tender and swollen joints by 14%, addition of fish oil gave a further significant reduction to 28% (tender joints) and 34% (swollen joints) (P < 0.01). Comparable reductions in the Western diet group on fish oil treatment were 11% and 22% respectively. Compared to baseline levels, higher enrichment of EPA in erythrocyte lipids, lower formation of LTB_4 and other prostaglandin metabolites were found in the anti-inflammatory diet group, especially when fish oil was given (Adam et al. 2003).

As in the study of Sundrarjun et al. (2004) (see 9.7.2), these studies demonstrate the additional efficacy of fish oil treatment with a low background n-6 fatty acid or AA intake: reduction of AA levels is a slow process (Adam 1995).

9.12 Limitations of human intervention studies with PUFAs

A number of factors have affected the quality of intervention studies with PUFAs in inflammatory arthritis (Belch & Hill 2000; Cleland & James 1997). Some of these issues have only emerged in recent years as a fuller understanding of the metabolism and biological effects of these fatty acids has developed (Belch & Hill 2000). Some factors that need to be taken into account when judging the outcome of trials are:

- Doses of PUFAs too low for an effect to be possible
- Trial not of sufficiently long duration for effects to be seen
- Use of an inappropriate (non-inert) placebo
- Genotype of subjects should be determined as it can affect treatment outcome (see 9.7.3 and 9.10)
- Background diet needs to be taken into consideration i.e. may be high in n-6 LA/AA
- Individuals have often had longstanding refractory disease
- Subjects are allowed to continue with their full disease-modifying antirheumatic drug (DMARD) or NSAID treatment regimens, making assessment of effects of PUFAs more difficult to see

With respect to the choice of placebo, this continues to present a problem. Olive oil (n-9 MUFA) was used as a placebo in early studies though it is now recognised to have anti-inflammatory effects. Other n-6 oils such as corn oil or sunflower oil may be somewhat pro-inflammatory. It is possible that any MUFA or PUFA has

Table 9.4 Dietary intake of PUFAs associated with beneficial effects in inflammatory arthritis studies.

Dietary treatment	Amount PUFA mg/kg bwt/d	Amount PUFA for 70 kg individual (g)	Restrictions on daily n-6 intake
GLA	14–40	1–2.8	—
EPA/DHA	43	3.0*	—
EPA/DHA + reduced n-6	30	2.1	< 90 mg/d AA
EPA/DHA + reduced n-6	40	2.8	< 10 g/d n-6 PUFA

* Cleland & James (2000) recommend 3–6 g/d EPA + DHA; Kremer (2000) recommends 3 g/d EPA + DHA or 3–6 g/d n-3 PUFA

significant potential immune effects and therefore the ideal placebo has not yet been identified (Belch & Hill 2000; Darlington & Stone 2001).

9.13   Recommendations for PUFA intake in inflammatory arthritis

From the studies quoted in the previous sections, it is possible to summarise approximate amounts of various PUFAs associated with beneficial effects. These are shown in Table 9.4. Note that some studies also restricted intakes of total n-6 PUFAs or AA in an attempt to favour incorporation of the n-3 PUFAs into membranes and their subsequent metabolism to less inflammatory products. *A priori*, this would seem to be a sensible idea.

Though GLA appears in this table, note that there have been many fewer studies using GLA from which to draw conclusions. Increasing GLA intake is only possible by taking a supplement, of which there are many available. There is some indication that the combination of EPA/DHA and GLA may be more effective against inflammation than either alone (Calder & Zurier 2001).

The following sections will attempt to explain how the level of intake of n-3 PUFA shown in Table 9.4 can be achieved and how intake of n-6 PUFAs, particularly of AA, can be reduced.

Our suggestion is that if such dietary alterations do not show a beneficial effect on symptoms or disease activity in a particular individual after a period of around six months, assuming compliance with treatment has been good, then the individual's genotype (or other factor such as high n-6 content of the diet) may be such as to preclude benefit from such a dietary change (see 9.7.3 and 9.10). There is thus little point in continuing what is likely to be a costly regime (however, see 9.17). A worsening in condition may be due to the same cause and clearly the dietary supplement should be stopped.

9.14   Current intakes of PUFAs

To understand the practicality of the amounts of fatty acid intake being suggested, the typical composition and amounts of normal dietary sources of n-3 fatty acids needs to be clarified.

Though total n-3 PUFA intakes are similar for vegans, vegetarians, and omnivores (< 1–3 g/d), there is great variability between these groups in terms of intakes of the long-chain PUFAs, EPA and DHA (Davis & Kris-Etherton 2003). As oily fish and eggs are the richest dietary sources of EPA and DHA, consumption of these fatty acids by omnivores varies according to fish and egg intake, with average daily consumption in the 100–150 mg range (Davis & Kris-Etherton 2003). Vegans consume negligible amounts of EPA and DHA while vegetarians consume minimal EPA (< 5 mg/d) and varying amounts of DHA, depending on their egg consumption. Vegan and vegetarian populations have a considerably higher consumption of n-6 PUFAs than omnivores, resulting in an elevated n-6 to n-3 ratio in USA vegans (14–20:1) and lacto-ovo-vegetarians (10–16:1) compared with omnivores (< 10:1) (Davis & Kris-Etherton 2003).

In the US diet, daily intake of n-6 PUFAs (LA) is around 13 g while that of n-3 PUFAs (largely ALA and DHA) is only 1.4 g (MacLean et al. 2004). Mean EPA plus DHA intake has been measured as 85–110 mg/d, depending whether NHANES III (third National Health and Nutrition Examination, 1988–94) or CSFII (Continuing Food Survey of Intakes by Individuals 1994–98) data were used (MacLean et al. 2004). Fats and oils provide 87% of total ALA, primarily as soya bean and canola (rapeseed) oil used in food preparation. The food group 'meat, poultry, fish and mixtures' provides around 90% of the EPA and DHA in the diet, largely reflecting fish consumption, though eggs are also a source (Kris-Etherton et al. 2000).

In the UK, as in most westernised countries, intakes of the n-6 PUFA, LA, have risen over the last 30 years as vegetable oils and spreads have replaced the traditional butters and lards: intake of LA in men has risen from around 10 g/d to 15 g/d (BNF 1999). To a lesser extent, changes in processing procedures and farming methods (feeding n-6-rich grain as opposed to n-3–rich pasture to cattle) have also contributed to this rise. Those who consume high amounts of meat, French fries, fast foods and foods fried in n-6–rich vegetable oils will have a raised consumption of n-6 PUFAs resulting in a high n-6:n-3 ratio. Table 9.5 shows the wide variation in intakes of n-3 and n-6 fatty acids between European countries, reflecting different dietary habits, notably fish eating in Iceland, Finland and the Scandinavian countries where in consequence, the ratio of n-6:n-3 is lowest.

In the UK, the average adult intake of oily fish is currently one-third of a portion per week but 70% of adults eat no oily fish (SACN 2004). In free living older people in the UK, fish intake provides 20–25% of total n-3 intake (Finch et al. 1998). Table 9.6 shows the sources of n-3 PUFAs in the diets of the UK elderly.

Where made, recommendations for the normal population with regard to intake of LC PUFAs are around 500 (range 200–1430) mg EPA + DHA/d (BNF 1999; Kris-Etherton et al. 2000) though these have been formulated with regard to reducing cardiovascular risk rather than inflammatory joint disease. However, from the above data, it seems likely that in most Western countries, with the exception of those that have a tradition of fish consumption, mean intakes of EPA + DHA may be well below that modest target, let alone the 3 g/d level associated with anti-inflammatory effects (see Table 9.4).

Table 9.5 Intakes of essential fatty acids (g/day) in 14 Western European countries, ranked lowest to highest n-6:n-3 ratio (adapted from Hulshof et al. 1999).

Country	Linoleic acid (LA) (g)			α-Linolenic acid (ALA) (g)			Ratio of n-6:n-3
	Men	Women	Men and women	Men	Women	Men and women	
Iceland	10.2	6.9	—	2.5	1.4	—	4.4
Finland	8.1	5.8	—	1.8	1.3	—	4.5
Denmark	12.0	9.0	—	2.2	2.1	—	4.9
Sweden	6.7	5.3	—	1.4	1.0	—	5.0
Norway	12.2	7.8	—	1.6	1.0	—	7.7
UK	—	—	11.4	—	—	1.4	8.1
Belgium	16.6	12.8	—	1.7	1.4	—	9.5
Germany	9.3	8.0	—	0.9	0.7	—	10.8
Netherlands	19.0	13.2	—	1.7	1.2	—	11.0
France	8.3	6.8	—	0.6	0.5	—	13.7
Greece	9.3	9.9	—	0.6	0.7	—	14.8
Portugal	12.1	—	—	0.7	—	—	17.3
Italy	—	—	14.5	—	—	0.8	18.0
Spain	—	—	21.6	—	—	0.8	27.0

Table 9.6 Percentage contributions of foods to intakes of n-3 fatty acids in free-living older people (over 65 years) in the UK (adapted from Finch et al. 1998).

Food	Males %	Females %
Fish and fish dishes	25	20
Vegetables, potatoes and savoury snacks (e.g chips and fried potatoes)	21	22
Meat and meat products	14	14
Cereals and cereal products	13	13
Fat spreads	10	10
Milk and milk products	5	6
Miscellaneous	5	7
Dietary supplements	3	3
Eggs and egg dishes	2	2
Fruit and nuts	2	4
Average daily intake (g)	**1.75**	**1.33**

9.15   How to achieve an anti-inflammatory intake of PUFAs

9.15.1   Oily fish

Marine algae and phytoplankton synthesise long-chain n-3 PUFAs, which is how these fatty acids are introduced into the food chain (Farrell 1998). Oily fish, such

Table 9.7 Typical n-3 fatty acid content of fish, fish oil and seafood (BNF 1999; BNF 2005; Simopoulos & Robinson 1999).

Food	Portion size (g)*	Total n-3 per portion (g)	Total long chain n-3 per portion (g)**
Cod	120	0.30	0.30
Haddock	120	0.19	0.19
Plaice	130	0.42	0.39
Herring	119	2.18	1.56
Mackerel	160	4.46	3.09
Kippers	130	4.37	3.37
Salmon	100	2.50	2.20
Trout	160	2.03	1.84
Tuna (fresh)	100	—	1.3
Tuna (in brine, drained)	45	0.08	0.08
Tuna (in oil, drained)	45	0.50	0.17
Pilchards (canned in tomato sauce)	110	3.16	2.86
Sardines (canned in tomato sauce)	100	2.02	1.67
Salmon (canned in brine)	100	1.85	1.55
Crab (canned)	85	0.91	0.85
Mussels (boiled)	40	0.26	0.24
Cod liver oil	5 ml	1.2	1.0
Cod liver oil capsules***	1 capsule ~ 500 mg	0.12–0.16	0.08–0.14
Fish oil concentrate***	1 capsule ~ 500 mg	0.13–0.30	0.11–0.21

* Portion sizes are based on those for average/medium servings (Ministry of Agriculture Fisheries and Food 1993)
** Chain length 20 carbons or more: includes 20:5 (EPA), 22:5 and 22:6 (DHA)
*** Based on selected products on the market in 2004; capsule size and quantity contained are variable

as mackerel are the richest source of EPA and DHA and make the largest contribution to their intake (BNF 1999). Fish found in cold water typically have a higher n-3 content than those in warm water. Freshwater fish, other than farmed fish, are a poorer source of EPA and DHA than marine fish (Farrell 1998). The n-3 fatty acid composition of different varieties of fish is shown in Table 9.7. A more comprehensive table showing the fatty acid composition of varieties of fish and shellfish, particularly suitable for US readers, can be found in Simopoulos and Robinson (1999).

Values given in Table 9.7 are subject to variation owing to differences in diet of the fish, fluctuation in food availability, location, stage of maturity, sex and size of the fish, season, seasonal variations in zooplankton that the fish consume, water temperature and preparation methods (e.g. canning) (Bell et al. 2003; BNF 1999; Farrell 1998; Kris-Etherton et al. 2000). Wild fish show greater variation in their composition than farmed fish: over a year, the fat content of herring and mackerel may range from 1% to 30% (BNF 1999).

Whether fish are farm raised or caught in the wild can affect their fatty acid content as this is dependent on their diet (Kris-Etherton et al. 2000). Currently salmon produced by aquaculture (farmed) are fed with diets containing only fish oils, but the use of fish oils for this purpose is increasing and cannot be sustained long-term (Bell et al. 2003). However, if vegetable oil replaces more than 66% of the added fish oil in the feed, considerable reductions in long-chain fatty acids are seen (Bell et al. 2003). Consumers need to be aware of this possibility.

From the information in Table 9.7, it is simple to calculate the number of servings of a particular oily fish needed per week, based on the minimum recommended intake of 3 g EPA + DHA/d for an anti-inflammatory effect (see Table 9.4). Taking the example of salmon, and assuming a constant level of 3.25 g long-chain n-3 PUFAs (EPA + DHA) per average 150 g serving, then 6–7 portions will be required per week. If the upper level of intake suggested by some researchers – 6 g/d – is desired, the number of portions per week would rise to 13.

Between six and 13 portions of fish per week is an unrealistic target and may be associated with excessive levels of intake of toxic contaminants (see section 9.18), so other means must also be used to increase tissue levels of long-chain n-3 PUFAs. Fish oil supplements are clearly an effective route by which intake of long-chain n-3 fatty acids can be increased, either as an adjunct to dietary intake (BNF 1999) or as an optional strategy. Alternatively, the intake of the short-chain n-3 PUFA, ALA, can be increased with the expectation of converting it to EPA, though as will be seen from 9.15.4, this is an inefficient process.

9.15.2   Fish oil supplements

A very large choice of n-3 fatty acid supplements in various formats is now available to consumers. As a generalisation, marine oils come from the fish flesh and contain around 180 mg EPA and 120 mg DHA per 1 g capsule (i.e. a ratio of 3:2), whereas cod liver oil comes from the fish liver and contains considerably lower quantities of EPA and DHA but also contains vitamins A and D (Kris-Etherton et al. 2000). EPA-enriched capsules of fish oil containing a higher ratio of EPA to DHA (4:1) are also on sale but at a premium price. Vitamin E is generally also added to reduce the risk of lipid peroxidation of these highly unsaturated oils. High strength or high potency oils are now available that are more concentrated sources of EPA and DHA and therefore require fewer capsules per day to achieve an effective dose. Typically in a 1 g capsule, these high strength oils contain around 310 mg EPA and 210 mg DHA.

The dose required per day will depend upon the composition of the supplement and on the n-3 PUFA content of the remainder of the diet. If no oily fish is eaten, 40 high strength capsules per week would provide the required dose of 21 g long-chain n-3 PUFAs, that is, approximately six capsules/d. Based on an intake of two portions of an oily fish like salmon per week (see section 9.15.1) giving an intake of 6.5 g EPA + DHA/week, an additional 14.5 g of long-chain PUFAs would be needed, which would be supplied by an intake of 28 high strength capsules per week, that is four capsules/d. Additional consumption of ALA would reduce the requirement (see 9.15.4).

Cod liver oil is a supplement that is commonly taken within this patient group. Though a less concentrated source of long-chain n-3 fatty acids, it does provide other important nutrients – vitamins A, D and E. Vitamin D status is often low in the elderly and is a particularly important nutrient for the OA patient group in order to reduce the risk of disease progression (see Chapter 8). Cod liver oil (1 g/d) has shown efficacy in OA, in terms of slowing cartilage destruction, pain and inflammation (see 9.7.5). However, because the n-3 content is quite low (often no more than 170 mg EPA + DHA per 1 g cod liver oil), a large amount would be required to produce straightforward anti-inflammatory effects in RA patients who would probably do better on fish body oils. In a 1 g dose, 800–1600 µg vitamin A and 5–8 µg vitamin D might be provided. Since it is thought that it may be unsafe to consume more than 25 µg/d vitamin D (risk of hypercalcaemia and hypercalciuria) or 1.5 mg (1500 µg ≡ 5000 IU)/d of vitamin A (increased risk of hip fracture) on a long-term basis (UK Expert Group on Vitamins and Minerals 2003), it may be unsafe to consume more than 1 g/d cod liver oil on a long-term basis, depending on the product. In particular, pregnant women should avoid using cod liver oil as a means of controlling inflammation owing to the known teratogenic effects of vitamin A which may become apparent at intakes of 3 mg/d (3000 µg ≡ 10 000 IU) (UK Expert Group on Vitamins and Minerals 2003).

9.15.3   Animal sources of n-3 PUFAs: grass-fed meat and game

The fatty acid composition of meat, milk and eggs is dependent on the nutrient composition of the animal's diet, whether the animal was wild or farmed and whether, for example, animals were fed flaxseed, grass or fish meal.

ALA accounts for more than 50% of the fat in green leaves, therefore meat from animals fed on grass will reflect this in the composition of their fat. Livestock raised on pasture produce meat that is high in n-3 fatty acids (Simopoulos & Robinson 1999; Wood et al. 1999). Starting in the 1950s, the meat industry began to fatten animals on grain resulting in a drop in n-3 fatty acid content and an increase in n-6 content resulting in a blander taste (Wood et al. 1999). Bulls fed on grain diets (concentrates) had much higher concentrations of LA (18:2n-6) and long-chain PUFAs of the n-6 series than those fed on grass which had more ALA (18:3n-3) and its long-chain n-3 derivatives (Wood et al. 1999). Though uncommon in most countries, it is still possible to obtain grass-fed beef and lamb, though unfortunately at a premium price. Sources can be found on the web. A steak of grass-fed beef is claimed to have two to six times more n-3 PUFAs than steak from a grain-fed cow (see Figure 9.6). Similarly, cows living on pasture produce milk that has a higher proportion of n-3 fats. Grass-based dairies can provide milk with an equal ratio of n-3:n-6 fatty acids (16.5 mg/g n-3 and 16.6 mg/g n-6) (Simopoulos & Robinson 1999) though the current preference for semi-skimmed milk makes this a less important source of n-3 PUFAs.

Owing to its wild origins, game such as venison and buffalo also tends to contain a higher proportion of n-3 fatty acids. Wild game meat is low in total (1–7%) and saturated fat but relatively rich in PUFA (Broadhurst et al. 2002; Mann 2000). It has a significantly higher content of EPA than grain-fed domestic meat (Miller 1986, see Figure 9.6). Tissue lipids of North American and African

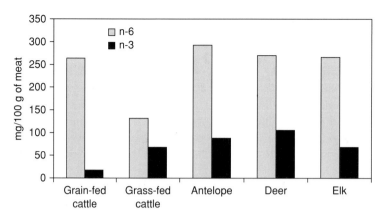

Figure 9.6 Essential fatty acid composition of meat from grain- and grass-fed cattle, antelope, deer and elk (reproduced with permission from Miller 1986).

ruminants were found to be similar to those of pasture-fed cattle {e.g. n-6/n-3 = 2.3–2.6 (muscle); n-6/n-3 = 2.3–3.0 (adipose tissue)} but dissimilar to grain-fed cattle (Cordain et al. 2002). The long-chain PUFAs are mainly present in small quantities as membrane phospholipids in lean tissue rather than being concentrated in adipose tissue (Broadhurst et al. 2002).

From Figure 9.6 it can be seen that beef from grass-fed cattle provides around 65 mg n-3 PUFA/100 g beef, whereas grain-fed beef provides less than 20 mg/100 g. Wild game such as deer or antelope (venison) provides a higher level at 90–100 mg n-3 PUFA/100 g. Grain-fed beef has a much higher ratio of n-6 to n-3 fatty acids (14:1) than wild game or grass-fed beef (approximately 2:1). An 8 oz (230 g) grass-fed beef steak would therefore provide approximately 150 mg n-3 PUFA but also around 130 mg *less* of n-6 PUFA than would meat from a grain-fed animal.

9.15.4   Sources of short-chain n-3 PUFA

If consumption of oily fish or supplement use is not possible owing to allergy, food preference or concern about fish stocks, sources of short-chain n-3 fatty acids may be consumed in the expectation of some degree of conversion to their long-chain analogues. Prolonged intake of ALA has been shown to result in appreciable levels of EPA (Adam 1995; Mantzioris et al. 1995). The conversion process from ALA to EPA and DHA is of great importance to vegans, vegetarians or those with no EPA or DHA sources in their diet. Vegetarians are advised by Davis and Kris-Etherton (2003) to double their intake of ALA so that more than 1% of their dietary energy comes from ALA (or 1.1 g/1000 cal).

The primary sources of ALA are selected seeds, nuts and legumes and the green leaves of plants, including sea plants – phytoplankton and algae (Davis & Kris-Etherton 2003). It is likely that ALA-rich cooking oils will provide the greatest contribution to ALA intake. As the ALA content of plants varies depending on factors such as season, climate, growing region and variety, any products produced from plants will vary accordingly. Flaxseeds (otherwise known as linseeds) are the richest sources of short-chain n-3 PUFA (Kris-Etherton 2003) but flaxseed (linseed) oil is not suitable for heating/frying as it is very unstable. Fresh, ground linseeds can be added to cereals as a vegetable source of n-3 fats, albeit a less potent source than EPA in fish oil (Cleland & James 2000). Table 9.8 shows the amount of ALA in various rich plant sources of n-3 fatty-acids, the total number of grams of ALA per serving and the n-6:n-3 ratio where available. A more comprehensive list of ALA sources can be found in Simopoulos and Robinson (1999).

Foods enriched with ALA – cooking oil, margarine, salad dressing and mayonnaise – helped to increase the intake of n-3 fatty acids in a study by Mantzioris and colleagues (2000) on healthy volunteers. Another dietary intervention study (Caughey et al. 1996) gave healthy volunteers flaxseed oil (content 56% ALA + 18% LA) and a spread consisting of flaxseed oil and butter in a 2:1 ratio (content 23% ALA + 8% LA) in place of their usual cooking oils and spreads and advised them to avoid foods high in n-6 fats. After four weeks of an average daily ingestion of 13.7 g/d ALA, an increment of 0.4% of the total fatty acid content in mononuclear cell EPA was observed. Though this is a low amount, the fact that TNF-α and IL-1β production fell by approximately 30% showed that this small increment had a beneficial effect (Caughey et al. 1996).

As evidenced by the study quoted above, rates of conversion of ALA to the long-chain n-3 PUFAs are low. Gerster's review of the subject (1998) describes a 1996 study by Valsta and colleagues that showed that a daily intake of 50 g of rapeseed oil containing 4.8 g ALA (BNF 1999) was estimated to be equivalent in terms of EPA generation to a weekly consumption of only 50–100 g fatty fish. *In vivo* studies with deuterated fatty acids have shown that if the intake of ALA is 2 g/d (0.6% of energy) and that of LA is 15 g/d (5% of energy), around 15% of dietary ALA is converted to long-chain n-3 PUFAs, of which there are five in number (for reference, see Gerster 1998, Kris-Etherton et al. 2000). This yields around 300 mg of long-chain n-3 PUFAs. However, if the intake of LA is increased to 30 g/d, conversion of ALA to long-chain PUFAs is decreased by around 40%, yielding only 180 mg (Kris-Etherton et al. 2000). In healthy individuals, some 5–10% of ALA is converted to EPA, and around 2–5% to DHA (de Deckere et al. 1998; Davis & Kris-Etherton 2003). It appears to be more difficult to get conversion to DHA than to EPA, though this is of less concern in arthritis where EPA is believed to be the active fatty acid.

Conversion is dependent on several factors including genetics, age, overall health and dietary intake. Several population groups are at greater risk of poor fatty acid conversion (or incorporation into tissue lipids) – those with diabetes (or other metabolic disorders where conversion enzymes may be compromised), neurological disorders, schizophrenia, premature infants, the elderly and chronic alcoholics (de Deckere et al. 1998; Davis & Kris-Etherton 2003). Alcohol is said to inhibit the activity of the Δ-5- and Δ-6-desaturases and to deplete tissues of long-chain n-3 fatty acids, presumably because both enzymes are needed for the conversion of ALA to long-chain products (Davis & Kris-Etherton 2003).

Table 9.8 ALA and LA content of selected plant foods (Davis & Kris-Etherton 2003; BNF 1999).

Food	Serving size (g)	Content ALA (g/100 g)	% fat as ALA	% fat as LA	ALA (g/serving)	n-6/n-3	Comment
Flaxseed oil	14	—	57	16	8.0	0.28	Richest known ALA source, highly unstable, should not be heated
Flaxseed, whole	24	—	57	16	5.2	0.28	Keeps well at room temperature
Flaxseed, ground	24	—	57	16	3.8	0.28	Best kept refrigerated or frozen
Greens (mixed)	56	—	56	11	0.1	0.19	Not significant contributors to intake because total fat is so low
Spinach (boiled)	90	0.25	—	—	0.23	—	—
Mushrooms	40	0.27	—	—	0.11	—	—
Hempseed oil	14	—	19	57	2.7	3.1	Also contains GLA (1.7%)
Walnuts*	28	—	14	58	2.6	4.1	Highest ALA content of any common nut
Walnuts[†]	20	7.47	—	—	1.49	—	
Walnut oil	11	11.5	—	—	1.27	—	
Canola/rapeseed oil*	14	—	11	21	1.6	2.0	Excellent n-6:n-3 ratio
Canola/rapeseed oil[†]	11	9.6	—	—	1.06	—	
Soya bean oil*	14	—	7	51	0.9	7.0	Not the best choice because of high n-6 content
Soya oil[†]	11	7.3	—	—	0.80	—	
Soya beans (cooked)	172	—	7	50	1.0	7	Can make a significant contribution to total ALA intake
Tofu (firm)	126	—	7	50	0.7	7	As for soya beans

* Davis & Kris-Etherton 2003
[†] BNF 1999

Table 9.9 Nutritional composition of the medium Columbus egg (www.columbuseggs.com).

Nutrient	Per 100 g	Per egg ($\cong$ 56 g)
Energy (kcal)	145 (63.8)	81
(kJ)	601	337
Protein (g)	12.5 (5.5)	7
Carbohydrate (g)	Trace	Trace
Fat (g)	10.5 (4.6)	5.9
saturates (g)	2.5 (1.1)	1.4
monounsaturates (g)	3.7 (1.6)	2.1
PUFA (g)	2.5 (1.1)	1.4
n-3/Omega-3 (g)	1.2 (0.5)	0.7
n-6/Omega-6 (g)	1.3 (0.6)	0.7
Sodium (mg)	100 (44)	0.1
Selenium (µg)	70.0	39.0
Vitamin E (mg)	20 (8.8)	11.0

9.15.5 Direct long-chain n-3 PUFA sources for vegetarians or non-fish eaters

There are very few vegetarian sources of long-chain n-3 fatty acids. Some possible sources are discussed below.

Eggs: Eggs are widely accepted, cheap, rich nutritional sources suitable for those who dislike fish and for lacto-ovo-vegetarians. Eggs provide some DHA (< 50 mg/egg) but very little EPA (Davis & Kris-Etherton 2003). It is well known that the composition of fatty acids in egg yolk can be altered (Farrell 1998). Many supermarkets sell DHA-enriched eggs that have a DHA content 2–3 times greater than conventional eggs. Eggs produced from chickens fed with flax/flax oil generally provide 60–100 mg DHA per egg while those from chickens fed microalgae provide rather more, 100–150 mg/egg (Davis & Kris-Etherton 2003).

In Europe, Columbus eggs, produced from chickens fed on cereals, soya, pulses and flaxseed oil are widely available and have the composition shown in Table 9.9 (www.columbuseggs.com) where the n-3 PUFA is DHA. While some back conversion to EPA is possible in humans, these enriched eggs are unlikely to be a satisfactory source of anti-inflammatory PUFAs.

Farrell (1998) showed that it was possible to enrich eggs with EPA as well as DHA by feeding hens diets enriched with fish oil or a combination of fish and vegetable oils. He studied the effects of consuming seven enriched eggs per week for 24 weeks in a group of 60 male and female participants. Participants were allocated to one of four groups as shown below, each of which received eggs from hens fed with diets enriched by different oils.

F   50 g fish oil/kg diet (1.25:1 :: n-6:n-3)
FL   30 g fish oil, 10 g linseed oil/kg (n-6:n-3 :: 1.5:1)
FLR   20 g fish oil, 10 g linseed oil, 10 g rapeseed (canola) oil/kg diet (n-6:n-3 :: 1.8:1)
C   control – 40 g sunflower oil/kg diet (25.8:1 :: n-6:n-3)

There was a five-fold increase in EPA and a twelve-fold increase in DHA in eggs from the F group compared to the amount in the control eggs. A 60 g egg from the FL group provided 430 mg n-3 PUFAs of which DHA, DPA and EPA accounted for 290 mg. Significant increases in EPA, DHA and total n-3 PUFAs were found in subjects consuming the enriched eggs compared with controls. In addition, the ratio of n-6 to n-3 PUFAs in plasma was significantly reduced, from 12.2:1 to 6.5–7.7:1. Neither blood cholesterol nor triacylglycerol levels of participants was increased. Untrained volunteers could not distinguish between the taste of the ordinary and enriched eggs. Though consumption of one enriched egg per day contributed substantially to n-3 intake, the amounts of long-chain PUFAs required for anti-inflammatory effects (3 g/d) would require the consumption of around 10 eggs/d, clearly an unrealistic and undesirable target.

Microalgae and seaweed: These are the only plant sources of long-chain n-3 fatty acids though they are not concentrated sources because of their extremely low total fat content. Supplements of DHA-rich microalgae are exceptions, however, providing 10–40% dry weight of DHA. Supplements of blue-green algae that are available include Spirulina, rich in GLA (n-6) although low in long-chain n-3 fatty acids, and *Aphanizomenon flos-aquae* a concentrated ALA source. Both of these seem to have a very high conversion rate to long-chain fatty acids compared to other plants (Davis & Kris-Etherton 2003).

Seaweed (macroalgae) is a source of EPA (~ 100 mg/100 g serving) but little DHA. However, seaweed would have to be consumed in some quantity to make much of a contribution to EPA intake, as may be the case in Japan and other parts of Asia (Davis & Kris-Etherton 2003). Hijiki seaweed should be avoided, owing to its high content of inorganic arsenic (FSA 2004).

Purslane: This vegetable (Figure 9.7), originating in India, is the richest ALA source of any green, leafy vegetable and is unusual in also being a source of EPA (Kris-Etherton et al. 2000). Though found worldwide, including in all 50 states of the USA, it is mainly consumed by populations in the Mediterranean basin and in the Middle East. It has succulent, reddish, wedge-shaped leaves, and both the leaves and the stalks can be used in salads, soups, stews and vegetable dishes. It has a mild sweet-sour flavour with a chewy texture (Brill 2004).

Novel foods: Several research groups have explored the use and practicality of novel (fortified) foods, with the aim of increasing individual consumption of long-chain n-3 fatty acids (James et al. 2003; Kris-Etherton et al. 2000; Metcalf et al. 2003; Mantzioris et al. 2000). Foods including bakery products, milk powders or salad dressings are fortified with oils and powders enriched with either EPA or DHA. Through these novel foods, researchers have managed to achieve long-chain n-3 intakes of 0.9–2.3 g EPA + DHA/d. The availability of a greater range of n-3-enriched novel food products (e.g. fish-oil-enriched sausages, milk, margarine and dips) would enable patients to increase their intake of long-chain n-3 PUFAs without having to alter their diets in unsustainable ways (James et al. 2003). 'Omega-3' enriched milk is now on sale in a number of countries including the UK, where the well known retailer, Marks & Spencer, has recently introduced a 'super milk' produced from cows that have been fed an 'omega-3-rich diet' which supplies DHA + EPA at a level of 48 mg per 250 ml. However, this is a poor

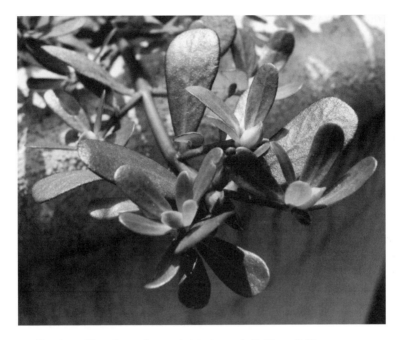

Figure 9.7 Purslane (*Portulaca oleracea*) (photograph © Steve Brill).

source of long-chain n-3 PUFAs compared with one portion of fatty fish e.g. salmon, which contains 3.25 g (EPA + DHA) per average 150 g serving.

In the longer term, the introduction of candidate genes that regulate the production of lipids in appropriate plant species may be used to manipulate ALA, EPA and DHA content of foods such as seeds and seed oils. This approach could complement classical genetic section programmes used to modify nutritional composition (Kris-Etherton et al. 2000).

9.15.6 Practical guidelines for vegetarians

Davis and Kris-Etherton (2003) suggest some ways in which vegans and vegetarians can optimise their long-chain n-3 PUFA status:

(1) Aim for no more than a 4:1 ratio of n-6:n-3 fatty acids in terms of calorie intake.
(2) If using concentrated fats and oils, choose olive, canola (rapeseed) or nut (e.g. walnut) oils. Do not use n-6-rich oils for cooking i.e. safflower oil, grapeseed oil, sunflower oil, corn oil, cottonseed oil or soya bean oil.
(3) Choose MUFAs as the primary source of fat, i.e. nuts (except butternuts), peanuts (a legume), avocado, olives, olive oil, canola (rapeseed) oil.
(4) Ensure sufficient ALA intake (for EPA and DHA conversion). Rich ALA sources include flaxseeds, hempseeds, canola (rapeseed) oil, soy, walnuts and green leaves from vegetables.
(5) Incorporate a direct DHA/EPA source if possible.

Table 9.10   n-6 content of cooking oils (information mainly from Davis & Kris-Etherton 2003).

Cooking oil	n-6 PUFA content
Safflower oil	75%
Grapeseed oil	70%
Sunflower oil	65%
Corn oil	57%
Cottonseed oil	52%
Soybean oil	51%
Canola/rapeseed oil	21%
Olive oil	8%

NB Flaxseed oil is 16% n-6 PUFA but is unsuitable for cooking

(6)   Limit intake of processed, deep fried and snack foods that are likely to be prepared with n-6 fats.

9.16   Reducing n-6 PUFAs in the diet

A number of studies have attempted to reduce the intake of n-6 PUFAs, including AA, while increasing the intake of n-3 PUFAs for greater effect (Adam et al. 2003; Caughey et al. 1996; Mantzioris et al. 2000; Sundrarjun et al. 2004). N-6 fats containing LA are abundant in products based on polyunsaturated vegetable oils such as soy, corn, sunflower, safflower and others and though their conversion to AA is very limited (Adam 1995; Adam et al. 2003; Broadhurst et al. 2002) they can inhibit the incorporation of dietary EPA into tissue phospholipids (Mantzioris et al. 1995). The percentage of n-6 fatty acids in cooking oils, in descending order of n-6 fatty acid content (Davis & Kris-Etherton 2003), is shown in Table 9.10. Those high in n-6 PUFAs should be avoided and substituted by oils low in n-6 PUFAs and rich in monounsaturated fats such as canola (rapeseed) and olive oils. Margarine/spreads prepared with monounsaturated fats such as olive oil or n-3 sources are already on the market and it is to be hoped that the range of such products will continue to rise.

As AA is the direct precursor of inflammatory eicosanoids, one German study (see 9.11) investigating the effect of an 'anti-inflammatory diet' on RA patients, attempted to reduce the dietary content of AA to less than 90 mg/d (Adam et al. 2003). This can be compared with a normal AA content that has been estimated in another country – Australia – to be around 130 mg/d for males and 96 mg/d for females (Mann et al. 1995). Foods with the highest AA content are egg yolks, particularly from duck and quail, organ meats (e.g. kidney, liver and liver pâté), Atlantic salmon, duck, turkey, tropical fish and shellfish, with lesser quantities from pork, chicken, lamb and beef (Broadhurst et al. 2002; Mann et al. 1995). Table 9.11 gives the AA content of a number of foods purchased in Australia. The EPA content and n-6:n-3 ratio (Li et al. 1998; Mann et al. 1995) have also been included as it is clearly important to balance the undesirability of a substantial amount of AA in any food source with the benefit to be obtained from a significant amount of EPA in that same source.

Table 9.11 n-6 and n-3 fatty acid content of selected Australian foodstuffs and the n-6:n-3 ratio (Li et al. 1998; Mann et al. 1995).

Food	AA (20:n-4)	EPA (20:5n-3)	Total n-6	Total n-3	n-6/n-3
		(mg/100 g edible food)			
Beef sirloin (lean)	30	11	125	45	2.8
Rump steak (lean)	35	19	136	74	1.8
T-bone steak (lean meat)	28	—	—	—	1.6
Lamb leg steak (lean)	41	25	212	123	1.7
Lamb fillet (lean)	49	17	233	93	2.5
Lamb chop (lean meat)	39	—	—	—	1.8
Pork leg steak (lean)	56	6	328	35	9.4
Pork chop (lean meat)	54	—	—	—	13.9
Chicken breast (no skin)	31	6	179	44	4.1
Chicken legs (no skin)	56	6	456	69	6.6
Chicken drumstick (lean meat)	43	—	—	—	9.6
Turkey drumstick (lean meat)	74	—	—	—	10.8
Turkey composite (with skin)	63	4	839	74	11.3
Turkey composite (no skin)	75	4	419	48	8.7
Cold turkey loaf (brand A)	50	2	409	34	12.0
Cold turkey loaf (brand B)	37	0	1084	70	15.5
Duck drumstick (lean meat)	99	—	—	—	10.7
Lamb kidney	153	77	335	213	1.6
Ox liver	294	138	759	610	1.2
Kangaroo	62	26	230	98	2.3
Emu	130	3	408	19	21.5
Chicken pâté (brand A)	142	15	1509	271	5.6
Chicken pâté (brand B)	160	18	1927	308	6.3
Duck pâté	311	0	2218	233	9.5
Chicken egg yolk	390	0	3536	381	9.3
Duck egg yolk	891	46	2965	705	4.2
Barramundi	26	10	40	47	0.9
Atlantic salmon (no skin)	100	537	676	2526	0.3

9.17 Collateral benefits of increasing the intake of long-chain n-3 PUFAs

9.17.1 Reduced risk of cardiovascular mortality

Mortality rates are increased in RA largely owing to an increased prevalence of cardiovascular disease (CVD) (James et al. 2003). Prevention of CVD should therefore be an explicit aim in the treatment of RA (James et al. 2003).

N-3 PUFA supplementation has consistently been associated with a decrease in plasma triglycerides, VLDL cholesterol (Ariza-Ariza et al. 1998) and a lowered risk of cardiac arrhythmia (Harris 2004). Oily fish/fish oil is not only protective against inflammation in RA, but also against cardiac death and sudden death (James et al. 2003) except in men with angina (Burr et al. 2003). Cardiovascular benefits have been noted at levels lower than those required for anti-inflammatory effects i.e. at EPA + DHA intakes of less than 1 g/d (Cleland & James 2000).

9.17.2   Reduced requirement for NSAIDs or other drugs

A number of studies have shown that supplementation with n-3 PUFA may allow a reduction in NSAID use (described in Cleland & James 1997, Lau 1993 and Kremer 2000). Thus n-3 fatty acids may constitute a real alternative in situations in which anti-inflammatory drugs are difficult to handle, such as old age, renal impairment or a high risk of severe gastrointestinal bleeding (Ariza-Ariza et al. 1998).

9.18   Safety issues

9.18.1   Contraindications for cod liver oil supplements

Pregnant women should not use cod liver oil supplements owing to the vitamin A they contain (see 9.15.2). They are also contraindicated for those who consume liver frequently owing to the levels of vitamin A provided by liver.

9.18.2   Side effects of n-3 PUFAs

Side effects noted from studies with n-3 PUFAs include gastrointestinal symptoms, such as nausea, flatulence, diarrhoea and headaches and a fishy taste or odour (MacLean et al. 2004).

Very high intakes of n-3 fatty acids may reduce blood clotting time. The US Food and Drug Administration (FDA) has advised that no significant increase in blood clotting time would be expected at total daily intakes of EPA and DHA of 3 g or less. Taking into account intake of EPA and DHA from the diet, the US FDA recommended that supplemental intake of these fatty acids should be no more than 2 g/day. People with clotting disorders or on blood thinning medication such as warfarin should *not* take n-3 fatty acids unless prescribed by a doctor (Simopoulos & Robinson 1999).

9.18.3   Peroxidation issues related to increased n-3 PUFA intake

As an increased n-3 PUFA intake from either plant or marine origin is accompanied by an increased susceptibility of LDL oxidation *in vitro*, sufficient amounts of antioxidants such as vitamin E should accompany high n-3 PUFA containing foods to minimise lipid peroxidation (de Deckere et al. 1998). This is why vitamin E is regularly added to fish oil supplements. Simopoulos advises that a supplement of at least 100 IU (67 mg d-α-tocopherol or 100 mg dl-α-tocopherol acetate)/d vitamin E should be consumed with an n-3 PUFA-rich diet unless seven or more servings of fruit and vegetables are being consumed daily (Simopoulos & Robinson 1999).

Fish that is not very fresh should be avoided and frozen fish should be consumed as soon as possible as undesirable products arising from peroxidation, such as cytotoxic aldehydes, develop with exposure to air at room temperature and even at home freezer temperatures over time (personal communication, Professor Nazlin Howell, 2005).

9.18.4   Effects on immunity of increased n-3 PUFA

N-3 PUFA will downregulate the anti-inflammatory response, which is advantageous in RA, but the suppression of immune function may decrease the host's resistance to infection. However, according to the report of an expert workshop by de Deckere and colleagues (1998), no adverse effects of marine n-3 PUFA on infection in humans have been reported.

9.18.5   Contamination with dioxins and dioxin-like PCBs

Dioxins and dioxin-like PCBs (polychlorinated biphenyls) are persistent chemicals, formed during combustion processes and as by-products in the manufacture of certain chemicals. They do not break down easily and so are widespread in low concentrations in the environment. Dioxins are believed to disrupt endocrine systems in humans, and cause developmental effects in young children. One specific dioxin, 2,3,7,8-TCDD, may cause cancer in humans.

These chemicals are found in low concentrations in many foods, especially fat-containing foods such as oily fish, meat and milk. They are known to accumulate in fish, which therefore make a significant contribution to the estimated dietary exposure to dioxins and PCBs in some countries with high levels of fish consumption (MAFF 1999). Larger oily fish contain more dioxins than the smaller varieties; herring contains greater amounts, salmon and mackerel contain moderate amounts and trout contains much smaller concentrations.

The risks and benefits of eating fish were recently investigated by a joint subgroup of the UK Committee on Toxicity of Chemicals in Food, Consumer Products and the Environment (COT) and the Scientific Advisory Committee on Nutrition (SACN) (www.food.gov.uk/multimedia/pdfs/fishreport2004full.pdf). The group recommended ranges of oily fish consumption that would give clear nutritional benefits while maintaining intakes of dioxins and dioxin-like PCBs below a tolerable daily intake (TDI) established by the COT of 2 pg World Health Organization toxic equivalent (WHO-TEQ)/kg bodyweight per day:

- For women of reproductive age and girls: 1–2 portions of fish per week based on protecting against adverse effects on fetal development
- For women past reproductive age, men and boys: 1–4 portions of fish per week

The above advice does not take into account consumption of fish-oil supplements, which can also be a source of dioxins and PCBs: their use may potentially affect the amount of oily fish that should be consumed. However, the UK Food Standards Agency is currently unable to advise on maximum safe combinations of oily fish and fish oil supplements. This is because intakes of dioxins and PCBs from fish oil supplements vary greatly from product to product, depending on the concentrations of dioxins and PCBs present and the amount of the oil consumed per daily dose of the supplement. Fish oils are subject to a Europe wide dioxin limit of 2 pg/g and manufacturers should test raw materials and final products to ensure that this limit is not exceeded, thus toxic effects from dioxins should not be a problem for those taking supplements (FSA 2002). However, there is currently no regulatory limit for dioxin-like PCBs. This question is currently being considered by the European Commission with a view to establishing a limit. Manufacturers should be able to supply certificates of analysis for their fish oils, which should be carefully scrutinised by those proposing to take significant quantities of fish oil supplements.

Although there is still concern regarding the concentration of dioxins and dioxin-like PCBs in the diet, it seems that overall, levels are falling owing to controls that are in place to regulate emissions of dioxins and PCBs from industrial processes and correct disposal of PCBs. Long-term monitoring of herring in the Baltic Sea has seen a reduction in PCB concentration of 6.3–13% per year since 1978.

9.18.6   Fish contamination with mercury

Fish is the major source of mercury in the diet, accounting for around 25% of total mercury intake in the UK in 1994 (Reilly 2002). More than 75% of fish mercury is present as methyl mercury, a potent neurotoxin, particularly for the fetus (Reilly 2002). Absorbed organic mercury is retained for a long time. Accumulation in fish is related to size: higher amounts of methyl mercury are found in fish higher up in the food-chain such as, shark, swordfish, pike, mackerel and tuna. Large tuna over 60 kg in weight may have levels of organic mercury up to 1 mg/kg in muscle, though higher levels of total mercury have been found in South American tuna (Reilly 2002). To limit the danger from fish sources, health authorities have set maximum permitted levels in fish as shown below (Reilly 2002).

Australia   0.5 mg/kg in most fresh fish and molluscs
             1.0 mg/kg for larger predators including tuna and shark
UK   0.5 mg/kg in fresh fish
             1.0 mg/kg for tuna, shark, swordfish and halibut
US FDA   1 mg/kg methyl mercury in fresh fish

Current dietary intakes are around the levels shown below (Reilly 2002).

UK adults   5 µg/d, upper range 9 µg/d
US adults   8 µg/d
Spain   18 µg/d (Basque region – fish consumption is high)
Egypt   78 µg/d (high levels are attributed to industrial pollution)

The FAO/WHO Joint Expert Committee on Food Additives (JECFA) advises that intake should not exceed 5 µg/kg bodyweight/week, giving an upper limit in adults of some 280–380 µg/week, though some agencies believe that this level has been set too high, believing the limit should be 0.7 µg/kg bw/week, which would limit consumption to around 40–50 µg/week (Reilly 2002).

The UK Total Diet Study of 1991 found an average level of mercury in fresh fish of 0.054 mg/kg (54 µg/kg) which, even at the lower recommended level of safe intake, would allow the consumption of up to seven fish meals per week if there were no other sources of mercury contamination in the diet. However, owing to the particular effects on the fetus and young child, pregnant women, those intending to become pregnant and breastfeeding mothers have been advised by the UK Food Standards Agency (FSA) to restrict their intake of some fish. Current advice for these women (and those under 16 years) is to avoid shark, swordfish and marlin and to restrict their intake of tuna to two medium cans (140 g each drained) or one fresh portion per week (FSA 2003). This in practical terms translates to six rounds of tuna sandwiches or three tuna salads per week. Others should be aware of the potential toxicity associated with high intakes of such fish.

Fish oils from reputable sources should have levels of mercury that do not exceed 1 µg/g, allowing the safe consumption of 40–50 1 g capsules/week (6–8/ day), assuming no other sources of mercury contamination in the diet.

Consumption of adequate levels of selenium appears to be protective against mercury toxicity (Ganther et al. 1972): selenium binds mercury very firmly in a 1:1 inert complex which is only excreted very slowly but appears to cause no harm when stored in the body (Suzuki et al. 1998). As fish is a major source of selenium in the diet, and the molar concentration of selenium in fish generally exceeds that of mercury by more than an order of magnitude (calculated as 18:1 from data in Ysart et al. 1999) the methyl mercury ingested may be less harmful than anticipated. This may explain the lack of evidence of neurological damage in children born to mothers in the Seychelles who regularly eat mercury-contaminated fish (Reilly 2002).

9.19 Ethical issues: fish stocks

Many fish stocks are depleted and some people believe it to be irresponsible to eat fish while this situation exists. If there is an increased demand for oily fish or derived supplements, fish stocks may be further depleted. Aquaculture is a fast growing technique and it is possible that the expected increase in fish consumption will be met in the long term by this process (Kris-Etherton et al. 2000). However, as explained by Bell and colleagues (2003), aquaculture currently uses more than 60% of global fish production and by 2010, more than 85% will be consumed in aquaculture feeds, a level that cannot be sustained. Though it is possible to use blends of rapeseed oil, linseed oil and fish oil in the seawater phase of the salmon growth cycle, fish oil feed needs to be given in a period before harvest to ensure adequate long-chain fatty acid concentrations. Those unhappy with this state of affairs should consume short-chain n-3 fatty acids (flaxseed products), grass-fed beef, lamb or game and restrict n-6 intake as described in section 9.16, though this is a less effective strategy for increasing the concentration of long-chain n-3 PUFAs.

9.20   Conclusion

We have cited evidence that certain fatty acids, most notably long-chain n-3 fatty acids, can suppress the production of inflammatory mediators and may impede cartilage destruction. However, human interventions with fish oil have been somewhat disappointing in their ability to provide significant improvement in arthritic symptoms other than morning stiffness and tender joint count. Some possible explanations for this have already been discussed (section 9.12), notably the effect of a background diet high in n-6 fatty acid sources. We have also pointed out that polymorphisms in cytokine genes may provide an explanation as to why some people benefit from fish oil supplementation whereas others do not, leading to a non-significant overall effect.

Patients suffering from RA and moderate to severe OA should be recommended to increase their intake of n-3 fatty acids (particularly of EPA sources where possible), and reduce their intake of n-6 fatty acids, at least for a trial period. We have not stipulated a ratio of n-6:n-3 to be achieved because, as explained by de Deckere and colleagues (1998), plant and marine n-3 PUFAs show different effects and because a decrease in n-6 intake does not produce the same effects as an increase in n-3 PUFA intake. In this chapter, we have explored the various ways in which an increased intake of n-3 fatty acids can be achieved and have suggested options for vegetarians.

Though examination of the risks associated with increased intake of fatty fish/fish oils has been reassuring, the use of fish oils as an adjunct to traditional treatment has been limited. This is probably partly due to ignorance among clinicians of the positive benefits of fish oils, to the proactive promotion by the pharmaceutical industry of anti-inflammatory and antirheumatic drugs, to the fact that patented fish oils are unavailable and to the difficulty of achieving dietary intervention or change (James et al. 2003). Clear dietary handouts and greater availability of n-3-fat-enriched products are required to enable patients to realise the potential of this safe method of ameliorating symptoms, reducing disease progression and improving their quality of life.

References

Adam O (1995) Anti-inflammatory diet in rheumatic diseases. *European Journal of Clinical Nutrition* **49**, 703–17.

Adam O, Beringer C, Kless T, Lemmen C, Adam A, Wiseman M, Adam P, Klimmek R, Forth W (2003) Anti-inflammatory effects of a low arachidonic acid diet and fish oil in patients with rheumatoid arthritis. *Rheumatology International* **23**, 27–36.

Arita M, Bianchini F, Aliberti J, Sher A, Chiang N, Hong S, Yang R, Petasis NA, Serhan CN (2005) Stereochemical assignment, antiinflammatory properties, and receptor for the omega-3 lipid mediator resolvin E1. *Journal of Experimental Medicine* 7, 201(5), 713–22.

Ariza-Ariza R, Mestanza-Peralta M, Cardiel MH (1998) Omega-3 fatty acids in rheumatoid arthritis: an overview. *Seminars in Arthritis and Rheumatism* **27**(6), 366–70.

Belch JJ, Hill A (2000) Evening primrose oil and borage oil in rheumatologic conditions. *American Journal of Clinical Nutrition* **71**(1 Suppl), 352S–6S.

Bell J, Tocher DR, Henderson RJ, Dick JR, VO Crampton (2003) Altered fatty acid compositions in Atlantic salmon (Salmo salar) fed diets containing linseed and rapeseed oils can be partically restored by a subsequent fish oil finishing diet. *Journal of Nutrition* **133**, 2793–801.

Berbert A, Kondo C, Almendra C, Matsuo T, Dichi I (2005) Supplementation of fish oil and olive oil in patients with rheumatoid arthritis. *Nutrition* **21**, 131–36.

BNF (1999) *Briefing Paper N-3 fatty acids and health*. British Nutrition Foundation.

Brill (2004) www.wildmanstevebrill.com

British Nutrition Foundation (BNF) (2005) *Cardiovascular Disease: Diet, Nutrition and Emerging Risk Factors. Report of the British Nutrition Task Force* (Sara Stanner, ed.) Oxford, Blackwell Publishing.

Broadhurst CL, Wang Y, Crawford MA, Cunnane SC, Parkington JE, Schmidt WF (2002) Brain-specific lipids from marine, lacustrine, or terrestrial food resources: potential impact on early African *Homo sapiens*. *Comparative Biochemistry and Physiology B: Biochemistry and Molecular Biology* **131**(4), 653–73.

Burr M, Ashfield-Watt P, Dunstan F, Fehily A, Breay P, Ashton T, Zotos P, Haboubi N, Elwood P (2003) Lack of benefit of dietary advice to men with angina: results of a controlled trial. *European Journal of Clinical Nutrition* **57**, 193–200.

Calder PC (1997) n-3 Polyunsaturated fatty acids and cytokine production in health and disease. *Annals of Nutrition and Metabolism* **41**, 203–34.

Calder PC, Field, CJ (2002) Fatty acids and the immune system. In: *Nutrition and the Immune System* (PC Calder, CJ Field, HS Gill, eds) Wallingford, CABI, pp. 57–92.

Calder PC, Zurier RB (2001) Polyunsaturated fatty acids and rheumatoid arthritis. *Current Opinion in Clinical Nutrition and Metabolic Care* **4**, 115–21.

Caughey GE, Mantzioris E, Gibson RA, Cleland LG, James MJ (1996) The effect of human tumor necrosis factor a and interleukin 1b production of diets enriched in n-3 fatty acids from vegetable oil or fish oil. *American Journal of Clinical Nutrition* **63**, 116–22.

Cleland LG, James MJ (1997) Rheumatoid arthritis and the balance of dietary n-6 and n-3 essential fatty acids. *British Journal of Rheumatology* **36**, 513–14.

Cleland LG, James MJ (2000) Fish oil and rheumatoid arthritis: antiinflammatory and collateral health benefits. *Journal of Rheumatology* **27**, 2305–7.

Cleland LG, James MJ, Proudman SM (2004) Food inflammation and the anti-inflammatory aspects of food. *Asia Pacific Journal of Clinical Nutrition* **13**(Suppl), S26.

Cordain L, Watkins BA, Florant GL, Kelher M, Rogers L, Li Y (2002) Fatty acid analysis of wild ruminant tissues: evolutionary implications for reducing diet-related chronic disease. *European Journal of Clinical Nutrition* **56**(3), 181–91.

Curtis CL, Rees SG, Little CB, Flannery CR, Hughes CE, Wilson C, Dent CM, Otterness IG, Harwood JL, Caterson B (2002a) Pathological indicators of degradation and inflammation in human osteoarthritic cartilage are abrogated by exposure to n-3 fatty acids. *Arthritis and Rheumatism* **46**(6), 1544–53.

Curtis CL, Rees SG, Cramp J, Flannery CR, Hughes CE, Little CB, Williams R, Wilson C, Dent CM, Harwood JL, Caterson B (2002b) Effects of n-3 fatty acids on cartilage metabolism. *Proceedings of the Nutrition Society* **61**(3), 381–89.

Curtis CL, Harwood JL, Cent CM, Caterson B (2004a) Biological basis for the benefit of neutrachemical supplementation in arthritis. *Drug Discovery Today* **9**, 165–72.

Curtis C, Rees S, Evans R, Dent CM, Caterson B, Harwood JL (2004b) The effects of n-3 polyunsaturated fatty acids on cartilage metabolism in patients with osteoarthritis: the results of a pilot clinical trial. *Proceedings of the third European Federation for the Science and Technology of Lipids*. Edinburgh, 5–8 September, p. 216.

Darlington LG, Stone TW (2001) Antioxidants and fatty acids in the amelioration of rheumatoid arthritis and related disorders. *British Journal of Nutrition* **85**(3), 251–69.

Davis BC, Kris-Etherton PM (2003) Achieving optimal essential fatty acid status in vegetarians: current knowledge and practical implications. *American Journal of Clinical Nutrition* **78**(3 suppl), 640S–646S.

de Deckere EA, Korver O, Verschuren PM, Katan MB (1998) Health aspects of fish and n-3 polyunsaturated fatty acids from plant and marine origin. *European Journal of Clinical Nutrition* **52**(10), 749–53.

Farrell DJ (1998) Enrichment of hen eggs with n-3 long-chain fatty acids and evaluation of enriched eggs in humans. *American Journal of Clinical Nutrition* 68, 538–44.

Finch S, Doyle W, Lowe C, Bates C, Prentice A, Smithers G, Clark P (1998) *National Diet and Nutrition Survey: People aged 65 years and over*, Volume 1. London, The Stationery Office.

Fortin PR, Lew RA, Liang MH, Wright EA, Beckett LA, Chalmers TC, Sperling RI (1995) Validation of a meta-analysis, The effects of fish oil in rheumatoid arthritis. *Journal of Clinical Epidemiology* 48(11), 1379–90.

FSA (2002) Food Standards Agency. *Survey of Dioxins and Dioxin-like PCBs in Fish Oil Supplements* (Number 26/02). www.food.gov.uk/science/surveillance/fsis-2002/26diox

FSA (2003) *Mercury in imported fish and shellfish, UK farmed fish and their products* (40/03). www.food.gov.uk/science/surveillance/fsis-2003/fsis402003

FSA Food Standards Agency (2004) *Arsenic in seaweed.* www.food.gov.uk/multimedia/pdfs/arsenicseaweed.pdf

Ganther HE, Goudie C, Sunde ML, Kopecky MJ, Wagner P (1972) Selenium: relation to decreased toxicity of methylmercury added to diets containing tuna. *Science* 175(26), 1122–24.

Gerster H (1998) Can adults adequately convert alpha-linolenic acid (18:3n-3) to eicosapentaenoic acid (20:5n-3) and docosahexaenoic acid (22:6n-3)? International *Journal for Vitamin and Nutrition Research* 68(3), 159–73.

Grimble RF, Howell WM, O'Reilly G, Turner SJ, Markovic O, Hirrell S, East JM, Calder PC (2002) The ability of fish oil to suppress tumor necrosis factor alpha production by peripheral blood mononuclear cells in healthy men is associated with polymorphisms in genes that influence tumor necrosis factor alpha production. *American Journal of Clinical Nutrition* 76(2), 454–59.

Harris WS (2004) Are omega-3 fatty acids the most important nutritional modulators of coronary heart disease risk? *Curr Atheroscler Rep* 6(6), 447–52.

Horrobin DF (1987) Low prevalences of coronary heart disease, psoriasis, asthma and rheumatoid arthritis in Eskimos: are they caused by high dietary intake of eicosapentaenoic acid, a genetic variation of essential fatty acid metabolism or a combination of both? *Med Hypotheses* 22, 227.

Hulshof KF, van Erp-Baart MA, Anttolainen M, Becker W, Church SM, Couet C, Hermann-Kunz E, Kesteloot H, Leth T, Martins I, Moreiras O, Moschandreas J, Pizzoferrato L, Rimestad AH, Thorgeirsdottir H, van Amelsvoort JM, Aro A, Kafatos AG, Lanzmann-Petithory D, van Poppel G (1999) Intake of fatty acids in western Europe with emphasis on trans fatty acids: the TRANSFAIR study. *European Journal of Clinical Nutrition* 53(2), 143–57.

James MJ, Gibson R, Cleland LG (2000) Dietary polyunsaturated fatty acids and inflammatory mediator production. *American Journal of Clinical Nutrition* 71(suppl), 343S–8S.

James MJ, Proudmann SM, Cleland LG (2003) Dietary n-3 fats as adjunctive therapy in a prototypic inflammatory disease: issues and obstacles for use in rheumatoid arthritis. *Prostaglandins, Leukotrienes and Essential Fatty Acids* 68, 399–405.

Kremer J, Lawrence D, Petrillo G, Litts L, Mullaly P, Rynes R, Stocker R, Parhami N, Greenstein N, Fuchs B, Mathur A, Robinson D, Sperling R, Bigaouette J (1995) Effects of high-dose fish oil on rheumatoid arthritis after stopping non-steroidal anti-inflammatory drugs. *Arthritis and Rheumatism* 38(8), 1107–14.

Kremer JM (2000) n-3 fatty acid supplements in rheumatoid arthritis. *American Journal of Clinical Nutrition* 71(suppl), 349S–51S.

Kris-Etherton PM, Taylor DS, Yu-Poth S, Huth P, Moriarty K, Kishell V, Hargrove RL, Zhao G, Etherton TD (2000) Polyunsaturated fatty acids in the food chain in the United States. *American Journal of Clinical Nutrition* 71, 179–88.

Lau CS, Morley KD, Belch JJF (1993) Effects of fish oil supplementation on non-steroidal anti-inflammatory drug requirement in patients with mild rheumatoid arthritis- a double-blind, placebo-controlled study. *British Journal of Rheumatology* 32, 982–89.

Leventhal LJ, Boyce EG, Zurier RB (1993) Treatment of rheumatoid arthritis with gamma linolenic acid. *Annals of Internal Medicine* 119(9), 867–73.

Leventhal LJ, Boyce EG, Zurier RB (1994) Treatment of rheumatoid arthritis with blackcurrant seed oil. *British Journal of Rheumatology* 33, 847–52.

Li D, Ng A, Mann NJ, Sinclair AJ (1998) Contribution of meat fat to dietary arachidonic acid. *Lipids* 33, 437–40.

MacLean CH, Mojica WA, Morton SC, Pencharz J, Hasenfeld Garland R, Tu W, Newberry SJ, Jungvig LK, Grossman J, Khanna P, Rhodes S, Shekelle P (2004) Effects of omega-3 fatty acids on lipids and glycemic control in Type II diabetes and the metabolic syndrome and on inflammatory bowel disease, rheumatoid arthritis, renal disease, systemic lupus erythematosus, and osteoporosis. *Summary, Evidence Report/Technology Assessment No. 89.* (Prepared by the Southern California/RAND Evidence-based Practice Center, Los Angeles, CA.) AHRQ Publication No. 04-E012-1. Rockville, MD: Agency for Healthcare Research and Quality, March 2004.

MAFF (1999) Dioxins and PCBs in UK and imported marine fish, No. **184**. www.defra.gov.uk/

Mann MJ, Johnson LG, Warrick GE, Sinclair AJ (1995) The arachidonic acid content of the Australian diet is lower than previously estimated. *Journal of Nutrition* **125**, 2528–35.

Mann N (2000) Dietary lean red meat and human evolution. *European Journal of Nutrition* **39**, 71–79.

Mantzioris E, Cleland LG, Gibson RA, Neumann MA, Demasi M, James MJ (2000) Biochemical effects of a diet containing foods enriched with n-3 fatty acids. *American Journal of Clinical Nutrition* **72**, 42–48.

Mantzioris E, James MJ, Gibson RA, Cleland LG (1995) Differences exist in the relationships between dietary linoleic and alpha-linolenic acids and their respective long-chain metabolites. *American Journal of Clinical Nutrition* **61**(2), 320–24.

Metcalf RG, James MJ, Mantzioris E, Cleland LG (2003) A practical approach to increasing intakes of n-3 polyunsaturated fatty acids: use of novel foods enriched with n-3 fats. *European Journal of Clinical Nutrition* **57**(12), 1605–12.

Miller GJ (1986) Lipids in wild ruminant animals and steers. *Journal of Food Quality* **9**, 331–43.

Ministry of Agriculture, Fisheries and Food (1993) *Food Portion Sizes*, 2nd edn. London, HMSO.

Pawlosky RJ, Hibbeln JR, Lin Y, Goodson S, Riggs P, Sebring N, Brown GL, Salem N Jr (2003) Effects of beef- and fish-based diets on the kinetics of n-3 fatty acid metabolism in human subjects. *American Journal of Clinical Nutrition* **77**(3), 565–72.

Reilly C (2002) *Metal Contamination of Food*. Oxford, Blackwell Science.

SACN (2004) Scientific Advisory Committee on Nutrition. *Advice to FSA: on the benefits of oily fish and fish consumption.* SACN www.sacn.gov.uk

Simopoulos AP, Robinson J (1999) *The Omega Diet*. New York, Harper Perennial.

Simopoulos AP (1999) Essential fatty acids in health and chronic disease. *American Journal of Clinical Nutrition* **70**(suppl) 560S–9S.

Sundrarjun T, Komindr S, Archararit N, Dahlan W, Puchaiwatananon O, Angthararak S, Udomsuppayakul U, Chuncharunee S (2004) Effects of n-3 fatty acids on serum interleukin-6, tumour necrosis factor-alpha and soluble tumour necrosis factor receptor p55 in active rheumatoid arthritis. *Journal of International Medical Research* Sep–Oct; **32**(5), 443–54.

Suzuki KT, Sasakura C, Yoneda S (1998) Binding sites for the (Hg-Se) complex on selenoprotein P. *Biochimica et Biophysica Acta* **1429**(1), 102–12.

UK Expert Group on Vitamins and Minerals (2003) Safe Upper Levels for Vitamins and Minerals London, Food Standards Agency, May 2003, ISBN 1-904026-11-7. www.food.gov.uk/multimedia/pdfs/vitmin2003.pdf

Volker D, FitzGerald P, Major G, Garg M (2000) Efficacy of fish oil concentrate in the treatment of rheumatoid arthritis. *Journal of Rheumatology* **27**(10), 2343–46.

Wood JD, Enser M, Fisher AV, Nute GR, Richardson RI, Sheard PR (1999) Manipulating meat quality and composition. *Proceedings of the Nutrition Society* **58**, 363–70.

Yaqoob P, Pala HS, Cortina-Borja M, Newsholme EA, Calder PC (2000) Encapsulated fish oil enriched in alpha-tocopherol alters plasma phospholipid and mononuclear cell fatty acid compositions but not mononuclear cell functions. *European Journal of Clinical Investigation* **30**(3), 260–74.

Yaqoob P (2003) Lipids and the immune response: from molecular mechanisms to clinical applications. *Current Opinion in Clinical Nutrition and Metabolic Care* **6**(2), 133–50.

Ysart G, Miller P, Crews H, Robb P, Baxter M, De L'Argy C, Lofthouse S, Sargent C, Harrison N (1999) Dietary exposure estimates of 30 elements from the UK Total Diet Study. Food Additives and Contaminants **16**(9), 391–403.

Zurier RB, Rossetti RG, Jacobson EW, DeMarco DM, Liu NY, Temming JE, White BM, Laposata M (1996) Gamma-linolenic acid treatment of rheumatoid arthritis. A randomized, placebo-controlled trial. *Arthritis and Rheumatism* **39**(11), 1808–17.

10 Glucosamine and chondroitin in osteoarthritis

10.1 Introduction

Glucosamine and chondroitin are natural substances manufactured in the body that are required for joint health. In recent years, the use of supplements of these substances by osteoarthritis sufferers has increased significantly, to the point where they are now *'top sellers in a $26 billion annual market'* (McAlindon 2001a). While many studies have indicated that glucosamine sulphate has a beneficial structural effect in OA, some more recent trials have been unable to confirm such an effect, raising the question of whether oral treatment, even with pharmacological doses of these compounds, can benefit the joints. We will review the evidence in the hope of clarifying recommendations that should be given to patients.

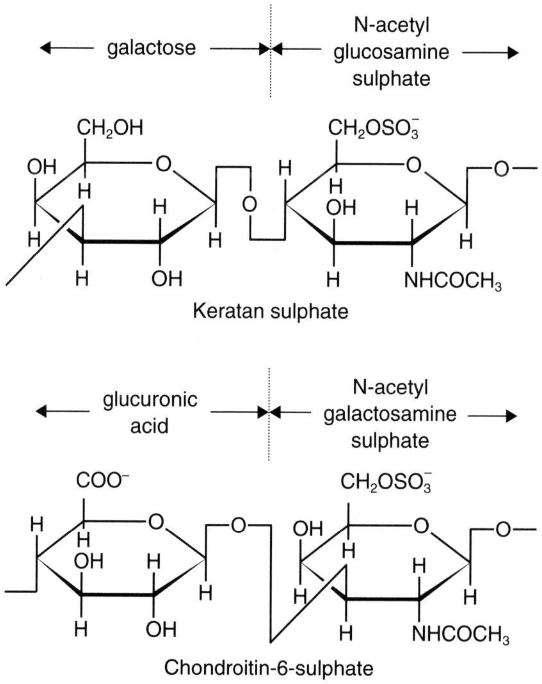

Figure 10.1 Repeating disaccharide units of the glycosaminoglycan molecules, keratan sulphate and chondroitin sulphate: it can be seen that the amino-sugar in keratan sulphate is N-acetyl glucosamine sulphate ('glucosamine').

10.2   What are glucosamine and chondroitin?

Glucosamine and chondroitin are components of cartilage and connective tissue. Glucosamine is an amino sugar (2-amino-deoxyglucose) that when bound to a second sugar, makes up one of the repeating disaccharide units that constitute glycosaminoglycans, the building blocks of connective tissue (Stryer 1988). The glucosamine derivative N-acetylglucosamine sulphate is one of the sugars that makes up the disaccharide unit in keratan sulphate, a component of cartilage (Stryer 1988) (Figure 10.1). Chondroitin sulphate is similar to keratan sulphate but with the repeating disaccharide unit made from N-acetylgalactosamine sulphate and glucuronic acid (Das & Hammad 2000) (Figure 10.1).

These long-chain polymers of chondroitin sulphate or keratan sulphate are the major glycosaminoglycans in cartilage (Das & Hammad 2000). When covalently attached to a polypeptide backbone called the core protein, chondroitin sulphate chains (100–150 per monomer) and keratin sulphate chains (30–60 per monomer) make up a structure known as an aggrecan monomer, or simply as 'aggrecan'. Around 140 of these aggrecan monomers are bound through the protein backbone to a very long filament of hyaluronate to give a proteoglycan aggregate as shown schematically in Figure 2.4 (section 2.3.2). Glucosamine is also an intermediate substrate in the synthesis of mucopolysaccharides and glycoproteins in synovial fluid (Setnikar & Rovati 2001).

10.3   Sources of glucosamine and chondroitin

The common starting materials for glucosamine and chondroitin supplements are lobster, crab and prawns (crustaceans). These are sources of chitin that, when hydrolysed with an acid, form glucosamine or chondroitin salts. Glucosamine is available in many different forms: glucosamine sulphate, glucosamine hydrochloride, N-acetyl-glucosamine and glucosamine chlorohydrate salt. These forms differ in the acid used to hydrolyse the chitin, for example, glucosamine sulphate is hydrolysed by sulphuric acid. It has been suggested that the form of glucosamine supplemented makes no difference, because the hydrochloric acid in the stomach will always form glucosamine hydrochloride (Curtis et al. 2004).

Glucosamine sulphate is the theraputic agent that has most frequently been studied. It normally contains glucosamine, sulphate, sodium (or potassium) and chloride ions in the ratio of 2:1:2:2 respectively. Indeed the Rotta (an Italian-based company) formulation, a pure substance synthesised from chitin, has been used in around 75% of glucosamine studies (Reginster et al. 2001; Setnikar & Rovati 2001; Towheed et al. 2005).

10.4   Bioavailability

While 88.7% of an oral dose of glucosamine sulphate was absorbed through the gastrointestinal (GI) tract in 120 hours, the absolute bioavailability of glucosamine was estimated as 44% (Setnikar & Rovati 2001). This was assessed by comparing the area under the plasma concentration time curve after oral administration of ^{14}C-crystalline glucosamine sulphate with the corresponding area after intravenous administration of the same substance. Absorption of chondroitin sulphate is much lower because of its size – macromolecules are not normally absorbed in the GI tract (Barthe et al. 2004). *In vitro* studies with radiolabelled chondroitin sulphate showed that low amounts were transported across the small intestine in the intact form but in the distal GI tract the molecule is effectively degraded to disaccharides (Barthe et al. 2004). Absorption rates from 8–15% are quoted, depending on the source, suggesting that large doses may be needed.

10.5   Postulated mechanism of action

The mechanism by which glucosamine and chondroitin work has not yet been fully elucidated, but there are a number of theories, the most popular of which is that they may provide substrates for cartilage repair.

Glucosamine seems to be capable of increasing proteoglycan synthesis (anabolic activity) in intact cartilage and decreasing catabolic activities such as those of metalloproteases, thus benefiting articular cartilage structure and joint tissues (Reginster et al. 2001). Experiments on cultured human chondrocytes have shown an increased production of aggrecans (Bassleer et al. 1998). This may explain the significant reduction in joint space narrowing (JSN) associated with glucosamine supplementation in some studies (see section 10.6). Furthermore, there is increasing evidence that glucosamine reverses some of the negative effects of interleukin 1β on cartilage metabolism (Pavelka et al. 2002) reducing the formation of nitric oxide and interleukin 6 (Shikhman et al. 2001).

Chondroitin sulphate is said to have similar chondroprotective effects. It is believed to act by a number of mechanisms that include contribution to the pool of glycosaminoglycans (GAGs) in cartilage, inhibition of synovial degradative enzymes and stimulation of GAG and collagen synthesis by chondrocytes (Das & Hammad 2000). It is able to cause an increase in mRNA synthesis by chondrocytes, which appears to correlate with an increase in the production of proteoglycans and collagen (McAlindon 2001a). Both compounds have an affinity for articular cartilage and synovial fluid (Das & Hammad 2000). The combination of glucosamine and chondroitin sulphate is thought to be synergistic, having a significantly greater effect than that of the two individual compounds added together: while glucosamine stimulates GAG production, chondroitin sulphate inhibits its degradation (Das & Hammad 2000).

Glucosamine sulphate has also been shown to have mild anti-inflammatory activity in its own right (Das & Hammad 2000), thereby explaining short-term symptom improvements in OA. This may relate to its ability to inhibit both superoxide radical generation and inducible nitric oxide (NO) synthesis (Reginster et al. 2001), in the latter case by suppressing inducible NO-synthase (iNOS) protein expression in activated macrophages and many tissues (Meininger et al. 2000). Inhibition of inducible NO synthesis at the time of induction of arthritis in rats has been shown to reduce profoundly synovial inflammation, joint swelling and tissue damage (for references, see Meininger et al. 2000).

It is possible that glucosamine may act as an immunosuppressant through its ability to suppress cells involved in immune responses i.e. T-cells and dendritic cells (Ma et al. 2002). Glucosamine has been shown to prolong allogenic allograft survival in mice. This effect has prompted Ma and colleagues (2002) to suggest that the beneficial effects of glucosamine could be explained by the suppression of immune activity. This could allow synovial tissue to regenerate unimpeded in the absence of soluble mediators of inflammation and pain generated by immune cells at the site of cartilage erosion (Ma et al. 2002).

Hoffer and colleagues (2001) have hypothesised that it is the sulphate in glucosamine sulphate, the form of glucosamine most frequently supplemented, that is the active component. The basis for this is the fact that sulphate is needed for GAG synthesis, which is inhibited when animals are depleted of sulphate, and the observation that large oral doses of glucosamine do not affect serum glucosamine concentrations. In support of his hypothesis, a study in a group of seven healthy subjects showed that glucosamine sulphate did indeed increase inorganic sulphate concentration in the synovial fluid (Hoffer et al. 2001). Sodium sulphate, though providing twice the amount of sulphate as glucosamine sulphate, showed no increase in sulphate concentration. This suggests that intestinal absorption of sulphate may be improved when it is ingested as the glucosamine salt (Hoffer et al. 2001). Consuming protein-containing food with glucosamine sulphate may further increase serum sulphate concentration owing to sulphur-amino-acid catabolism (Hoffer et al. 2001). However, such an hypothesis is not supported by the beneficial effects of glucosamine hydrochloride in some studies (Das & Hammad 2000; Leffler et al. 1999; Clegg et al. 2006).

10.6 Trials of glucosamine and chondroitin and their efficacy in OA

10.6.1 Meta-analyses of glucosamine and chondroitin trials

The number of small trials of glucosamine and chondroitin in OA has prompted a number of investigators to carry out meta-analyses, as described below.

A thorough, well explained and executed meta-analysis and quality review of studies that tested oral or parenteral glucosamine sulphate, glucosamine hydro-chloride, or chondroitin sulphate in knee and hip OA from 1966–99 was carried out by McAlindon and colleagues (2000). A total of 57 studies was identified, 15 of which matched the inclusion criteria set (e.g. minimum four-week trial, placebo-controlled, double-blind and randomised) and reported sufficient numerical results to permit data extraction. These studies included from 17 to 329 participants. The results of each study were allocated a quality value and an outcome value, i.e. how effective they were compared to placebo.

Effect sizes were calculated from the studies reviewed: moderate treatment effect sizes were found for glucosamine supplementation (0.44; 95% CI 0.24, 0.64) and

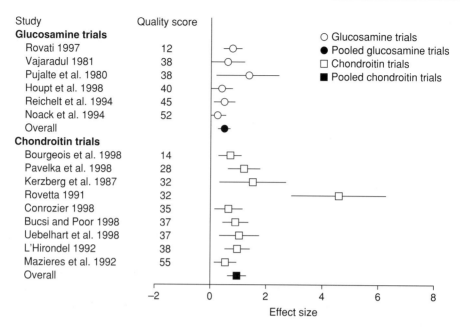

Figure 10.2 Forest plot of effect sizes for trials and pooled (reproduced with permission from McAlindon et al. 2000).

large treatment effects were seen for chondroitin supplementation (0.78; 95% CI 0.60, 0.90). The quality scores given to these papers ranged from 12.3% to 55.4% (100% being the highest quality). The effect sizes and quality scores from individual and grouped effects of chondroitin and glucosamine trials are shown in Figure 10.2. When only those high quality or large-scale trials were included, effect sizes for both chondroitin and glucosamine diminished: glucosamine sulphate studies above the median quality score had a low to moderate effect size.

Although methodological issues relating to trial quality and size and publication bias have led to exaggerated estimates of benefit, McAlindon and colleagues (2000) concluded at that time that:

'Some degree of efficacy appears probable for these preparations.'

Richy and colleagues included chondroitin in addition to glucosamine in their high quality, conservative, meta-analysis published in 2003. Their analysis included some long-term influential studies (see below) not available at the time of the McAlindon meta-analysis. They looked at the symptomatic and structural effects of both oral glucosamine sulphate and chondroitin sulphate in knee osteoarthritis in 15 studies published between 1980 and 2002. Data from 1775 patients were analysed and the quality of the studies was assessed. The quality scores ranged from 60–100%, averaging 78.4%. This meta-analysis confirmed the results of previous meta-analyses, the data providing evidence of a structural efficacy of glucosamine on Western Ontario and McMaster Universities (WOMAC) index and joint space narrowing, the latter being highly significant (P < 0.001) with a low to moderate effect size (0.41; 95% CI 0.21, 0.60). The effect size was alternatively described as a minimal difference in joint space narrowing of 0.27 mm (95% CI 0.13, 0.41 mm) between placebo and active drug groups after three years of daily administration of 1500 mg of glucosamine sulphate (Richy et al. 2003). This can be compared with typical joint space narrowing in knee OA which ranges from 0.06–0.6 mm per year (Reginster et al. 2001). While the chondroitin studies also showed significant benefit, in particular on the Lequesne Index, visual analogue scale pain, mobility and treatment response, data on structural effects were too restricted for analysis.

These authors (Richy et al. 2003) also attempted to determine whether there was any evidence of publication bias (i.e. more positive trials published) by carrying out a funnel plot graph for responders, which, in the absence of publication bias, displays a symmetrical inverted funnel. They concluded that while the asymmetry was statistically significant (p = 0.08), publication bias was not the only source of funnel plot asymmetry, there being other possible contributors.

A meta-analysis dealing only with chondroitin studies was carried out by Leeb and colleagues (2000). They looked at the possible efficacy of chondroitin sulphate treatment on pain and function in OA patients. Seven studies were identified covering a total population of 703 patients between 1991 and 1998. Although the findings were not significant, they concluded that chondroitin sulphate may benefit pain relief and function in OA. The study length and participant numbers were major drawbacks in these studies. A dose of 2000 mg/day did not appear to be superior to 800 mg/day.

The largest and most recent of the meta-analyses is the updated Cochrane review of randomised controlled trials (RCTs) of the effect of glucosamine in OA by Towheed and colleagues (2005) which includes a further four RCTs. Twenty double-blind, randomised, parallel group trials that reported results between 1980 and 2004 were included in the meta-analysis. The studies encompassed a total group size of 2596 adults with a mean age of 61 years, 67% of whom were female. The average study length was 23.7 weeks but would have been nine weeks if the two three-year trials had been excluded.

Seventeen of the 20 studies compared glucosamine to placebo while four compared it to a non-steroidal anti-inflammatory drug (NSAID). One study compared it to both placebo and an NSAID. The route of administration and doses used varied from study to study but 16 of the studies administered glucosamine orally at a dose of 1500 mg/d. Thirteen of the studies used the Rotta preparation of glucosamine sulphate. The type and site of OA evaluated differed in the 20 trials: 16 RCTs evaluated the knee exclusively while two evaluated multiple sites and two did not specify location. Outcome variables included pain (20 studies), range of motion (6 studies), functional status (15 studies) and radiographic assessment for changes in cartilage thickness (2 studies).

Collectively, the 20 identified studies found glucosamine to be better than placebo with a significant (28% change from baseline) improvement in pain (effect size −0.61; 95% CI −0.95, −0.28; see Figure 10.3) and a significant (21%) improvement in function as measure by the Lequesne Index (effect size −0.51; 95%

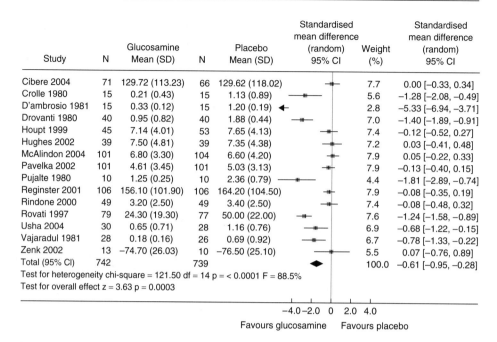

Study	N	Glucosamine Mean (SD)	N	Placebo Mean (SD)	Standardised mean difference (random) 95% CI	Weight (%)	Standardised mean difference (random) 95% CI
Cibere 2004	71	129.72 (113.23)	66	129.62 (118.02)		7.7	0.00 [−0.33, 0.34]
Crolle 1980	15	0.21 (0.43)	15	1.13 (0.89)		5.6	−1.28 [−2.08, −0.49]
D'ambrosio 1981	15	0.33 (0.12)	15	1.20 (0.19)		2.8	−5.33 [−6.94, −3.71]
Drovanti 1980	40	0.95 (0.82)	40	1.88 (0.44)		7.0	−1.40 [−1.89, −0.91]
Houpt 1999	45	7.14 (4.01)	53	7.65 (4.13)		7.4	−0.12 [−0.52, 0.27]
Hughes 2002	39	7.50 (4.81)	39	7.35 (4.38)		7.2	0.03 [−0.41, 0.48]
McAlindon 2004	101	6.80 (3.30)	104	6.60 (4.20)		7.9	0.05 [−0.22, 0.33]
Pavelka 2002	101	4.61 (3.45)	101	5.03 (3.13)		7.9	−0.13 [−0.40, 0.15]
Pujalte 1980	10	1.25 (0.25)	10	2.36 (0.79)		4.4	−1.81 [−2.89, −0.74]
Reginster 2001	106	156.10 (101.90)	106	164.20 (104.50)		7.9	−0.08 [−0.35, 0.19]
Rindone 2000	49	3.20 (2.50)	49	3.40 (2.50)		7.4	−0.08 [−0.48, 0.32]
Rovati 1997	79	24.30 (19.30)	77	50.00 (22.00)		7.6	−1.24 [−1.58, −0.89]
Usha 2004	30	0.65 (0.71)	28	1.16 (0.76)		6.9	−0.68 [−1.22, −0.15]
Vajaradul 1981	28	0.18 (0.16)	26	0.69 (0.92)		6.7	−0.78 [−1.33, −0.22]
Zenk 2002	13	−74.70 (26.03)	10	−76.50 (25.10)		5.5	0.07 [−0.76, 0.89]
Total (95% CI)	742		739			100.0	−0.61 [−0.95, −0.28]

Test for heterogeneity chi-square = 121.50 df = 14 p = < 0.0001 F = 88.5%
Test for overall effect z = 3.63 p = 0.0003

−4.0 −2.0 0 2.0 4.0
Favours glucosamine   Favours placebo

Figure 10.3 Pooled results from 15 RCTs that compared glucosamine and placebo with respect to pain reduction, where pain was measured by a number of different methods (reproduced with permission from Towheed et al. 2005).

CI −0.96, −0.05). WOMAC pain, function and stiffness outcomes did not reach statistical significance. Furthermore, when only the eight studies that had adequate concealment of treatment allocation were included in the analysis, there was no benefit on pain or WOMAC function. In the four trials that compared the Rotta glucosamine to NSAID treatment, glucosamine was superior in two and equivalent in two. In two trials using the Rotta preparation, radiological progression of knee OA was significantly reduced over a three year period. In terms of numbers of reported adverse reactions, glucosamine was equivalent to placebo but much superior to NSAIDs.

The authors concluded that studies that evaluated the Rotta preparation showed glucosamine to be superior to placebo in the treatment of pain and functional impairment of symptomatic OA. However, using the WOMAC outcomes of pain, stiffness and function, no benefit over placebo was seen for any glucosamine preparation.

10.6.2 Long-term glucosamine trials

A recent study included in the Richy et al. (2003) and Towheed et al. (2005) meta-analyses that has had particular influence is that of Reginster and colleagues (2001) published in *The Lancet*. McAlindon (2001b) has referred to this trial as 'a landmark in OA research'. This was a well conducted, long-term (three year), randomised, double-blind, placebo-controlled trial of 212 patients with mild to moderate knee OA, assigned to receive either 1500 mg oral glucosamine sulphate or placebo. Outcome measures in this study included joint structural changes, (assessed by radiology at baseline, one, and three years) mean joint space width, disease-specific scores to assess joint pain and stiffness and physical function, rescue medication use (NSAID, analgesics) and adverse side effects (noted daily by patients). In the glucosamine sulphate group, 36% of patients did not complete the three year study, with a similar number of non-completers (33%) in the placebo group. There were no significant differences in reasons for withdrawal. The trial found no loss of joint space width in patients receiving glucosamine sulphate compared to those in the placebo group who saw a significant narrowing at three years. Significant improvements in pain and physical function were also seen in the glucosamine sulphate group compared to the placebo group. However, no significant differences were noted in joint stiffness between the groups. Thus it appears that joint structural changes in OA can be prevented with the use of glucosamine sulphate, and significant improvements in symptoms can be achieved. A later subgroup analysis of the same data (Bruyere et al. 2003) suggested that joint structure modification by glucosamine sulphate might be more effective in patients with less severely affected joints. This Reginster study has since been criticised by McAlindon in not having relevant radiographic data (e.g. osteophytosis, global severity).

This criticism cannot be levelled against another long-term trial included in the later meta-analyses that showed similar benefits of glucosamine supplementation on knee joint structure. Pavelka and colleagues (2002) supplemented 200 subjects with mild to moderate severity OA with glucosamine sulphate or placebo for a three year period. The dropout rate in the placebo group was 46% over three years and 35% in the glucosamine sulphate-treated patients. There were no significant differences between the groups in the reasons for dropping out. While subjects on placebo experienced significant joint space narrowing, those in the glucosamine sulphate group had no change. The difference between the groups on intention to treat analysis was significant ($p = 0.001$). Symptoms improved significantly in the glucosamine sulphate group compared to the placebo group, as measured by the Lequesne Index and the WOMAC total index and pain, function and stiffness subscales. This trial also looked at secondary radiographic features of osteoathritis, i.e. atlas osteophyte scores, finding a significant improvement in the glucosamine sulphate group compared to the placebo group ($p = 0.03$).

A subsequent pre-planned analysis of data from 319 postmenopausal women who had participated in one or other of the above studies (Pavelka et al. 2002; Reginster et al. 2001) showed that over a period of three years, there was no joint space narrowing in the glucosamine group, whereas participants in the placebo group experienced a narrowing of 0.33 mm ($p < 0.0001$, between groups) (Bruyere et al. 2004). Percent changes in the WOMAC Index over three years showed an improvement in the glucosamine sulphate group {-14.1% (95% CI $-22.2, -5.9$)} and a trend for worsening in the placebo group ($p = 0.003$, between groups). The

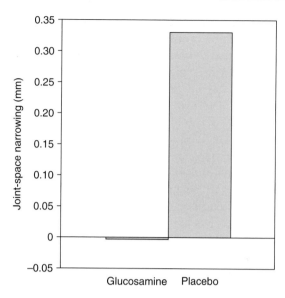

Figure 10.4   Mean joint space narrowing after three years in glucosamine sulphate and placebo groups (data taken from Bruyere et al. 2004).

prevention of joint space narrowing with glucosamine treatment is a significant finding in terms of halting disease progression (see Figure 10.4).

10.6.3   Combination trials including manganese

Das and Hammad (2000) and Leffler and colleagues (1999) added another nutritional factor in their studies. They investigated the efficacy of a combination of daily glucosmine hydrochloride (2000 mg and 1500 mg respectively), chondroitin sulphate (1600 mg and 1200 mg respectively) with manganese ascorbate (304 mg and 228 mg respectively). The rationale for the use of manganese is that this trace mineral is required for glycosaminoglycan synthesis and its intake is thought to be low in around 37% of the American population (Das & Hammad 2000). Leffler et al. (1999) studied a small group – 34 men – with degenerative joint disease of the lower back or knee, whereas Das and Hammad (2000) studied a larger group of 93 patients with knee OA. Leffler and colleagues (1999) found significant improvement in outcome measures of knee OA at 16 weeks as did Das and Hammad (2000) at four and six months. However, the latter did not find any benefit, as measured by the Lequesne Index, in patients with radiographically severe OA (n = 21). The authors assert that the fact that those with severe OA did not improve is not surprising since the proposed mechanism of action depends of the existence of cartilage in the arthritic joint (Das & Hammad 2000). The encouraging results of this excellent study that only had a 4% dropout rate, with no serious side effects, suggest that further study of this combination therapy is needed.

10.6.4   Glucosamine trials with negative findings

Although the earlier meta-analyses and studies quoted above show good support for the use of glucosamine, in the later meta-analysis with a higher number of studies (Towheed et al. 2005), the benefit was attenuated and indeed a number of trials have not shown glucosamine to have any advantage over placebo. Five such trials are described below.

Houpt and colleagues (1999) carried out a two-month RCT of glucosamine hydrochloride in 118 participants with knee OA. While they found trends in favour of the active treatment, they found no significant change in the WOMAC pain scale that was their primary endpoint.

The RCT of Rindone and colleagues (2000) also found that 1500 mg glucosamine (Applehart Laboratories, Bedford, NH; form unspecified), administered over a two month period, did not perform any better than placebo in reducing knee pain, as measured on a visual analogue scale, in 98 veteran patients who had suffered from arthritis for a mean of 12 (glucosamine group) to 14 (placebo group) years.

Hughes and Carr (2002) similarly showed no benefit of supplementation with 1500 mg/d of glucosamine sulphate in a good quality six month UK trial in patients with a wide range of degrees of severity of OA, including some with Kellgren and Lawrence grade 4 disease. Eighty patients with knee OA were randomised in a double-blind, placebo-controlled manner to receive either 1500 mg glucosamine sulphate or placebo. This study found no differences between placebo and glucosamine sulphate in patients' global pain assessment and therefore as a symptom modifier, active supplementation was no more effective than placebo. However, the authors note that their patients had, on average, considerably more severe OA than those in the trial of Reginster and colleagues (2001), where beneficial results of glucosamine supplementation were seen.

McAlindon and colleagues (2004) recruited 205 subjects with symptomatic knee OA over the Internet to a 12 week RCT with glucosamine, partly to test the feasibility of performing a RCT online. They found no difference between treatment or placebo groups with respect to pain score, stiffness, physical function, overall score and analgesic use. This trial can be criticised, however, on a number of counts: the agent was changed from glucosamine sulphate (1.5 g/d) to glucosamine hydrochloride (1.5 g/d) part way through the trial; the groups were not well matched at baseline, differing in sex, NSAID use, and body mass index. Participants tended to be taking NSAIDs or other analgesics and had more severe disease than participants in positive glucosamine trials (McAlindon et al. 2004).

Another of the studies included in the Towheed meta-analysis differed from the others in being a glucosamine discontinuation trial (Cibere et al. 2004). Recruited subjects had to have been using glucosamine for at least one month prior to randomisation and had to have experienced at least moderate relief from knee pain. They ware randomised to glucosamine sulphate (1500 mg/d) or placebo. The primary outcome measure was the proportion of disease flares experienced in the glucosamine and placebo groups. During the follow-up period of up to six months, disease flare was seen in 42% of placebo patients and 45% of glucosamine patients. No differences were found in severity of disease flare or other secondary outcomes between placebo and glucosamine patients. Adjustment of the model (Cox regression analysis) for radiographic OA severity did not significantly affect the results. Analysis of serum and urine from trial subjects showed no effect of glucosamine sulphate on biomarkers of cartilage type II collagen degradation (Cibere et al. 2005).

10.7 Possible reasons for conflicting trial results

Several methodological and other factors may contribute to the different results seen in glucosamine trials. These include:

- Differences in arthritis severity between trials at baseline
- Differences in study design
- Differences in study length
- Differences in study endpoints
- Lack of standardisation of OA diagnosis
- Different composition and quality of the supplement
- Extent of concurrent NSAID treatment
- Publication bias, i.e. small trials with negative results are unlikely to be reported.

Differences in study design, length, endpoints and methodology make direct comparison of these trials difficult. For instance, of six glucosamine trials reviewed by McAlindon and colleagues (2000), five had inadequate evidence of allocation concealment.

Results of some trials suggest that glucosamine may only be effective in mild to moderate OA. For instance, no benefit was found in patients with radiographically severe (Kellgren and Lawrence grade 4, see section 2.5.2) OA in the trial of Das and Hammad (2000), despite significant improvement in those with mild to moderate arthritis. The two high quality long-term studies of glucosamine supplementation (Pavelka et al. 2002; Reginster et al. 2001), both of which showed significant benefit in pain, physical function and joint structure compared to placebo, only included patients with mild to moderate arthritis (Kellgren and Lawrence grades 2 and 3). According to Das and Hammad (2000), the mechanism of action of glucosamine depends on the existence of cartilage in the arthritic joint, which may no longer be the case in those with radiographically severe disease. This would imply that patients recommended to try treatment with glucosamine should have OA of mild to moderate severity only. However, not all studies support such a hypothesis: Cibere et al. (2005) found no significant effect on their results when adjustment was made for radiographic OA severity.

Glucosamine and chondroitin sulphate are both obtained from shellfish or animal tissue sources and quality can vary widely depending on extraction techniques and quality control. As dietary supplements, their manufacture is not regulated, as is the case for drugs. Independent laboratory analyses have shown that many products do not contain the amounts nor meet the purity stated on the label (Das

& Hammad 2000). The form or quality of glucosamine used is not specified in some trials (e.g. Rindone et al. 2000). While most of the trials cited used glucosamine sulphate of pharmaceutical quality, this has not always been the case, leading to some uncertainty about the dose administered. A few trials have used glucosamine as the hydrochloride rather than the sulphate. A number of these have had positive results (Das & Hammad 2000; Leffler et al. 1999), suggesting that the presence of sulphate is probably not a requirement for a beneficial effect as suggested by Hoffer and colleagues (2001).

Often within glucosamine studies, rescue treatments for analgesia – commonly NSAIDs or paracetamol – are allowed, but this varies between studies and consumption may be inconsistent between and within participants. While supplementation with glucosamine sulphate increases serum sulphate concentration, ingestion of paracetamol reverses this effect as paracetamol is metabolised by sulphation (Hoffer et al. 2001). Since sulphate depletion inhibits GAG synthesis, concurrent use of paracetamol could confound results. No study has taken account of this effect. In the opinion of Pavelka and colleagues (2002), consumption of analgesics is not a valid outcome measure in OA trials.

10.8 Topical treatment

Though oral glucosamine and chondroitin appear to have beneficial structural and symptomatic effects, evidence shows that the dose reaching the articular cartilage is a fraction of the percentage of the oral dose (Cohen et al. 2003). Cohen and colleagues (2003) therefore studied the efficacy of a topical glucosamine and chondroitin cream. The cream contained 30 mg/g glucosamine sulphate, 50 mg/g chondroitin sulphate, 140 mg/g shark cartilage, 10–30% of which is chondroitin sulphate, 32 mg/g camphor and 9 mg/g peppermint oil. Chondroitin sulphate has been shown to be effective as a transfer agent for dermal drugs. Fifty-nine subjects with knee OA completed the eight-week, placebo-controlled trial, the placebo being a simple cosmetic cream with a lesser amount of peppermint oil included to ensure that both preparations had a similar smell. On average, taking into account transdermal absorption (20–40%), between 60–120 mg glucosamine sulphate and 156–300 mg of chondroitin sulphate was delivered daily through topical application. This application was found to have a significant effect in relieving knee OA pain, with improvements evident within four weeks. Adverse events were equally distributed between treatment and placebo groups. While it is possible that peppermint oil and camphor may have been partly responsible for the analgesic effect, this study shows the potential benefit of topical creams. This is a fruitful area for research.

10.9 Comparison with NSAIDs

A number of studies have compared glucosamine sulphate and chondroitin sulphate to NSAIDs in terms of pain relief. In the Cochrane Review of Towheed et al. (2005) comparison of glucosamine sulphate with NSAIDs (mostly ibuprofen) in four trials showed glucosamine to be superior in two and equivalent in two. Adverse events and dropout rates were much higher in the NSAID treatment groups than in the glucosamine sulphate groups (McAlindon 2001a; Towheed et al. 2005) showing the superior tolerance to glucosamine treatment. Chondroitin sulphate was compared to diclofenac by Morreale and colleagues (1996) in 146 patients with knee OA. At days 60 and 90, reduction of pain was greater in the chondroitin group.

10.10   Safety issues

10.10.1   Adverse events

Glucosamine sulphate and chondroitin both appear to be safe to use (McAlindon et al. 2000). Side effects that have been reported can be classified into three types (US General Accounting Office 2001):

- Gastrointestinal: stomach ache, nausea, indigestion, constipation, heartburn and diarrhoea
- Neurological: headache and drowsiness
- Dermatological: rash, itch and flushing

Peer reviewed trials of glucosamine and chondroitin to date include around 1500 participants who have taken oral glucosamine or chondroitin, some for up to three years. Adverse event rates reported in the treatment groups show no significant difference from those of the placebo groups (Richy et al. 2003). In the four major studies that provided details on serious adverse events, the observed rates were low and statistically identical between treatment and placebo groups (Richy et al. 2003).

Studies comparing glucosamine with NSAIDs show that it is substantially safer, particularly with respect to GI toxicity (McAlindon 2001a).

10.10.2   Contraindications

People who have an allergy to shellfish should avoid these supplements. Although chitin is a carbohydrate derived from this source and no protein should be present, allergic reactions may still occur. Pregnant and lactating women should also avoid these supplements owing to a lack of clinical studies in this patient group.

Some studies have indicated that patients with prostate cancer have increased concentrations of chondroitin in prostate cancer tissue. High levels are predictive of poor prognosis, thus supplements containing chondroitin should not be used (Ricciardelli et al. 1997, 1999).

10.10.3   Caution with usage

Chondroitin has a similar structure to heparin (an anticoagulant). If these two products are taken in combination, an increase in bleeding time may be seen in some individuals. It is therefore important that any individual taking chondroitin (or a related substance, dermatan sulphate, sometimes called chondroitin B sulphate) alongside heparin or daily aspirin should frequently have their blood clotting times checked (US General Accounting Office 2001).

It has been suggested that patients with diabetes mellitus should exercise caution when using glucosamine. Glucosamine is widely used to increase flux through the hexosamine phosphate pathway and may therefore affect insulin secretion or action (Monauni et al. 2000). Monauni and colleagues (2000) acutely infused glucosamine at a low and high dose into 10 healthy subjects. They found a mild dysfunction in β-cell secretion and at a higher dose, impairment in glucose utilisation under hyperglycaemic or hyperinsulinaemic conditions. Rovati et al. (1999), however, cast doubt on the relevance of this observation, saying that the majority of correlations drawn are based on animal studies or have used glucosamine infusions giving considerably higher blood concentrations of glucosamine than those that can be achieved therapeutically by the oral route (Rovati et al. 1999).

A tendency for fasting blood glucose to *decrease* with glucosamine was seen in the long-term (three year) study by Reginster and colleagues (2001) that recruited 212 participants. In the three year trial of Pavelka and colleagues (2002) that randomised 200 participants, four subjects developed diabetes mellitus during the study but three were in the placebo group. Scroggie and colleagues (2003) also demonstrated that oral glucosamine does not result in clinically significant alterations in glucose metabolism. Their study showed that among 38 patients given either 1500 mg glucosamine sulphate and 1200 mg chondroitin sulphate or placebo over 90 days, mean Haemoglobin A_1c (HBA$_1$c, a long-term indicator of glycaemic control) concentrations did not change significantly.

Clinical trial data on 3063 human subjects involved in glucosamine trials were reviewed by Anderson and colleagues (2005). They found no evidence that glucosamine affected glucose metabolism and concluded that glucosamine is safe under current conditions of use. Thus it appears that fears of adverse effects on glycaemic control are unfounded.

There is a possibility that users of glucosamine may be at risk from subtle compromises of immune response, and immune activity should be assessed in long-term studies (Ma et al. 2002).

10.11 Further studies

Though it is encouraging that a number of trials with these agents have had positive outcomes, particularly for mild to moderate arthritis, conflicting results show the need for large scale, long-term, rigorous studies, all authors agreeing on this. It is also of some concern that studies that have been associated with positive findings have largely been those with pharmaceutical sponsorship. Clear, clinically relevant, endpoints are required to determine the optimal dose and route of administration of glucosamine and chondroitin sulphate if they are shown to have beneficial effects in OA.

Further research should address several unanswered questions raised by Towheed et al. (2005) before glucosamine (and chondroitin) can become a first line treatment for osteoarthritis:

- What is the long-term safety and efficacy of glucosamine and chondroitin?
- Is there any further benefit of mixed glucosamine preparations such as those including chondroitin sulphate?
- Are the different glucosamine preparations equally effective? (Their content and purity need to be established)
- Is glucosamine hydrochloride equivalent to glucosamine sulphate?
- Is glucosamine helpful for all of those with osteoarthritis or is the efficacy dependent on joint involvement, disease severity and genetic factors?
- What is the optimal dose and route of administration to maximise efficacy and minimise toxicity?
- How do glucosamine and chondroitin work?
- Can glucosamine modify disease progression?

10.12   Preliminary results from GAIT

At the time of writing (October 2005), a preliminary report of the first stage of a large, long-term, US trial has appeared in abstract form. The Glucosamine/chondroitin Arthritis Intervention Trial (GAIT) is sponsored by the US National Institutes of Health (NIH) and initiated by two of its institutes, the National Center for Complementary and Alternative Medicine (NCCAM), and the National Institute of Arthritis and Musculoskeletal and Skin Diseases (NIAMS). The study was set up to assess short-term effectiveness (24 weeks) on pain and joint function and long-term (a further 18 months) effects on progression of knee OA, in comparison with a Cox-2 inhibitor. This multicentre trial randomised 1583 male and female participants of ≥ 40 years of age with knee pain of at least six months' duration and X-ray evidence of knee OA (Kellgren–Lawrence grades 2 or 3). Participants were randomly assigned (double blind) to receive treatment for 24 weeks with 50% continuing on treatment for an additional 18 months. The five treatment groups were:

- Glucosamine hydrochloride alone, 500 mg three times a day (G)
- Sodium chondroitin sulphate alone (CS), 400 mg three times a day
- Glucosamine hydrochloride and chondroitin sulphate at the above doses (G + CS)
- Celecoxib 200 mg daily (COX, an NSAID)
- Placebo (P)

All patients were allowed to use up to 4000 mg acetaminophen (paracetamol) daily as rescue analgesia, except within 24 hours of study visits. The primary outcome measure was a 20% improvement from baseline in WOMAC pain at week 24.

Baseline characteristics of recruited subjects were as follows: mean age 58.6 years, BMI 31.7 kg/m^2, OA symptoms 10 years, 64% female, summed mean WOMAC Pain 236 ± 73 mm, 59% Kellgren–Lawrence Grade 2, 78% in 125–300 mm WOMAC Pain stratum and were evenly distributed across all arms.

Table 10.1 Response rates in GAIT by treatment group and pain stratum (adapted from Clegg et al. 2005).

Treatment	All patients (%)	WOMAC pain 125–300 mm (%)	WOMAC pain 301–400 mm (%)
P	60.1	61.7	54.3
Cox-2	70.1[1]	70.3[3]	69.4[4]
G	64.0	63.6	65.7
CS	65.4	66.5	61.4
G + CS	66.6[2]	62.9	79.2[5]

[1] p = 0.008, Treatment vs. P; [2] p = 0.09, Treatment vs. P; [3] p = 0.04, Treatment vs. P; [4] p = 0.06, Treatment vs. P; [5] p = 0.002, Treatment vs. P

The first, 24-month, phase of the study was completed by 1258 subjects, 80% of those randomised. Results of the 'intention to treat' analysis from the first phase are summarised in Table 10.1.

While the placebo response was high – 60% of all patients showing a 20% improvement from baseline in WOMAC Pain – responses significantly better than placebo were seen both with celecoxib and with the combination of glucosamine and chondroitin, but the latter only reached significance in the group with severe pain at baseline, i.e. WOMAC Pain 301–400 mm. In patients with less severe pain (WOMAC Pain 125–300 mm), the improvement seen was not significantly different from that with placebo. In the group with more severe pain at baseline, secondary outcomes of 50% WOMAC Pain response, WOMAC Stiffness, WOMAC Function, health assessment questionnaire, patient assessments and use of rescue acetaminophen all demonstrated changes consistent with the primary outcome. Adverse events were mild and evenly distributed among treatment groups. The authors concluded that combination of glucosamine hydrochloride and chondroitin sulphate is effective in treating moderate to severe pain in OA. They suggest that the lack of response in those with mild pain may be due to a floor effect that limits the ability to detect response.

We await with interest the full published report of this trial and the results from the longer-term phase which will investigate the effect of glucosamine and chondroitin on progression of knee OA. This trial will make a significant contribution to the evidence base for the use of these supplements.

10.13 Conclusions and recommendations for glucosamine and chondroitin use

Although recommendations will need to be modified in the light of new data, on balance the current evidence suggests that a therapeutic trial of supplementation with glucosamine and chondroitin sulphate is warranted, at least in individuals with moderate to severe knee pain obliged to resort to NSAIDs. The possible benefits with respect to pain and disease progression and lack of apparent side effects even in long-term studies, suggest that the only risk is to the pocket.

Table 10.2 Composition of some glucosamine and chondroitin supplements available in the UK.

Product	GS + CS per capsule/tablet	Other ingredients	Dose per day	Recommended daily dose provides
Healthspan, Chondromax	GS 500 mg + CS (marine) 400 mg	—	3 per day	1500 mg GS 1200 mg CS
Pharma Nord, Bio-glucosamine Plus	GS 250 mg + CS 200 mg	—	2–3 twice a day with food	1000–1500 mg GS 400–600 mg CS
Lamberts, GS 750 mg	GS 750 mg	—	2 per day	1500 mg GS
Lamberts, Vegetarian Glucosamine	GHCl 750 mg	—	2 per day	1500 mg GHCl
Lamberts, GS and CS Complex	GS 500 mg + CS (marine) 100 mg	—	3 per day	1500 mg GS 300 mg CS
Holland and Barrett, High strength C/G Complex	500 mg GS + 400 mg CS	Manganese 1.67 mg Vitamin C 167 mg	3 per day	1500 mg GS 1200 mg CS
Holland and Barrett, GS 1000 mg	1000 mg GS	—	1–2 per day	1000–2000 mg GS
Holland and Barrett, Advance C-Jointin	GS 1000 mg + CS 200 mg	Vitamin E 6.7 mg Vitamin C 60 mg Manganese 1 mg Boron 1.5 mg EPO 250 mg MSM 750 mg	3 per day	1000 mg GS 200 mg CS

GS: glucosamine sulphate; GHCl: glucosamine hydrochloride; CS: chondroitin sulphate; EPO: Evening Primrose Oil; MSM: methylsulphonylmethane.

From the quoted studies, it seems that a daily dose of 1500 mg glucosamine (sulphate or hydrochloride) should be recommended for patients with OA (no research has been carried out in RA patients) and should be taken for a minimum of one month, although a few studies showed effects in as little as two weeks (Richy et al. 2003). There is little evidence on effective dose in the case of chondroitin sulphate though 1200 mg is often used (Deal & Moskowitz 1999; Leeb et al. 2000). The combination of 1500 mg glucosamine (as hydrochloride) and 1200 mg chondroitin sulphate taken daily for six months showed significant benefits in those with moderate to severe knee pain compared to either agent alone (Clegg et al. 2006), suggesting synergistic effects. Section 10.14 outlines the factors that should be considered if choosing to supplement with glucosamine or chondroitin.

Those wishing to increase their manganese intake can do so by drinking tea, the richest source of manganese in the UK diet.

10.14 Supplements of glucosamine sulphate and chondroitin available

In the UK and USA, glucosamine and chondroitin are considered as food supplements as opposed to being classed as drugs as they are in many European countries. This has a number of drawbacks, the most notable being that dietary supplements are far more variable in their composition than drug formulations, thus potential benefits will vary depending on the composition of the glucosamine sulphate supplement (McAlindon et al. 2001b). In fact, studies in the USA have revealed that a number of preparations claiming to contain certain doses of glucosamine or chondroitin sulphate have significantly less (or none) of the dosages described (Deal & Moskowitz 1999). Though glucosamine sulphate is the form that has been used in most studies, the beneficial results seen in GAIT, the largest study to date, were achieved with glucosamine hydrochloride, suggesting that it is the glucosamine part of the molecule that matters and not the associated anion. Doses may vary between supplements, as may their form (liquid, capsule or pill). The best advice is to try to find a pharmaceutical grade product rather than one marketed as a nutritional supplement, or at the very least to ask the manufacturer for quality assurance data on the product you plan to recommend or take. A 1500 mg dose of glucosamine sulphate of the drug formulation manufactured by Rotta, as described in 10.3, has been approved for once daily prescription treatment for OA in many European countries and elsewhere in the world (Reginster et al. 2001). In Australia, the Australian Therapeutic Goods Administration regulates glucosamine products to acceptably high levels of purity (Cumming 1999). Supplements may also incorporate other ingredients e.g. n-3 fatty acids, chondroitin, vitamin A, C and E.

Table 10.2 shows some examples of readily available glucosamine and chondroitin products in the UK, though whether any of these contains pharmaceutical grade chondroitin sulphate is unknown: potential users are advised to check.

References

Anderson JW, Nicolosi RJ, Borzelleca JF (2005) Glucosamine effects in humans: a review of effects on glucose metabolism, side effects, safety considerations and efficacy. *Food and Chemical Toxicology* 43(2), 187–201.

Bassleer C, Rovati L, Franchimont P (1998) Stimulation of proteoglycan production by glucosamine sulfate in chondrocytes isolated from human osteoarthritic articular cartilage *in vitro*. *Osteoarthritis and Cartilage* 6(6), 427–34.

Barthe L, Woodley J, Lavit M, Przybylski C, Philibert C, Houin G (2004) *In vitro* intestinal degradation and absorption of chondroitin sulfate, a glycosaminoglycan drug. *Arzneimittel Forschung* 54(5), 286–92.

Bruyere O, Honore A, Ethgen O, Rovati LC, Giacovelli G, Henrotin YE, Seidal L, Reginster JY (2003) Correlation between radiographic severity of knee osteoarthritis and future disease progression. Results from a 3-year prospective, placebo-controlled study evaluating the effect of glucosamine sulphate. *Osteoarthritis and Cartilage* 11(1), 1–5.

Bruyere O, Pavelka P, Rovati LC, Deroisy R, Olejarova M, Gatterova J, Giacovelli G, Reginster JY (2004) Glucosamine sulphate reduces osteoarthritis progression in postmenopausal women with knee osteoarthritis: evidence from two 3-year studies. *Menopause* 11, 138–43.

Cibere J, Kopec JA, Thorne A, Singer J, Canvin J, Robinson DB, Pope J, Hong P, Grant E, Esdaile JM (2004) Randomized, double-blind, placebo-controlled glucosamine discontinuation trial in knee osteoarthritis. *Arthritis and Rheumatism* 51(5), 738–45.

Cibere J, Thorne A, Kopec JA, Singer J, Canvin J, Robinson DB, Pope J, Hong P, Grant E, Lobanok T, Ionescu M, Poole AR, Esdaile JM (2005) Glucosamine sulfate and cartilage type II collagen degradation in patients with knee osteoarthritis: randomized discontinuation trial results employing biomarkers. *Journal of Rheumatology* 32(5), 896–902.

Clegg DO, Reda DJ, Harris CL, Klein MA, O'Dell JR, Hooper MM, Bradley JD, Bingham CO 3rd, Weisman MH, Jackson CG, Lane NE, Cush JJ, Moreland LW, Schumacher HR Jr, Oddis CV, Wolfe F, Molitor JA, Yocum DE, Schnitzer TJ, Furst DE, Sawitzke AD, Shi H, Brandt KD, Moskowitz RW, Williams HJ (2006) Glucosamine, chondroitin sulfate, and the two in combination for painful knee osteoarthritis. *New England Journal of Medicine* 354, 795–808.

Cohen M, Wolfe R, Mai T, Lewis D (2003) A randomised, double-blind, placebo-controlled trial of a topical cream containing glucosamine sulfate, chondroitin sulfate and camphor for osteoarthritis of the knee. *Journal of Rheumatology* 30(3), 523–28.

Cumming A (1999) Glucosamine in osteoarthritis, Letter to the Editor. *The Lancet* 354, 1640–41.

Curtis CL, Harwood JL, Cent CM, Caterson B (2004) Biological basis for the benefit of neutrachemical supplementation in arthritis. *Drug Discovery Today* 15, 9(4), 165–72.

Das A Jr, Hammad TA (2000) Efficacy of a combination of FCHG49 glucosamine hydrochloride TRH122 low molecular weight sodium chondroitin sulphate and manganese ascorbate in the management of knee osteoarthritis. *Osteoarthritis and Cartilage* 8(5), 343–50.

Deal CL, Moskowitz RW (1999) Nutraceuticals as theraputic agents in osteoarthritis. The role of glucosamine, chondroitin sulfate, and collagen hydrolysate. *Rheumatology Disease Clinics of North America* 25(2), 379–95.

Hoffer LJ, Kaplan LN, Hamadeh MJ, Grigoriu AC, Baron M (2001) Sulfate could mediate the therapeutic effect of glucosamine sulfate. *Metabolism* 50(7), 767–70.

Houpt JB, McMillan R, Wein C, Paget-Delio SD (1999) Effect of hydrochloride in the treatment of pain of osteoarthritis of the knee. *Journal of Rheumatology* 26, 2423–2430.

Hughes R, Carr A (2002) A randomized, double-blind, placebo-controlled trial of glucosamine sulphate as an analgesic in osteoarthritis of the knee. *Rheumatology* 41(3), 279–84.

Leeb BF, Schweitzer H, Montag K, Smolen JS (2000) A metaanalysis of chondroitin sulphate in the treatment of osteoarthritis. *Journal of Rheumatology* 27(1), 205–11.

Leffler CT, Philippi AF, Leffler SG, Mosure JC, Kim PD (1999) Glucosamine, chondroitin, and manganese ascorbate for degenerative joint disease of the knee or low back: a randomised, double-blind, placebo-controlled pilot study. *Military Medicine* 164(2), 85–91.

Ma L, Rudert WA, Harnaha J, Wright M, Machen J, Lakomy R, Qian S, Lu L, Robbins PD, Trucco M, Giannoukakis N (2002) Immunosuppressive effects of glucosamine. *Journal of Biological Chemistry* 18, 277(42), 39343–49.

McAlindon TE, LaValley MP, Gulin JP, Felson DT (2000) Glucosamine and chondroitin for treatment of osteoarthritis – a systematic quality assessment and meta-analysis. *Journal of the American Medical Association* 283(11), 1469–75.

McAlindon TE (2001a) Glucosamine and chondroitin for osteoarthritis? In: *Bulletin on the Rheumatic Diseases* vol 50, no 7 (DL Conn, ed) Atlanta, The Arthritis Foundation, ISSN 0007 5248.

McAlindon TE (2001b) Glucosamine for osteoarthritis: dawn of a new era? *The Lancet* 357(9252), 247–48.

McAlindon TE, Formica M, LaValley M, Lehmer M, Kabbara K (2004) Effectiveness of glucosamine for symptoms of knee osteoarthritis: results from an internet-based randomized double-blind controlled trial. *American Journal of Medicine* 117, 643–49.

Meininger CJ, Kelly KA, Li H, Haynes TE, Wu G (2000) Glucosamine inhibits inducible nitric oxide synthesis. *Biochemical and Biophysical Research Communications* **279**, 234–39.

Monauni T, Zenti MG, Cretti A, Daniels MC, Targher G, Caruso B, Caputo M, McClain D, Del Prato S, Giaccari A, Muggeo M, Bonora E, Bonadonna RC (2000) Effects of glucosamine infusion on insulin secretion and insulin action in humans. *Diabetes* **49**, 926–35.

Morreale P, Manopulo R, Galatti M, Boccanera L, Saponati G, Bocchi L (1996) Comparison of the anti-inflammatory efficacy of chondroitin sulphate and diclofenac sodium in patients with knee osteoarthritis. *Journal of Rheumatology* **23**, 1385–91.

National Center for Complementary and Alternative Medicine (2001) Glucosamine/chondroitin Arthritis Intervention Trial www.nccam.nih.gov/nccam/fi/concepts

Pavelka K, Gatterova J, Olejarova M, Machacek S, Giacovelli G, Rovati LC (2002) Glucosamine sulphate use and delay of progression of knee osteoarthritis; a 3-year, randomised, placebo-controlled, double-blind study. *Archives of Internal Medicine* **14**, 162(18), 2113–23.

Reginster JY, Deroisy R, Rovati LC, Lee RL, Lejeune E, Bruyere O, Giacovelli G, Henrotin Y, Dacre JE, Gossett C (2001) Long-term effects of glucosamine sulphate on osteoarthritis progression: a randomized, placebo-controlled clinical trial. *The Lancet* **357**, 251–56.

Ricciardelli C, Mayne K, Sykes PJ, Raymond WA, McCaul K, Marshall VR, Tilley WD, Skinner JM, Horsfall DJ (1997) Elevated stromal chondroitin sulfate glycosaminoglycan predicts progression in early-stage prostate cancer. *Clinical Cancer Research* **3**, 983–92.

Ricciardelli C, Quinn DI, Raymond WA, McCaul K, Sutherland PD, Stricker PD, Grygiel JJ, Sutherland RL, Marshall VR, Tilley WD, Horsfall DJ (1999) Elevated levels of peritumoral chondroitin sulfate are predictive of poor prognosis in patients treated by radical prostatectomy for early-stage prostate cancer. *Cancer Research* **59**, 2324–28.

Richy F, Bruyere O, Ethgen O, Cucherat M, Henrotin Y, Reginster (2003) Structural and symptomatic efficacy of glucosamine and chondroitin in knee osteoarthritis: a comprehensive meta-analysis. *Archives of Internal Medicine* **163**(13), 1514–22.

Rindone JP, Hiller D, Collacott E, Nordhaugen N, Arriola G (2000) Randomized, controlled trial of glucosamine for treating osteoarthritis of the knee. *Western Journal of Medicine* **172**, 91–94.

Rovati LC, Annefeld M, Giacovelli G, Schmid, Setnikar I (1999) Correspondence: Glucosamine in osteoarthritis. *The Lancet* **354**, 1640.

Scroggie DA, Albright A, Harris MD (2003) The effect of glucosamine-chondroitin supplementation of glycosylated hemoglobin levels in patients with type 2 diabetes mellitus: a placebo-controlled, double-blinded, randomised clinical trial. *Archives of Internal Medicine* **163**(13), 1587–90.

Setnikar I, Rovati L (2001) Absorption, distribution, metabolism and excretion of glucosamine sulphate. *Arzneim Forsch Drug Res* **51**(II), 699–725.

Shikhman AR, Kuhn K, Alaaeddine N, Lotz M (2001) N-acetylglucosamine prevents IL-1 beta-mediated activation of human chondrocytes. *Journal of Immunology* **166**, 5155–60.

Stryer L (1988) *Biochemistry*, 3rd edition. New York, WH Freeman and Co p. 276.

Towheed TE, Maxwell L, Anastassiades TP, Shea B, Houpt J, Robinson V, Hochberg M, Wells G (2005) Glucosamine therapy for treating osteoarthritis. *The Cochrane Database of Systematic Reviews*, Issue **2**. Art No, CD002946.pub2.DOI, 10. 1002/14651858.CD002946.pub2.

US General Accounting Office (GAO) (2001) GAO-01-1129 'Anti-Aging' Health Products, Appendix II, Known Claims, Adverse Effects, Contraindications, and Interactions of Herbal and Speciality Supplements, pp. 28–35. US General Accounting Office. www.ods.od.nih.gov/pubs/gao-01-1129.pdf

11 Other foods or supplements marketed for arthritis relief

11.1 Introduction

There are many supplements on the market – other than those discussed in previous chapters – that are claimed to help arthritis, but there is little evidence published in peer-reviewed journals to support their use. Patients often get their information on such supplements from the internet. However, most sites easily accessed by consumers are those of profit-based companies advertising alternative products with claimed efficacy that is often unsupported in peer-reviewed literature (Suarez-Almazor et al. 2001). Some foods or supplements that patients may well be using in the hope of improving their arthritis will be discussed below.

11.2 Green tea extracts

Green tea is an extract of the tea plant *Camellia sinensis*: unlike black tea, it is not fermented. It contains a group of polyphenols known as catechins, the most abundant of which is the gallate ester, epigallocatechin gallate (EGCG) (Adcocks et al. 2002). The catechins are both antioxidant and anti-inflammatory, being able to inhibit tumor necrosis factor (TNF) synthesis: they can also inhibit matrix metalloproteinases, limiting angiogenesis (Adcocks et al. 2002).

A polyphenolic fraction from green tea given orally to mice significantly reduced the incidence of collagen-induced arthritis and markedly reduced the expression of inflammatory mediators such as cyclo-oxygenase 2, IFN-γ and TNF-α in arthritic joints (Haqqi et al. 1999). In an *in vitro* system, micromolar concentrations of catechins (0.2–20 µmol/L), particularly those containing a gallate ester (e.g. ECCG and epicatechin gallate, ECG) were effective at inhibiting proteoglycan and type II collagen breakdown in human and bovine cartilage (Adcocks et al. 2002). The chondroprotective effect was distinct from the anti-inflammatory effect expressed through inhibition of cytokine synthesis. The authors speculate that an antiproteolytic effect may have been involved (Adcocks et al. 2002). This belief has been reinforced by subsequent work that has shown that catechin gallate esters from green tea, namely ECGC and ECG, can potently inhibit certain aggrecanases (ADAMTS-1, -4 and -5) that cause degradation of cartilage aggrecan, a large aggregating proteoglycan that, with type II collagen, is the major constituent of articular catrtilage (Vankemmelbeke et al. 2003). In fact, the catechin gallate esters were able to inhibit the aggrecanases ADAMTS-1, -4 and -5, at considerably lower concentrations (0.002–2 µmol/L) than required for the inhibition of the collagenases. As consumption of green tea can give plasma concentrations of the catechin gallate esters of 0.1–5 µmol/L with a half life of a few hours, this effect on aggrecanases, and to a lesser extent on the collagenases, may protect cartilage integrity if a similar concentration can reach the joint (Vankemmelbeke et al. 2003).

Thus there is potential significant benefit to arthritis sufferers from drinking green tea in the prevention of progression of cartilage damage and reduction of inflammation. Human trials, particularly in early OA, are warranted. In the meantime, as green tea infusions have been drunk for many centuries without harm, we can confidently recommend this course of action.

11.3 Ginger

Ginger (Zingiberaceae family) has been used in Ayurvedic and Chinese medicine for over 2000 years as an anti-inflammatory treatment for rheumatism and for nausea and travel sickness (Altman & Marcussen 2001). There are many forms of ginger extracts available, containing several hundred different constituents including gingeroles, β-carotene, capsaicin, caffeic acid, curcumin and salicylate (Altman & Marcussen 2001). The major pungent compounds in ginger are the gingerols, of which 6-gingerol appears to be responsible for the characteristic taste (Thorne Research 2003). These can be converted to shogaols, zingerone and paradol.

There are three main mechanisms through which ginger may influence OA and RA:

(1) Reduction of inflammation by inhibiting both the cyclooxygenase and lipoxygenase pathways and leukotriene synthesis (Altman & Marcussen 2001)
(2) By reducing the production of TNF-α through inhibition of gene expression (shown in human OA synoviocytes and chondrocytes) (Altman & Marcussen 2001)
(3) By analgesic effects of ginger components, 6-gingerol and 6-shogaol (Thorn Research 2003)

Studies have been carried out addressing the influence of ginger extract on rheumatism (Srivastava & Mustafa 1989, 1992). Although both showed that ginger afforded pain relief and reduced joint swelling in OA and RA, they were of poor scientific design. Three later studies have used a more rigorous study design (Altman & Marcussen 2001; Bliddal et al. 2000; Wigler et al. 2003).

Bliddal and colleagues (2000) studied the influence of ginger extract compared with ibuprofen and placebo treatments in 67 patients with OA of the knee and hip. The patients were involved in a three-way crossover study, with one-week washout between each treatment. Patients were treated three times a day with one of:

(1) 170 mg/d ginger extract
(2) Ibuprofen 400 mg
(3) Placebo

Fifty-six patients completed the study. Several outcome measures were assessed. A significantly better effect of ibuprofen and ginger than placebo was found, but only in the first treatment period and not in the study overall.

Wigler et al. (2003) studied the effects of 1000 mg/d ginger extract (Zintona EC) on 29 patients with symptomatic knee arthritis, in a six-month crossover design. There was a very high dropout rate, 65%, within this already small study. During the first three months of the study, the ginger extract was no better than placebo, but at the end of six months, three months after crossover, the ginger extract group showed a significant superiority over the placebo group in terms of pain and handicap assessed on a visual analogue scale (Wigler et al. 2003).

Altman and Marcussen (2001) studied a far larger patient group (261 OA patients) over a six-week treatment period, though 22% dropped out during the study. Patients were randomised to receive either a placebo (coconut oil) or one capsule containing 255 mg of ginger extract (EV.EXT 77 of *Zingiber officinale* and *Alpina galanga* rhizomes) twice daily. Outcome measures were assessed at baseline, two and six weeks. A significant reduction in knee pain on standing and after walking 50 feet was found in the group taking the ginger extract compared to the group taking placebo, but no influence was apparent upon quality of life or analgesic use.

Gastrointestinal effects, such as bad taste and dyspepsia, were noted by significantly more patients taking ginger than placebo (59 *vs.* 21) in the Altman and Marcussen study (2001). Similar side effects were seen in the study of Bliddal and colleagues (2000). These side effects were not deemed to be serious by the study investigators. Ginger is on the US Food and Drug Administration's 'generally recognised as safe' list, therefore ginger extracts should be considered to have a good safety profile. Though there are no known drug interactions, individuals on anticoagulant therapy should use ginger supplements with caution as ginger may have an effect on platelets (Thorne Research 2003).

According to the Thorne Research monograph (2003), a typical dose of ginger is 1–4 g/d taken in divided doses, though the form of ginger is not specified. Another internet source suggests a maximum dose of 2 g/d powdered ginger or 400 mg/d dry extract in three divided doses. Prospective users should be cautious, as there is no validated recommendation as to optimal dose or form.

Though at the moment there is insufficient evidence to support the use of ginger extract, further trials may be warranted.

11.4   New Zealand green-lipped mussel

The incidence of arthritis in New Zealand coastal dwelling Maoris is said to be very low owing to their anti-inflammatory diet of raw green-lipped mussels (NZGLM) *Perna canaliculus* (Cho et al. 2003). The active ingredients of the mussels have not yet been identified, though they contain some five to six types of n-3 polyunsaturated fatty acids (PUFAs), including eicosapentaenoic acid (EPA), docosahexaenoic acid (DHA), docosapentaenoic acid (DPA), plus sterols and antioxidants that together have an anti-inflammatory effect that has been demonstrated in both human and animal arthritis (Cho et al. 2003; Halpern 2000). A number of double-blind, randomised placebo-controlled trials in RA and OA were carried out in the 1980s with an extract of NZGLM known as Seatone (Darlington & Ramsey 1993). These trials had mixed results, some showing benefit while others showed no effect (Larkin et al. 1985). The most impressive results were achieved by Gibson and colleagues (1980). They carried out a placebo-controlled trial in 28 patients with RA and 38 patients with OA. Compared to the control groups, there was a net improvement of 37% in the rheumatoid group, which was significant with respect to articular and functional indices, and a net improvement of 36% in the osteoarthritic group, which was significant in terms of pain, functional index and time taken to walk 50 feet (Gibson & Gibson 1981). However, another well designed randomised placebo-controlled trial in 47 RA patients reported by Caughey et al. (1983), found no benefit of a dose of 1050 mg/d green-lipped mussel extract over placebo. After the first six weeks, during which naproxen was given in addition to the mussel extract, there was a very high dropout rate from both treatment and placebo groups.

A lipid-rich extract (Lyprinol®) prepared by supercritical extraction of freeze dried NZGLM with the addition of antioxidants has stabilised the activity and enabled more consistent results to be obtained. This extract has shown inhibition of leukotriene (LTB$_4$) biosynthesis by polymorphonuclear cells *in vitro* and of prostaglandin PGE$_2$ by activated macrophages (Halpern 2000). Rats treated orally with Lyprinol® were able to avoid an arthritic response to arthritis-inducing substances while human clinical studies have demonstrated significant anti-inflammatory activity (Halpern 2000).

More recently, Cho and colleagues (2003) studied the efficacy of Lyprinol® in a group of 60 Korean patients aged 40–75 with osteoarthritis. This was an open clinical trial with no placebo group. Only 43 of 60 enrolled participants completed the full eight-week trial. Although the study concluded that 80% of patients reported pain relief and improvement of joint function after eight weeks of treatment, the poor study design prevents clear conclusions being drawn.

A recent systematic review of the use of green-lipped mussel in clinical trials has concluded that there is little compelling evidence for its use in OA or RA (Cobb & Ernst 2005).

Well-designed studies with Lyprinol® and Seatone are required to establish its efficacy and safety. At the moment, there is insufficient evidence to recommend this supplement for use in either OA or RA patients.

11.5 Methylsulfonylmethane (MSM)

Methylsulfonylmethane (MSM) is a sulphur-containing compound made naturally in the body from sulphur-containing amino acids (Figure 11.1). It can also be found in foods such as fruit, alfalfa, corn, tomatoes, tea, coffee and milk (Parcell 2002). There is no recommended dietary allowance (RDA) or reference nutrient intake (RNI) for sulphur as we receive an adequate amount from dietary protein, largely in the form of the sulphur amino acids methionine and cysteine. Legumes are the only protein foods that have inadequate amounts of sulphur amino acids.

The rationale for using MSM in arthritis is presumably based on the requirement for sulphur in the formation of connective tissues. In section 10.2, we explained that cartilage proteoglycan was made up of keratan sulphate and chondroitin

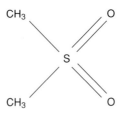

Figure 11.1   Structure of methylsulfonylmethane (MSM).

sulphate chains. Thus sulphate is important for cartilage formation, as shown by the fact that a reduction in sulphate concentration from 0.3 mM (physiological) to 0.2 mM in the medium resulted in a 33% reduction of glycosaminoglycan synthesis in human articular cartilage *in vitro* (van der Kraan et al. 1990). However, we now know that sulphur metabolism may be perturbed in arthritic disease: sulphur concentration in arthritic equine cartilage was found to be only one-third the level of that in normal cartilage (Rizzo et al. 1995). In patients with OA of the hip, levels of one of the disaccharide isomers of keratan sulphate were significantly lower in synovial fluid from patients with advanced disease than in those with early stage disease (Yamada et al. 2000).

Patients with established RA have an impaired ability to oxidise sulphur, which appears to predispose to persistent clinical disease, as evidenced by the following studies. In 114 patients with RA, 72% had poor capacity to oxidise sulphur-containing drugs compared with 37% of age matched healthy controls (Emery et al. 1992a). Sulphur oxidation capacity was tested in 54 patients with recent onset symmetrical polyarthritis who were followed up at one and four years (Emery et al. 1992b). The prevalence of poor sulphur oxidation in those with persistent disease was 69% at one year but had risen to 74% at four years, compared to 31% in those who were asymptomatic at this point (p < 0.01). In a later study, plasma inorganic sulphate was found to be significantly depressed in RA patients compared to controls with non-RA disease {85 (SD 36) *vs.* 604 (SD 412) µmol/L; p < 0.001} (Bradley et al. 1994). In the RA patients, synovial fluid sulphate was also significantly reduced compared to the level in non-RA controls {202 (SD 117) *vs.* 1041 (SD 700) µmol/L; p < 0.001} (Bradley et al. 1994). Interestingly, fasting cysteine levels were significantly raised in the RA patients compared to controls {50 (SD 20) *vs.* 17 (81) µmol/L; p < 0.001} suggesting that the conversion of cysteine to sulphate is faulty in RA subjects (Bradley et al. 1994).

There are two key enzymes (see Figure 11.2) involved in sulphate production from cysteine (Millard et al. 2003) the first of which is cysteine dioxygenase, which converts cysteine to cysteine sulphinate. It is this step that is suggested by Bradley and colleagues (1994) to be defective. Expression of cysteine dioxygenase, and therefore the capacity to form sulphate, is blocked by TNF-α which is often high in RA patients (Dr R. Waring, personal communication, 2005). The other key step is the conversion of sulphite to sulphate by the enzyme sulphite oxidase which requires a molybdenum cofactor (Sardesai 1993). Though deficiencies of both sulphite oxidase and molybdenum cofactor are known, these are rare inborn

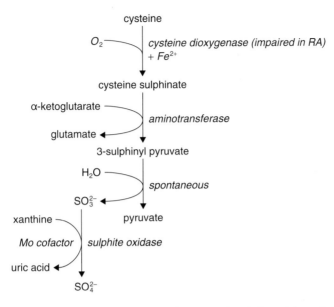

Figure 11.2   Metabolic production of sulphate from cysteine (adapted from Salway 1994).

errors of metabolism. According to Sardesai (1993), molybdenum deficiency is not found in free living humans, as most foods contain molybdenum, with legumes, dairy products, and meats being the richest sources. The Merck Manual of Diagnosis and Therapy (www.merck.com/mrkshared/mmanual/home.jsp) quotes the intake of molybdenum as 100–500 µg/day and a safe, adequate intake of molybdenum to be 75–250 µg/day for adults, suggesting that a molybdenum deficiency is unlikely.

Whether or not MSM might compensate for the apparent lack of ability to produce sulphate is questionable. According to Dr Kerry L Lang:

> 'The claim that MSM is an important source of dietary sulfur is unsupported by published research. One study that involved feeding MSM to guinea pigs found that the sulfur from MSM was absorbed rapidly into the bloodstream and was incorporated into methionine and cysteine of serum proteins. However, most of the sulfur appeared in the urine; less than 1% was incorporated into serum proteins. Increasing the dosage of MSM 100-fold increased the incorporation into serum proteins only threefold, indicating that the capacity to use MSM in this pathway is limited. Thus, while MSM is naturally present in small amounts in a variety of foods, its contribution to sulfur metabolism in humans is likely to be negligible.' (Kerry L Lang, www.quackwatch.org).

A Pub Med search of the scientific literature from 1966 to 2006 using the terms 'methylsulfonylmethane' or 'MSM' and 'arthritis', recovered only seven results, of which two were animal studies, one demonstrating low toxicity of MSM. Parcell (2002) reported one small double-blind, placebo-controlled study in 16 patients with degenerative arthritis. Ten of these patients were treated with 2.25 g MSM/d for six weeks while six patients received placebo capsules. Eight of the ten patients experienced some relief within this time while only one person on placebo showed minimal improvement. A more recent, larger, good quality study randomised 50 patients with knee OA to a double-blind trial of MSM (3 g twice a day) or placebo (Kim et al. 2006). Symptoms of pain and physical functioning were significantly improved at 12 weeks. Further studies are clearly warranted.

11.6   Noni juice

Morinda citrifolia (Noni) also known as Indian Mulberry or Nonu, is a knobbly, potato-like fruit found on a small evergreen shrub or tree in countries from India through south-east Asia to eastern Polynesia, which when mature is translucent white. The Noni fruit has been extensively used in folk medicine by Polynesians for over 2000 years as a tonic and medicine. It has been reported to have broad therapeutic effects, including anti-cancer and anti-arthritic activity, in both clinical practice and laboratory animal models, though the mechanism for these effects remains unknown (Wang & Su 2001).

The Scientific Committee on Food of the European Commission evaluated Tahitian Noni® Juice, a patented and readily available fruit juice based on noni fruit that has been marketed for several years in a number of countries (Scientific Committee on Food, 2002). They describe it thus:

'. . . *a fruit juice mixture of 89% Noni juice* (Morinda citrifolia L) *and 11% common grape and blueberry juice concentrates and natural flavours. Its composition in terms of macronutrients, vitamins and minerals is comparable to the ranges known for typical fruit juices . . .' {though} '. . . none of eight frequently occurring isoflavones could be detected in Tahitian Noni® Juice.'*

From the data supplied (by the manufacturers, Morinda Inc.) and the information available, the Committee concluded that though there were:

'. . . *no indications of adverse effects from laboratory animal studies on subacute and subchronic toxicity, genotoxicity and allergenicity . . .'* {neither was there any} '. . . *evidence for special nutritional benefits of Tahitian Noni® Juice which go beyond those of other fruit juices.' (Scientific Committee on Food 2002)*

There are a number of published *in vitro* studies suggesting that components of noni fruit may have anti-tumour effects, preventing cell transformation and angiogenesis, and an animal study that found that a polysaccharide-rich component of the fruit showed anti-tumour activity in a mouse model. However, there are no studies on the use of noni juice in arthritis and no published human studies in any disease. Such accounts as there are, are anecdotal and no basis for recommendation. A recent report of hepatotoxicity (Millonig et al. 2005) and an earlier one of hyperkalaemia (Mueller et al. 2000) associated with consumption of noni juice are not reassuring. Furthermore, the fact that the American Attorneys General of California, Arizona, New Jersey and Texas have taken legal action against Morinda

Inc. for unsubstantiated health claims about Tahitian Noni® Juice speaks for itself. There is no rationale for using this juice in arthritis.

11.7 Shark cartilage

The rationale for using shark cartilage in the treatment of arthritis may be based on the fact that it is a source of chondroitin sulphate (see Chapter 10.2) and may therefore be able to contribute to the pool of glycosaminoglycans (GAGs) in cartilage. Its main therapeutic application is, however, as an angiogenesis inhibitor in the treatment of cancer. Indeed, a standardised shark cartilage extract has been shown to inhibit the activity of matrix metalloproteinases *in vitro* and has been used in clinical trials in patients with advanced cancer (Shepherd 2001). Matrix metalloproteinases are required for the formation of new blood vessels without which cancer cannot progress and metastasise. It has been suggested that shark cartilage may also inhibit the vascularisation of human cartilage, which is likely to be beneficial in the therapy of rheumatoid arthritis (Grosios et al. 2004; see Chapter 2).

Despite these indications, there are no published studies in the peer reviewed scientific literature using shark cartilage in arthritis. There are, however, a number of indications of toxic effects associated with shark cartilage treatment. In 60 adult patients with advanced cancer treated orally with shark cartilage at 1 g/kg/d in divided doses, five were taken off study because of gastrointestinal toxicity or intolerance to shark cartilage (Miller et al. 1998). Of the 47 fully assessable patients, 21 adverse events (grade 1, eight events; grade 2, seven events; and grade 3, six events) were recorded, 14 of which were gastroenterologic (nausea, vomiting, constipation).

The US General Accounting Office in their advisory document on 'Anti-Aging' Health Products (2001) advises that use of this supplement could lead to thyroid hormone toxicity, may cause nausea, indigestion, fever, fatigue and dizziness and furthermore, that it may slow down the healing process in those recovering from surgery.

Thus there is no indication for the use of this supplement.

11.8 Herbal remedies

Herbal remedies have been used for thousands of years in the treatment of rheumatic diseases. While these are, strictly speaking, outside the scope of this book, a number of patients will be using such remedies and so a brief summary of those most commonly encountered or showing some efficacy will be given.

The use of herbal medications in OA was reviewed by Long and colleagues in 2001. At that time they found:

- Weak evidence – a single RCT with significant results – for mild to moderate relief with Reumalex (a herbal medicine), willow bark, common stinging nettle and the Ayurvedic herbal preparation, Articulin-F

- Promising evidence – two trials with favourable outcomes – for Devil's claw and ASU (avocado/soya bean unsaponifiables)
- Moderately strong evidence for phytodolor (a fixed herbal formulation) and capsaicin cream

Long and colleagues (2001) point out that the incidence of adverse effects for these herbal medicines appears to be low and therefore they may offer a much needed alternative for individuals with long-term chronic OA. A considerable number of additional trials have been carried out since then that are included in a more recent review by Setty and Sigal (2005) which summarises current evidence for the use of herbal medicines in rheumatology.

An interesting study that post-dates the Setty and Sigal review is that by Winther and colleagues (2005). Their randomised, double-blind, placebo-controlled, cross-over trial showed that daily treatment with 5 g of a powder made from seeds and shells of a rose-hip subspecies *(Rosa canina)* significantly reduced symptoms of knee and hip osteoarthritis and reduced the use of rescue medication. It is thought that the effect may be due to the presence of an anti-inflammatory galactolipid in this particular subspecies of rose-hip.

By far the largest number of studies and most peer reviewed published information relates to the use of *Harpagophytum procumbens* (Devil's claw), root tubers of which have been used in south and south-west Africa for centuries for the treatment of musculoskeletal complaints (Gagnier et al. 2004). A recent systematic review (Gagnier et al. 2004) found:

- Moderate evidence of benefit for the use of *Harpagophytum* powder at 60 mg harpagoside in the treatment of OA of the spine, hip and knee
- Moderate evidence of benefit for the use of an aqueous *Harpagophytum* extract at a daily dose of 100 mg harpagoside in the treatment of acute exacerbations of chronic non-specific low back pain
- Moderate evidence of benefit for the use of an aqueous extract of *Harpagophytum procumbens* at 60 mg harpagoside being non-inferior to 12.5 mg/d rofecoxib for chronic non-specific low back pain in the short term
- Strong evidence of benefit for the use of an aqueous *Harpagophytum* extract at a daily dose of 50 mg harpagoside in the treatment of acute exacerbations of chronic non-specific low back pain

In addition to Devil's claw, other herbs with anti-inflammatory properties that have been used successfully in the treatment of OA by qualified UK practitioners include meadowsweet, turmeric, cuaiacum gum, bogbean and white willow (personal communication, Dr Ann Walker 2005). Ginger is also given to improve circulation and dandelion root may be used to relieve constipation, if present. Other herbs commonly included in a prescription for OA in the UK include celery seed, black cohosh, licorice and wild yam (personal communication, Dr Ann Walker 2005).

Table 11.1 Herbal remedies used for arthritic conditions showing some efficacy in human trials.

Herb	Use	Proposed mechanism	Side effects Contraindications	Reference
Harpagophytum procumbens (Devil's claw)	OA	Anti-inflammatory action by altering eicosanoid biosynthesis Decreased production of cartilage-degrading MMPs	Side effects GI upset Contraindicated in gastric/duodenal ulcers, gallstones, diabetes	Long et al. 2001; Chrubasik et al. 2002; Chrubasik et al. 2004; Gagnier et al. 2004 (systematic review); Schulze-Tanzil et al. 2004; Setty & Sigal 2005
Boswellia	OA	Anti-inflammatory, analgesic and immuno-modulatory properties	Minor GI disturbances	Sander at al. 1998; Kimmatkar et al. 2003; Setty & Sigal 2005
Tripterygium wilfordii Hook F (Lei gong teng, Thunder god vine)	RA	Inhibits production of cytokines	Numerous side effects including osteoporosis, amenorrhoea Contraindicated in peptic ulcers	Tao et al. 2002; Setty & Sigal 2005
Uncaria tomentosa (Cat's claw)	RA	Decreases production of TNF-α	Nephrotoxic	Setty & Sigal 2005
Urtica diocia (Stinging nettle)	OA	Decreases production of TNF-α, may suppress MMP expression	Side effects: urticarial rash, mild GI upsets	Setty & Sigal 2005
Rosa canina (rose hip) sub-species	OA	Anti-inflammatory effect of galacto-lipid?	None	Winther et al. 2005
Willow bark especially that of *Salix alba*	OA	Constituent, salicin is oxidised to salicylic acid, analgesic and anti-inflammatory	Contraindications peptic ulcer, diabetes, hepatic or renal disorders, allergy to aspirin	Long et al. 2001; Setty & Sigal 2005
SKI 306X, an extract from *Tricosanthes kirilowii, Clematis mandshurica* and *Prunella vulgaris*	OA	Inhibits proteoglycan degradation		Choi et al. 2002

Table 11.2 Other supplements for which benefit has been claimed in arthritis.

	Description	Claims	Efficacy/ evidence	Side effects and contraindications	Suggested dose
Aloe vera	A succulent plant with fleshy leaves containing gel in which can be found vitamins, minerals, enzymes and amino acids	Anti-inflammatory, wound healing, antioxidant, antiseptic, analgesic, immunity boosting	No evidence in RA or OA	Laxative effects: choose those free from aloin and emodin. Do not take in pregnancy or lactation	None suggested for RA/OA
Bromelain	A digestive enzyme derived from pineapples	Powerful anti-inflammatory action, blood thinning	No evidence in RA or OA	None	250–500 mg three times per day
Feverfew	A plant belonging to the daisy family	Anti-inflammatory effects due to presence of tanetin, which interferes with inflammatory compounds. May reduce pain in arthritis	No evidence in OA or RA	Do not take in pregnancy or lactation, or if on anticoagulant drugs	125–250 mg, depending on extract strength
Maitake	An edible mushroom	Contains immune-stimulating substances known as beta-glucans	No evidence in RA/OA	No toxic side effects, however avoid during pregnancy and lactation	600 mg/d extracts, 1–7 g/d dried mushroom. Vitamin C aids absorption
Olive leaf	From the olive tree	Powerful antibacterial, anti-viral, anti-fungal, anti-parasitic substances and antioxidant activity	No evidence in RA/OA	No toxic effects seen. Do not use in pregnancy or lactation	500 mg twice to four times per day between meals
Sarsaparilla	Often known as Smilax, a group of climbing vines found in tropical and subtropical parts of the world. The roots contain hormone-like steroids and glycosides	Anti-inflammatory properties	No evidence in RA/OA	No serious long-term side effects although may cause indigestion; may lead to temporary kidney damage if taken in excess	250 mg three times per day
Wild yam	A Mexican vine, its roots are rich in steroidal saponins	Anti-inflammatory actions and antioxidant function	No evidence in RA/OA	Excess may cause nausea and diarrhoea. Do not use in pregnancy or lactation	250–500 mg/d

Studies with herbs or herbal preparations that have shown efficacy in arthritic conditions are summarised in Table 11.1. Interested readers are referred to the three reviews mentioned above.

11.9 Other supplements

Table 11.2 gives information about some other supplements for which claims have been made but for which any evidence of efficacy is lacking.

11.10 Conclusion

Of the alternative remedies and supplements discussed, green tea, ginger and perhaps NZGLM hold promise as potential treatments for arthritis. The same can probably be said of *Harpagophytum procumbens* (Devil's claw). One of the difficulties encountered in this research area is that studies are done with non-standard preparations making generic proof of their effectiveness difficult (Chrubasik et al. 2002).

References

Adcocks C, Collin P, Buttle D (2002) Catechins from green tea (*Camellia sinensis*) inhibit bovine and human cartilage proteoglycan and type II collagen degradation in vitro. *Journal of Nutrition* 132, 341–46.

Altman RD, Marcussen KC (2001) Effects of a ginger extract on knee pain in patients with osteoarthritis. *Arthritis and Rheumatism* 44 (11), 2531–38.

Bliddal H, Rosetzsky A, Schlichting P, Weidner MS, Andersen LA, Ibfelt HH, Christensen K, Jensen ON, Barslev J (2000) A randomized, placebo-controlled, cross-over study of ginger extracts and ibuprofen in osteoarthritis. *Osteoarthritis and Cartilage* 8(1), 9–12.

Bradley H, Gough A, Sokhi RS, Hassell A, Waring R, Emery P (1994) Sulfate metabolism is abnormal in patients with rheumatoid arthritis. Confirmation by *in vivo* biochemical findings. *Journal of Rheumatology* 21(7), 1192–96.

Caughey D, Grigor R, Caughey E, Young P (1983) *Perna Canaliculus* in the treatment of rheumatoid arthritis. *European Journal of Rheumatology and Inflammation* 6, 197–200.

Cho SH, Jung YB, Seong SC, Park HB, Byun KY, Lee DC, Song EK, Son JH (2003) Clinical efficacy and safety of Lyprinol®, a patented extract from New Zealand green-lipped mussel (*Perna canaliculus*) in patients with osteoarthritis of the hip and knee: a multicenter 2-month clinical trial. *European Annals of Allergy and Clinical Immunology* 35(6), 212–16.

Choi JH, Choi JH, Kim DY, Yoon JH, Youn HY, Yi JB, Rhee HI, Ryu KH, Jung K, Han CK, Kwak WJ, Cho YB (2002) Effects of SKI 306X, a new herbal agent, on proteoglycan degradation in cartilage explant culture and collagenase-induced rabbit osteoarthritis model. *Osteoarthritis and Cartilage* 10(6), 471–78.

Chrubasik S, Pollak S, Black A (2002) Effectiveness of devil's claw for osteoarthritis. *Rheumatology* 41(11), 1332–33; author reply 1333.

Chrubasik S, Conradt C, Roufogalis BD (2004) Effectiveness of *Harpagophytum* extracts and clinical efficacy. *Phytotherapy Research* 18(2), 187–89.

Cobb C, Ernst E (2005) Systematic review of a marine nutriceutical supplement in clinical trials for arthritis: the effectiveness of the New Zealand green-lipped mussel *Perna canaliculus*. *Clinical Rheumatology* 25, 275–84.

Darlington LG, Ramsey NW (1993) Clinical Review – Review of dietary therapy for rheumatoid arthritis. *British Journal of Rheumatology* 32, 507–14.

Emery P, Bradley H, Gough A, Arthur V, Jubb R, Waring R (1992a) Increased prevalence of poor sulphoxidation in patients with rheumatoid arthritis: effect of changes in the acute phase response and second line drug treatment. *Annals of the Rheumatic Diseases* **51**, 318–20.

Emery P, Bradley H, Arthur V, Tunn E, Waring R (1992b) Genetic factors influencing the outcome of early arthritis – the role of sulphoxidation status. *British Journal of Rheumatology* **31**, 449–51.

Gagnier JJ, Chrubasik S, Manheimer E (2004) *Harpagophytum procumbens* for osteoarthritis and low back pain: a systematic review. BMC *Complementary and Alternative Medicine* **15**, 4(1), 13.

Gibson R, Gibson S, Conway V, Chappell D (1980) *Perna canaliculus* in the treatment of arthritis. *Practitioner* **224**, 955–60.

Gibson R, Gibson S (1981) Green-lipped mussel extract in arthritis. *The Lancet* Feb 21, 439.

Grosios K, Wood J, Esser R, Raychaudhuri A, Dawson J (2004) Angiogenesis inhibition by the novel VEGF receptor tyrosine kinase inhibitor, PTK787/ZK222584, causes significant anti-arthritic effects in models of rheumatoid arthritis. *Inflammation Research* 2004 53(4), 133–42.

Halpern GM (2000) Anti-inflammatory effects of a stabilized lipid extract of *Perna canaliculus* (Lyprinol®). *Allergy and Immunology* (Paris) **32**(7), 272–78.

Haqqi T, Anthony D, Gupta S, Ahmad N, Lee M, Kumar G, Mukhtar H (1999) Prevention of collagen-induced arthritis in mice by a polyphenolic fraction from green tea. *Proceedings of the National Academy of Sciences USA* **96**, 4524–29.

Kimmatkar N, Thawani V, Hingorani L, Khiyani R (2003) Efficacy and tolerability of *Boswellia serrata* extract in treatment of osteoarthritis of knee – a randomized double-blind placebo-controlled trial. *Phytomedicine* **10**(1), 3–7.

Larkin JG, Capell HA, Sturrock RD (1985) Seatone in rheumatoid arthritis: a six-month placebo-controlled study. *Annals of the Rheumatic Diseases* **44**(3), 199–201.

Long L, Soeken K, Ernst E (2001) Herbal medicines for the treatment of osteoarthritis: a systematic review. *Rheumatology* **40**(7), 779–93.

Millard J, Parsons RB, Waring RH, Williams AC, Ramsden DB (2003) Expression of cysteine dioxygenase (EC 1.13.11.20) and sulfite oxidase in the human lung: a potential role for sulfate production in the protection from airborne xenobiotica. *Molecular Pathology* **56**(5), 270–74.

Miller DR, Anderson GT, Stark JJ, Granick JL, Richardson D (1998) Phase I/II trial of the safety and efficacy of shark cartilage in the treatment of advanced cancer. *Journal of Clinical Oncology* **16**(11), 3649–55.

Millonig G, Stadlmann S, Vogel W (2005) Herbal hepatotoxicity: acute hepatitis caused by a Noni preparation (*Morinda citrifolia*). *European Journal of Gastroenterology and Hepatology* **17**(4), 445–47.

Mueller BA, Scott MK, Sowinski KM, Prag KA (2000) Noni juice (*Morinda citrifolia*): hidden potential for hyperkalemia? *American Journal of Kidney Diseases* **35**(2), 310–12.

Parcell S (2002) Sulfur in human nutrition and applications in medicine. *Alternative Medicine Review* **7**(1), 22–44.

Rizzo R, Grandolfo M, Godeas C, Jones KW, Vittur F (1995) Calcium, sulfur, and zinc distribution in normal and arthritic articular equine cartilage: a synchrotron radiation-induced X-ray emission (SRIXE) study. *Journal of Experimental Zoology* 1, 273(1), 82–86.

Salway JG (1994) *Metabolism at a Glance.* Oxford, Blackwell Scientific Publications.

Sander O, Herborn G, Rau R (1998) Is H15 (resin extract of *Boswellia serrata*, 'incense') a useful supplement to established drug therapy of chronic polyarthritis? Results of a double-blind pilot study (Article in German). *Zeitschrift fur Rheumatologie* **57**(1), 11–16.

Sardesai VM (1993) Molybdenum: an essential trace element. *Nutrition in Clinical Practice* **8**, 277–81.

Schulze-Tanzil G, Hansen C, Shakibaei M (2004) Effect of a *Harpagophytum procumbens* DC extract on matrix metalloproteinases in human chondrocytes *in vitro* (article in German). *Arzneimittel Forschung* **54**(4), 213–20.

Scientific Committee on Food (2002) *Opinion of the Scientific Committee on Food on Tahitian Noni juice.* European Commission, 11 December 2002 http://europa.eu.int/comm/food/fs/sc/scf/out151_en.pdf

Setty AR, Sigal LH (2005) Herbal medications commonly used in the practice of rheumatology: mechanisms of action, efficacy, and side effects. *Seminars in Arthritis and Rheumatism* **34**(6), 773–84.

Shepherd FA (2001) Angiogenesis inhibitors in the treatment of lung cancer. *Lung Cancer* **34**, S81–S89.

Srivastava KC, Mustafa T (1989) Ginger (*Zingiber officinale*) and rheumatic disorders. *Medical Hypotheses* **29**(1), 25–28.

Srivastava KC, Mustafa T (1992) Ginger (*Zingiber officinale*) in rheumatism and musculoskeletal disorders. *Medical Hypotheses* **39**(4), 342–48.

Suarez-Almazor ME, Kendall CJ, Dorgan M (2001) Surfing the Net – information on the World Wide Web for persons with arthritis: patient empowerment or patient deceit? *Journal of Rheumatology* **28**, 185–91. Comment in: *Journal of Rheumatology* 2001 28(1), 1–2.

Tao X, Younger J, Fan FZ, Wang B, Lipsky PE (2002) Benefit of an extract of *Tripterygium wilfordii* Hook F in patients with rheumatoid arthritis: a double-blind, placebo-controlled study. *Arthritis and Rheumatism* **46**(7), 1735–43.

Thorne Research (2003) Monograph: *Zingiber officinale* (Ginger). *Alternative Medicine Review* **8**(3), 331–35.

US General Accounting Office (GAO) (2001) Health products for seniors. 'Anti-ageing' products pose potential for physical and economic harm. Appendix II. www.ods.od.nih.gov/pubs/gao-01-1129.pdf

van der Kraan PM, Vitters EL, de Vries BJ, van den Berg WB (1990) High susceptibility of human articular cartilage glycosaminoglycan synthesis to changes in inorganic sulfate availability. *Journal of Orthopaedic Research* **8**(4), 565–71.

Vankemmelbeke M, Jones G, Fowles C, Ilic M, Handley C, Day A, Knight G, Mort J, Buttle D (2003) Selective inhibition of ADAMTS-1, -4 and -5 by catechin gallate esters. *European Journal of Biochemistry* **270**, 2394–2403.

Wang MY, Su C (2001) Cancer preventive effect of *Morinda citrifolia* (Noni). *Annals of the New York Academy of Sciences* **952**, 161–68.

Wigler L, Grotto I, Caspi D, Yaron M (2003) The effects of Zintona EC (a ginger extract) on symptomatic gonarthritis. *Osteoarthritis and Cartilage* **11**, 783–89.

Winther K, Apel K, Thamsborg G (2005) A powder made from seeds and shells of a rose-hip subspecies (*Rosa canina*) reduces symptoms of knee and hip osteoarthritis: a randomized, double-blind, placebo-controlled clinical trial. *Scandinavian Journal of Rheumatology* **34**, 302–8.

Yamada H, Miyauchi S, Morita M, Yoshida Y, Yoshihara Y, Kikuchi T, Washimi O, Washimi Y, Terada N, Seki T, Fujikawa K (2000) Content and sulfation pattern of keratan sulfate in hip osteoarthritis using high performance liquid chromatography. *Journal of Rheumatology* **27**, 1721–24.

12 Assessment of level of evidence for nutritional recommendations and suggestions for the future

12.1 Summary of nutritional factors that may affect risk of RA and OA

We have presented evidence for nutritional factors having a role in the onset, progression and treatment of OA and RA. Obesity, even at a young age, correlates strongly with risk of developing OA and is also associated with risk of RA in some studies, though the evidence is weaker and there is no association with overweight (BMI 25–30 kg/m^2) as such (see section 3.6).

Though there is little evidence for an effect of dietary factors on susceptibility to OA, there is considerably more evidence for an effect in RA. Higher consumption of olive oil, fish, fruit, cooked vegetables, β-cryptoxanthin (largely from oranges) and vitamin C appear to protect against the development of RA, the strongest effects being seen for vitamin C and olive oil where high consumption reduced risk by a factor of three (see section 3.8). A high level of intake of both fish and β-cryptoxanthin reduced risk around twofold, while a low intake of vitamin D increased risk by a factor of around 1.5. By contrast, being in the top third of intake of red meat and meat products appeared to double the risk of developing inflammatory polyarthritis.

However, it needs to be pointed out that having a high red meat intake, or alternatively a high vitamin C or fruit and vegetable intake may be associated with other lifestyle behaviours that may affect risk. For example, protein is a very satiating nutrient and high meat eaters may consequently eat fewer fruits and vegetables and therefore fail to benefit from their protective effects.

12.2 Level of evidence for nutritional recommendations in RA and OA

We have categorised the nutritional factors that affect disease progression, symptoms or severity by strength of evidence – strong, moderate or weak. These have been categorised separately for OA and RA in Tables 12.1 and 12.2 respectively, which also give the section numbers where more detailed information can be found.

We hope that practitioners will use the evidence presented in this book and summarised in these tables to help patients take a measure of control over their

Table 12.1 Summary of nutritional approaches to OA according to level of evidence.

Level of evidence	Nutritional approach	Sections where covered	Treatment suggestion	Result	Caveats
Good	Body weight	3.6 5.2	Achieve normal BMI by weight loss if relevant.	Reduced inflammation and strain on joints.	
	Vitamin D	8.7 Figures 8.2–8.7 Tables 8.6, 8.7	Unless patients have a good intake of oily fish or spend considerable time in the sun, they should be advised to take supplements of vitamin D, up to a level of 25 µg/d, particularly if over 65 years, institutionalised, housebound, dark-skinned living at latitudes > 50°, if they wear enveloping clothing or are vegetarian.	Significantly reduced progression of knee and hip OA.	Avoid supplementing at a level above 25 µg/d except under medical guidance, owing to the risk of hypercalcaemia and hypercalciuria.
	Glucosamine and Chondroitin	Chapter 10 Tables 10.1, 10.2 Figures 10.1–10.4	Daily dose of 1500 mg glucosamine (as sulphate or chloride) preferably along with 1200 mg chondroitin sulphate. Use pharmaceutical grade or high quality supplements. Some trials included manganese (228/304 mg/d as manganese ascorbate), a co-factor in glycosaminoglycan synthesis (10.6.3). Topical application is an option (10.8).	Many published trials found significant beneficial effects of glucosamine on pain, stiffness, function and joint space narrowing. The largest, high quality trial showed a significant effect on pain only in combination with chondroitin and only in moderate to severe disease. Some studies show greater benefit in mild to moderate arthritis.	Avoid these supplements if allergic to shellfish, on heparin or daily aspirin or if suffering from prostate cancer. Also avoid if pregnant or lactating, owing to a lack of clinical studies in this patient group.
Moderate	Vitamin C	8.3 Appendix 3	Ensure dietary intake at least up to the RNI/RDA level by consuming a high level of fruit and vegetables with good vitamin C content or supplement up to 500 mg/d.	Threefold reduced risk of OA progression and development of knee pain seen at medium and high dietary intakes of vitamin C in the Framingham OA Cohort Study.	

Table 12.1 (cont'd)

Level of evidence	Nutritional approach	Sections where covered	Treatment suggestion	Result	Caveats
Weak	Selenium	8.4	Eat rich sources of selenium, such as Brazil nuts, offal or fish. In areas with selenium intake < 120 μg/d (e.g. Europe), supplement with 100–200 μg/d selenium.	Effect may be beneficial, as lower selenium status has been significantly associated with knee OA, most notably in women and African Americans.	Selenium is toxic, so keep total selenium intake from foods and supplement to ≤ 450 μg/d.
	Copper Zinc	8.5 Appendix 3	Ensure intake is up to RDA/RNI levels as both copper and zinc are required for synthesis and degradation of connective tissue and for CuZnSOD activity/structure.	May benefit connective tissue management and superoxide scavenging.	Avoid copper supplementation above the RDA/RNI and doses of zinc more than twice the RDA/RNI, which may impair copper absorption.
	Cod liver oil Oily fish Fish oil	9.7.5, 9.15–9.19	2 × 1000 mg capsules cod liver oil/d, containing a relatively low dose of EPA + DHA (e.g. 340 mg/d), plus vitamin A (1600–3200 μg/d) plus vitamin D (10–16 μg/d). Oily fish may represent a suitable alternative to cod liver oil as it also contains vitamin D. Alternatively supplement with fish oil (1 × 1 g capsule/d) and vitamin D (see above).	Cartilage-degrading enzymes were decreased and mediators of inflammation were downregulated in cartilage and joint tissue implying a beneficial effect of cod liver oil on disease progression. The vitamin D content may have added benefit.	It may be unsafe to consume more than 1 g/d cod liver oil on a long-term basis, owing to its content of vitamins A and D. Pregnant women should not consume cod liver oil owing to the known teratogenic effects of vitamin A.
	Ginger	11.3	A typical dose of ginger (form unspecified) is 1–4 g/d taken in divided doses.	Some evidence of pain relief, reduced handicap and joint swelling.	Care if on anti-coagulant therapy as ginger may have an effect on platelets.
	New Zealand green-lipped mussel	11.4	Food sources presumably limited to New Zealand. Stabilised extracts of NZGLM such as Lyprinol® may be preferable.	Pain and function improved in some studies perhaps owing to apparent anti-inflammatory effect.	Safety and efficacy not established. Well designed trials required.

Table 12.2 Summary of nutritional approaches to RA according to level of evidence (see table footnote, p. 223).

Level of evidence	Nutritional approach	Sections where covered	Treatment	Result	Caveats
Good	Oily fish, fish oil, n-3 PUFA	Chapter 9 Tables 9.4–9.11 Figures 9.5–9.7	Increase intake of n-3 PUFA, long chain if possible, and reduce intake of n-6 PUFA (with the exception of GLA/DGLA), replacing by n-9 (olive oil) products, at least for a trial period of 6 months. Aim for an intake of 3–6 g/d EPA + DHA (equivalent to 13 portions of oily fish per week) from fish, fish (body) oil supplements and other suitable sources.	Depending on individual genotype, n-6 content of diet and medication use, increased n-3 PUFA intake, particularly of EPA, can have significant beneficial effects on number of tender joints, duration of morning stiffness, pain and NSAID requirement by reducing inflammation and joint degradation.	Pregnant women should avoid shark, swordfish and marlin and restrict intake of tuna to two medium cans of tuna or one fresh portion per week. Fish-oil supplements must conform to requirements on level of toxic contaminants.
Moderate	Fasting	7.2	Fasting from food for 4–10 days, sometimes in preparation for a big event.	Relief of symptoms probably due to immunosuppression. However, symptoms recur on reintroduction of food.	Not recommended owing to risk of malnutrition.
	Food exclusion	7.2 Table 7.1 Appendix 4	Exclusion diet followed by reintroduction of foods one by one. Then, long-term avoidance of culprit foods based on individual food sensitivity.	Personally tailored elimination diets may be successful for up to 30–40% RA patients.	If improvement not seen within 3 weeks, abandon diet. Risk of weight loss. Only carry out under supervision of an appropriate health professional.
	Vegetarian or vegan diet	7.3	No meat or poultry. Avoidance of fish, shellfish, eggs and dairy products according to strictness of diet.	May benefit 25–45% RA patients. Benefit often associated with change in faecal flora.	Risk of weight loss and detrimental effects on nutritional status. Advice of a dietitian should be sought.
	Vitamin E	8.3 Appendix 3	A short period (up to 12 weeks) of vitamin E supplementation (say at 400 mg/d) could be tried. At the very least, adequate intake by dietary means should be advised.	As α-tocopherol appears to exert a significant analgesic effect in RA, a reduction in pain may be noticed and a concomitant reduction in NSAID dose might be achieved.	Need to consume adequate vitamin C to recycle active α-tocopherol.

Table 12.2 *(cont'd)*

Level of evidence	Nutritional approach	Sections where covered	Treatment	Result	Caveats
Moderate	Vitamin D	8.7 Figures 8.2–8.7 Tables 8.6, 8.7	As low dietary intakes and status are common in RA patients, increased consumption of vitamin D from oily fish or supplements is recommended, unless patients have considerable sun exposure.	Vitamin D may reduce disease activity by modulating the hyperactive T-cell immunity of RA and acting as an immunosuppressant.	Avoid supplementing at a level above 25 µg/d except under medical guidance, owing to the risk of hypercalcaemia and hypercalciuria.
	Selenium	8.4 Figure 8.1 Tables 8.2–8.4	Eat rich sources of selenium such as Brazil nuts, offal or fish. In areas with selenium intake < 120 µg/d (e.g. Europe), supplement with selenium. Though studies that showed benefit used 200–600 µg/d for 3–8 months, supplementation should not exceed 300 µg/d and should preferably start at a lower level.	RA patients appear to have lower selenium status than healthy individuals. A number of double blind RCTs showed significant improvements in measurable parameters of disease activity on selenium supplementation but not all interventions showed benefit.	Selenium is toxic, so keep total selenium intake from foods and supplement to ≤ 450 µg/d.
	GLA	9.7, 9.9 Table 9.4	Supplement with GLA, 1–2.8 g/d, e.g. as evening primrose oil or blackcurrant seed oil, preferably in combination with long-chain n-3 PUFA (fish/fish oil).	Some evidence for anti-inflammatory effect: reduction in morning stiffness, number of swollen and painful joints and reduced use of NSAIDs.	
Weak	Mediterranean diet	7.4 Figure 7.1	Large amounts of fruit and vegetables, fish, olive oil and non-refined bread and cereals eaten. Meat and meat products replaced by fish or poultry or vegetarian dishes.	Improvement in physical functioning and decreased inflammation in one study.	

Weak					
Elemental diet	7.5	Hypoallergenic diet made up of food components such as amino acids, glucose, medium chain triglycerides, vitamins and minerals. Consumed as a powder dissolved in water.	Can improve RA symptoms in a sub-set of individuals but symptoms re-emerge when the normal diet is resumed.	Given the unpopularity of the elemental diet and the difficulty in sustaining it, use only on a temporary basis as a diet of last resort.
Vitamin C β-carotene	8.3 Appendix 3	Ensure intake is at least up to RDA/RNI levels owing to level of oxidative stress associated with RA.	Low serum levels of antioxidants are associated with elevated risk of RA.	
Copper Zinc	8.5 Appendix 3	Ensure intake is up to RDA/RNI levels as both copper and zinc are required for synthesis and degradation of connective tissue and for CuZnSOD activity/structure. Additionally, there is some evidence for zinc malabsorption in RA.	May benefit connective tissue management and superoxide scavenging.	Supplementation with copper above the RDA/RNI level should be avoided, while doses of zinc more than twice the RDA/RNI may impair copper absorption.
Iron	8.6 Table 8.5	Supplement only where clear iron deficiency has been measured.	Relief of symptoms of iron-deficiency anaemia.	If anaemia is the 'anaemia of chronic disease', iron supplementation is not appropriate and may worsen inflammation.
New Zealand green-lipped mussel	11.4	Food sources presumably limited to New Zealand. Stabilised extracts of NZGLM such as Lyprinol® may be preferable.	One trial showed improvement in articular and functional indices in 37% of RA patients, perhaps because of apparent anti-inflammatory effect.	Safety and efficacy not established. Well designed trials required.

NB: This table does not address the additional nutritional requirements of impaired nutritional status or malnutrition resulting from the RA disease process (see sections 2.4.8.7, 5.2.1, 5.3, 5.5) nor any additional requirements for supplements (e.g. of folic acid, calcium, vitamin D) associated with drug treatment for RA (see sections 2.4.10, 4.2, 5.6).

own state of health by dietary means. We particularly recommend that patients, especially when presenting with early stage disease, should be informed that certain nutrients or supplements may be able to slow disease progression, notably vitamin D in OA.

12.3 Suggestions for the future

A number of suggestions for further research have been made in previous chapters. Human trials with green tea in early OA and well-designed studies with stabilised New Zealand green-lipped mussel (NZGLM) extracts are examples. In general, there are indications that studies on patients with less severe or early disease are more likely to be successful. It would seem wise to concentrate effort in this group of patients with a view to reducing disease progression, except where pain reduction is the primary aim of the intervention.

As illustrated by the interaction found between TNF genotype and effect of fish oil supplementation, it is important to consider possible genotype effects when altering diet or giving supplements. In particular, the effect of vitamin D may be dependent on polymorphisms known to exist in the vitamin D receptor gene (Keen et al. 1997; Garcia-Lozano et al. 2001). Future dietary interventions should include genetic testing where relevant polymorphisms may exist, or at the very least, samples should be laid down for DNA isolation and later testing wherever possible.

Though considerable consideration has been given to vitamin E, particularly in relation to RA, up to now, only α-tocopherol, the form of vitamin E in supplements and the main form in the UK diet, has been investigated. In fact, γ-tocopherol, the major form in the US diet, is potentially a more interesting component of vitamin E as both it and its major metabolite have much stronger anti-inflammatory properties than α-tocopherol (Jiang et al. 2000). Both γ-tocopherol and its major metabolite at physiologically relevant concentrations reduce the synthesis of PGE_2 by inhibition of cyclo-oxygenase activity in intact cells (Jiang et al. 2000). Competition with AA at the binding site of cyclo-oxygenase appears likely to be the possible mechanism for this effect. An intervention with γ-tocopherol in early RA is worthy of consideration.

References

Garcia-Lozano JR, Gonzalez-Escribano MF, Valenzuela A, Garcia A, Nunez-Roldan A (2001) Association of vitamin D receptor genotypes with early onset rheumatoid arthritis. *European Journal of Immunogenetics* **28**, 89–93.

Jiang Q, Elson-Schwab I, Courtemanche C, Ames BN (2000) Gamma-tocopherol and its major metabolite, in contrast to alpha-tocopherol, inhibit cyclo-oxygenase activity in macrophages and epithelial cells. *Proceedings of the National Academy of Sciences USA* **97**, 11494–99.

Keen RW, Hart DJ, Lanchbury JS, Spector TD (1997) Association of early osteoarthritis of the knee with a Taq I polymorphism of the vitamin D receptor gene. *Arthritis and Rheumatism* **40**, 1444–49.

Appendix 1
How to interpret the statistical data on studies quoted in this book

Written with the help of Alexander Thompson BSc, MRes, MPhil

Epidemiological studies are widely cited in the text and this Appendix has been compiled to help you understand the strength of the evidence quoted. Within epidemiology, the application of statistical methods allows an assessment of the degree of risk that someone with a particular exposure pattern, lifestyle or genetic profile has of contracting a specific disease or benefiting from a treatment. Different types of epidemiological study are subject to different sources of error or bias as explained below (section 1) and are weighted accordingly, with the highest level of evidence being the randomised, controlled trial.

The meaning of epidemiological or statistical terms used frequently throughout the book is explained in section 2. Further definitions that may clarify the meaning of these and other statistical terms are included in the Glossary.

1. Types of study mentioned in the text

Ecological study: A descriptive study that aims to identify associations between exposures and outcomes using population level rather than individual level data, e.g. per capita alcohol consumption and prevalence of heart disease in Europe. They are hypothesis-generating not hypothesis-testing studies.

Case control study: An analytic study in which subjects are recruited on the basis of their disease status (*cases = diseased, controls = healthy*) and are then compared with respect to the frequency of their exposure to a prior event or factor of interest, e.g. a dietary factor. Case control studies can be useful for examining rare diseases or for testing many exposures. Furthermore, they are relatively quick and cheap to conduct. However, because both the disease and exposure events have already occurred, this design is particularly susceptible to bias – perhaps due to the differential selection of cases and controls (selection bias) or the reporting of exposure information (information bias).

Prospective study: Any study design where participants are followed through time, and occurrences of the outcome of interest are ascertained, e.g. cohort studies.

Cohort study: An analytical study that recruits subjects who have been, currently are, or may in the future be exposed to the agent of interest. These individuals are then followed up for a period of time (frequently many years) and the incidence of events in the varying exposure groups compared. Because exposure status is determined before disease onset, selection bias is reduced and the temporal relationship between exposure and outcome can be observed. However, the large number of participants and many years of follow up that these studies invariably require can lead to participant withdrawal and loss to follow up. Differential loss to follow up or systematic errors in disease ascertainment can lead to bias.

Nested case control: A case control study that is conducted within another study – usually a cohort study. Individuals who develop the outcome of interest during follow up become the cases, and a sample of those who remain free of the outcome are used as the controls. Since this study design uses only a subset of the disease-free individuals in the analysis, it is particularly useful where measuring the exposure levels of every individual in the cohort would be impractical – perhaps for reasons of time or expense.

Randomised controlled trial (RCT): An experimental study that resembles a cohort study in that groups of individuals with differing exposure levels are followed up through time. Crucially, however, the exposure levels are randomly assigned by the investigator. The use of randomisation (in conjunction with an appropriate sample size) reduces bias and confounding to a greater extent than is possible in other observational study designs, with the result that the RCT can be regarded as the most valid and rigorous method of testing hypotheses in epidemiology.

2.   Statistical terms that are frequently used in this book

Risk: The probability that a specified event will occur. Risk is expressed as the number of times an event occurs as a proportion of the total number of events possible. For example, if in a group of 10 individuals six die and four do not, the risk of death is 6/10, or 0.6.

Relative risk/Risk ratio (RR): The ratio of two risks. If the risk of disease in the exposed group is $a/(a + b)$, and in the unexposed group $c/(c + d)$, then the risk ratio (relative risk) is $\{a/(a + b)\}/\{c/(c + d)\}$.

	Diseased	Healthy	
Exposed	a	b	a + b
Unexposed	c	d	c + d

A RR = 1 indicates a lack of an association between exposure status and disease, a RR < 1 implies that the exposure makes the outcome less likely, while a RR > 1 implies that the exposure makes the outcome more likely. RR is useful in the analysis of cohort studies.

Odds ratio (OR): The ratio of two odds; particularly useful when analysing a dichotomous (e.g. yes/no) exposure and a disease outcome – for example in a case control study:

	Cases	Controls
Exposed	a	b
Unexposed	c	d

The odds of being a case is a/b in the exposed group and c/d in the unexposed group. Therefore the odds ratio is $(a/b)/(c/d)$, which simplifies to ad/bc. An OR can range from zero to infinity. An OR = 1 indicates no association between exposure and outcome, an OR < 1 implies that the exposure makes the outcome less likely, while an OR > 1 implies that the exposure makes the outcome more likely.

Adjusted relative risk (RR): RR that has been statistically adjusted for other factors that are likely to affect risk e.g. cigarette smoking, age, body mass index.

Significance: Also known as *significance level*, this refers to whether an observed result has achieved *statistical significance* in the analyses conducted. A p value of 0.05 is commonly used as the cut-off for significance. A p value less than the cut-off suggests that the samples under comparison are more different, or the data under consideration more extreme than could be expected to have occurred by chance alone. It must be stressed, however, that statistical significance does not imply biological significance and one should always bear in mind the magnitude of the effect observed.

p value: In hypothesis testing, the probability of finding a result as extreme, or more extreme, than that observed in your study by chance alone. In most biological science, $p = 0.05$ (i.e. a 1 in 20 chance) is taken as the cut-off probability for declaring findings to be 'significant'. It is rarely sufficient to report the p value associated with a statistical test alone (although this is done frequently), since the 0.05 cut-off is arbitrary and not very informative by itself. A more informative approach is to report confidence intervals.

p trend: a p value derived from the application of statistical techniques to make and justify statements about trends in the data.

Confidence interval (CI): Loosely speaking, a statistical range with a specified probability (generally 95%) that a given parameter (e.g. a sample mean) lies within the range given. Wide confidence intervals indicate low precision, narrow intervals greater precision. For ORs and RRs, confidence intervals that do not span 1 (unity) indicate a significant association at the defined probability level.

Standard deviation: A measure of spread or variation associated with a sample mean. The standard deviation (SD) is calculated as the positive square root of the variance and gives an indication of the degree of dispersion of the data around an estimated mean. The more variable the data, the greater the SD.

Mean: Known more commonly as 'average', the arithmetic mean of a sample is calculated as the sum of all the values in a sample divided by the number of observations. The sample mean provides an estimate of the true population mean. The sample mean can be drastically affected by outliers.

Median: The median of a sample is the number that divides the data into two halves and is therefore the middlemost value when the data are ranked. The median provides a useful measure of centrality in place of the mean when the data contain outliers, as these extreme values tend not to greatly affect the position of the middlemost data.

Tertiles, quartiles, quintiles: The cut points that divide the data into three, four and five equal parts respectively. Although these terms strictly refer to the points that divide the data, in the literature, and in this book, they are commonly used to describe the thirds, quarters and fifths themselves e.g. thirds of body weight.

Correlation coefficient, r: A test statistic that describes the degree of correlation between two variables. If $r > 0$, there is a positive association between the two variables; if $r < 0$ it is negative. An $r = 0$ indicates no correlation whatsoever. Significance testing can determine whether r is significantly different from zero or not. The closer r is to +1 or –1 the greater the degree of association between the two variables. See also r^2.

Coefficient of determination, r²: The square of the correlation coefficient, r^2, ranges between 0 and 1, and describes the proportion of variation in the dependent variable that is explained by variation in the independent variable. For example, if in a correlation of height and weight, $r = 0.8$, then $r^2 = 0.64$. From this we would conclude that 64% of the variation in height can be explained by variation in weight. The r^2 statistic is particularly useful in that it prevents us attaching spurious importance to weak correlations that have only achieved statistical significance because of the large number of participants included.

Effect size: A statistical term that is a measure of the strength of an association between two variables. Examples include relative risks and odds ratios for categorical outcomes, and Cohen's d (among others) for differences in the means of continuous variables. Sometimes effect size is known as 'treatment effect' because it is often used when dealing with therapeutic interventions.

Intention to treat analysis: A strategy for analysing data in which all participants are included in the group to which they were assigned, regardless of whether they completed the intervention given to the group. Such analysis helps reduce bias that may be caused by loss of participants, which may disrupt the baseline equivalence established by random assignment and may reflect non-adherence to the protocol.

Meta-analysis: a statistical technique for combining the findings from independent studies. With reference to clinical trials, a meta-analysis provides an estimate of the overall treatment effect, giving due weight to the size of the different studies included.

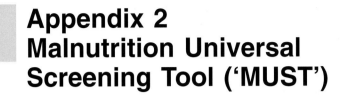

Appendix 2
Malnutrition Universal
Screening Tool ('MUST')

Reproduced with kind permission of BAPEN from *The 'MUST' Report. Nutritional Screening of Adults: A Multidisciplinary Responsibility. Development and Use of the Malnutrition Universal Screening Tool (MUST) for Adults*. Editor: Professor Marinos Elia. BAPEN, 2003. ISBN 1-899467-70-X.

'MUST'

'MUST' is a five-step screening tool to identify **adults**, who are malnourished, at risk of malnutrition (undernutrition), or obese. It also includes management guidelines which can be used to develop a care plan. It is for use in hospitals, community and other care settings and can be used by all care workers.

This guide contains:

- A flow chart showing the 5 steps to use for screening and management
- BMI chart
- Weight loss tables
- Alternative measurements when BMI cannot be obtained by measuring weight and height

The 5 'MUST' Steps

Step 1: measure height and weight to get a BMI score using chart provided. *If unable to obtain height and weight, use the alternative procedures shown in this guide.*

Step 2: note percentage unplanned weight loss and score using tables provided.

Step 3: establish acute disease effect and score.

Step 4: add scores from steps 1, 2 and 3 together to obtain overall risk of malnutrition.

Step 5: use management guidelines and/or local policy to develop care plan.

Please refer to *The 'MUST' Explanatory Booklet* for more information when weight and height cannot be measured, and when screening patient groups in which extra care in interpretation is needed (e.g. those with fluid disturbances, plaster casts, amputations, critical illness and pregnant or lactating women). The booklet can also be used for training. See *The 'MUST' Report* for supporting evidence. Please note that 'MUST' has not been designed to detect deficiencies or excessive intakes of vitamins and minerals and is of **use only in adults**.

Step 1: BMI score (and BMI)

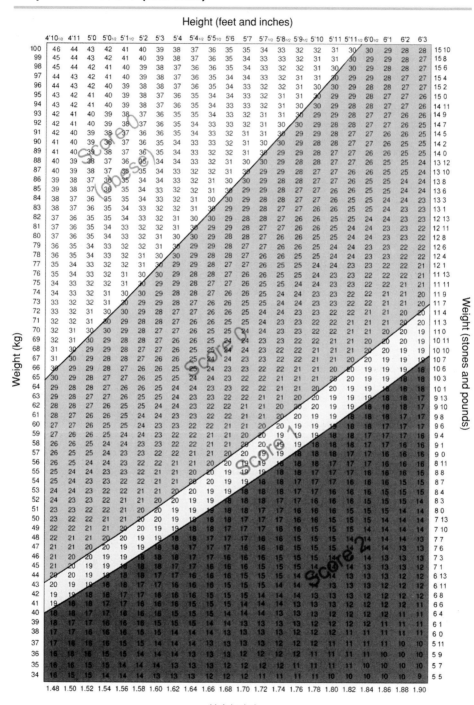

Height (feet and inches)

Height (m)

Weight (kg)

Weight (stones and pounds)

Note: The black lines denote the exact cut off points (30, 20 and 18.5 kg/m^2), figures on the chart have been rounded to the nearest whole number.

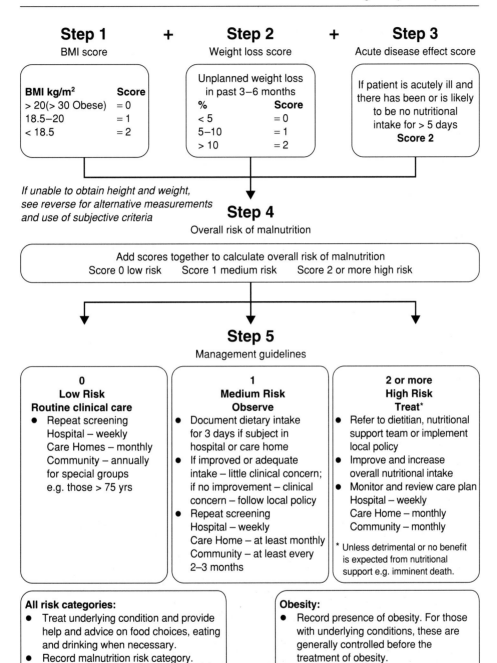

Step 1 + **Step 2** + **Step 3**

BMI score

BMI kg/m²	Score
> 20(> 30 Obese)	= 0
18.5–20	= 1
< 18.5	= 2

Weight loss score

Unplanned weight loss
in past 3–6 months

%	Score
< 5	= 0
5–10	= 1
> 10	= 2

Acute disease effect score

If patient is acutely ill and
there has been or is likely
to be no nutritional
intake for > 5 days
Score 2

*If unable to obtain height and weight,
see reverse for alternative measurements
and use of subjective criteria*

Step 4

Overall risk of malnutrition

Add scores together to calculate overall risk of malnutrition
Score 0 low risk   Score 1 medium risk   Score 2 or more high risk

Step 5

Management guidelines

0 **Low Risk** **Routine clinical care**	1 **Medium Risk** **Observe**	2 or more **High Risk** **Treat***
• Repeat screening Hospital – weekly Care Homes – monthly Community – annually for special groups e.g. those > 75 yrs	• Document dietary intake for 3 days if subject in hospital or care home • If improved or adequate intake – little clinical concern; if no improvement – clinical concern – follow local policy • Repeat screening Hospital – weekly Care Home – at least monthly Community – at least every 2–3 months	• Refer to dietitian, nutritional support team or implement local policy • Improve and increase overall nutritional intake • Monitor and review care plan Hospital – weekly Care Home – monthly Community – monthly * Unless detrimental or no benefit is expected from nutritional support e.g. imminent death.

All risk categories:
• Treat underlying condition and provide help and advice on food choices, eating and drinking when necessary.
• Record malnutrition risk category.
• Record need for special diets and follow local policy.

Obesity:
• Record presence of obesity. For those with underlying conditions, these are generally controlled before the treatment of obesity.

Re-assess subjects identified at risk as they move through care settings
See The 'MUST' Explanatory Booklet for further details and The 'MUST' Report for supporting evidence

Step 2: weight loss score

Weight before weight loss (kg)	Score 0 Wt Loss < 5%	Score 1 Wt Loss 5–10%	Score 2 Wt Loss > 10%	Weight before weight loss (st lb)	Score 0 Wt Loss < 5%	Score 1 Wt Loss 5–10%	Score 2 Wt Loss > 10%
34 kg	< 1.70	1.70–3.40	> 3.40	5st 4lb	< 4lb	4lb–7lb	> 7lb
36 kg	< 1.80	1.80–3.60	> 3.60	5st 7lb	< 4lb	4lb–8lb	> 8lb
38 kg	< 1.90	1.90–3.80	> 3.80	5st 11lb	< 4lb	4lb–8lb	> 8lb
40 kg	< 2.00	2.00–4.00	> 4.00	6st	< 4lb	4lb–8lb	> 8lb
42 kg	< 2.10	2.10–4.20	> 4.20	6st 4lb	< 4lb	4lb–9lb	> 9lb
44 kg	< 2.20	2.20–4.40	> 4.40	6st 7lb	< 5lb	5lb–9lb	> 9lb
46 kg	< 2.30	2.30–4.60	> 4.60	6st 11lb	< 5lb	5lb–10lb	> 10lb
48 kg	< 2.40	2.40–4.80	> 4.80	7st	< 5lb	5lb–10lb	> 10lb
50 kg	< 2.50	2.50–5.00	> 5.00	7st 4lb	< 5lb	5lb–10lb	> 10lb
52 kg	< 2.60	2.60–5.20	> 5.20	7st 7lb	< 5lb	5lb–11lb	> 11lb
54 kg	< 2.70	2.70–5.40	> 5.40	7st 11lb	< 5lb	5lb–11lb	> 11lb
56 kg	< 2.80	2.80–5.60	> 5.60	8st	< 6lb	6lb–11lb	> 11lb
58 kg	< 2.90	2.90–5.80	> 5.80	8st 4lb	< 6lb	6lb–12lb	> 12lb
60 kg	< 3.00	3.00–6.00	> 6.00	8st 7lb	< 6lb	6lb–12lb	> 12lb
62 kg	< 3.10	3.10–6.20	> 6.20	8st 11lb	< 6lb	6lb–12lb	> 12lb
64 kg	< 3.20	3.20–6.40	> 6.40	9st	< 6lb	6lb–13lb	> 13lb
66 kg	< 3.30	3.30–6.60	> 6.60	9st 4lb	< 7lb	7lb–13lb	> 13lb
68 kg	< 3.40	3.40–6.80	> 6.80	9st 7lb	< 7lb	7lb–13lb	> 13lb
70 kg	< 3.50	3.50–7.00	> 7.00	9st 11lb	< 7lb	7lb–1st 0lb	> 1st 0lb
72 kg	< 3.60	3.60–7.20	> 7.20	10st	< 7lb	7lb–1st 0lb	> 1st 0lb
74 kg	< 3.70	3.70–7.40	> 7.40	10st 4lb	< 7lb	7lb–1st 0lb	> 1st 0lb
76 kg	< 3.80	3.80–7.60	> 7.60	10st 7lb	< 7lb	7lb–1st 1lb	> 1st 1lb
78 kg	< 3.90	3.90–7.80	> 7.80	10st 11lb	< 8lb	8lb–1st 1lb	> 1st 1lb
80 kg	< 4.00	4.00–8.00	> 8.00	11st	< 8lb	8lb–1st 1lb	> 1st 1lb
82 kg	< 4.10	4.10–8.20	> 8.20	11st 4lb	< 8lb	8lb–1st 2lb	> 1st 2lb
84 kg	< 4.20	4.20–8.40	> 8.40	11st 7lb	< 8lb	8lb–1st 2lb	> 1st 2lb
86 kg	< 4.30	4.30–8.60	> 8.60	11st 11lb	< 8lb	8lb–1st 3lb	> 1st 3lb
88 kg	< 4.40	4.40–8.80	> 8.80	12st	< 8lb	8lb–1st 3lb	> 1st 3lb
90 kg	< 4.50	4.50–9.00	> 9.00	12st 4lb	< 9lb	9lb–1st 3lb	> 1st 3lb
92 kg	< 4.60	4.60–9.20	> 9.20	12st 7lb	< 9lb	9lb–1st 4lb	> 1st 4lb
94 kg	< 4.70	4.70–9.40	> 9.40	12st 11lb	< 9lb	9lb–1st 4lb	> 1st 4lb
96 kg	< 4.80	4.80–9.60	> 9.60	13st	< 9lb	9lb–1st 4lb	> 1st 4lb
98 kg	< 4.90	4.90–9.80	> 9.80	13st 4lb	< 9lb	9lb–1st 5lb	> 1st 5lb
100 kg	< 5.00	5.00–10.00	> 10.00	13st 7lb	< 9lb	9lb–1st 5lb	> 1st 5lb
102 kg	< 5.10	5.10–10.20	> 10.20	13st 11lb	< 10lb	10lb–1st 5lb	> 1st 5lb
104 kg	< 5.20	5.20–10.40	> 10.40	14st	< 10lb	10lb–1st 6lb	> 1st 6lb
106 kg	< 5.30	5.30–10.60	> 10.60	14st 4lb	< 10lb	10lb–1st 6lb	> 1st 6lb
108 kg	< 5.40	5.40–10.80	> 10.80	14st 7lb	< 10lb	10lb–1st 6lb	> 1st 6lb
110 kg	< 5.50	5.50–11.00	> 11.00	14st 11lb	< 10lb	10lb–1st 7lb	> 1st 7lb
112 kg	< 5.60	5.60–11.20	> 11.20	15st	< 11lb	11lb–1st 7lb	> 1st 7lb
114 kg	< 5.70	5.70–11.40	> 11.40	15st 4lb	< 11lb	11lb–1st 7lb	> 1st 7lb
116 kg	< 5.80	5.80–11.60	> 11.60	15st 7lb	< 11lb	11lb–1st 8lb	> 1st 8lb
118 kg	< 5.90	5.90–11.80	> 11.80	15st 11lb	< 11lb	11lb–1st 8lb	> 1st 8lb
120 kg	< 6.00	6.00–12.00	> 12.00	16st	< 11lb	11lb–1st 8lb	> 1st 8lb
122 kg	< 6.10	6.10–12.20	> 12.20	16st 4lb	< 11lb	11lb–1st 9lb	> 1st 9lb
124 kg	< 6.20	6.20–12.40	> 12.40	16st 7lb	< 12lb	12lb–1st 9lb	> 1st 9lb
126 kg	< 6.30	6.30–12.60	> 12.60				

Alternative measurements and considerations

Step 1: BMI (body mass index)

If height cannot be measured

- Use recently documented or self-reported height (if reliable and realistic).
- If the subject does not know or is unable to report their height, use one of the alternative measurements to estimate height (ulna, knee height or demispan).

If height and weight cannot be obtained

- Use mid upper arm circumference (MUAC) measurement to estimate BMI category.

Step 2: Recent unplanned weight loss

If recent weight loss cannot be calculated, use self-reported weight loss (if reliable and realistic).

Subjective criteria

If height, weight or BMI cannot be obtained, the following criteria which relate to them can assist your professional judgement of the subject's nutritional risk.

(1) BMI
   - Clinical impression – thin, acceptable weight, overweight. Obvious wasting (very thin) and obesity (very overweight) can also be noted.
(2) Unplanned weight loss
   - Clothes and/or jewellery have become loose fitting (weight loss).
   - History of decreased food intake, reduced appetite or swallowing problems over 3–6 months and underlying disease or psycho-social/physical disabilities likely to cause weight loss.
(3) Acute disease effect
   - No nutritional intake or likelihood of no intake for more than 5 days.

Further details on taking alternative measurements, special circumstances and subjective criteria can be found in *The 'MUST' Explanatory Booklet*. A copy can be downloaded at www.bapen.org.uk or purchased from the BAPEN office. The full evidence-base for 'MUST' is contained in *The 'MUST' Report* which is also available from the BAPEN office:

Secure Hold Business Centre, Studley Road, Redditch, Worcs BN98 7LG. Tel: 01527 457850.

Alternative measurements: instructions and tables

If height cannot be obtained, use length of forearm (ulna) to calculate height using tables below. *(See The 'MUST' Explanatory Booklet for details of other alternative measurements (knee height and demispan) that can also be used to estimate height).*

Estimating height from ulna length

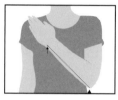

Measure between the point of the elbow (olecranon process) and the midpoint of the prominent bone of the wrist (styloid process) (left side if possible).

HEIGHT (m)														
Men(< 65 years)	1.94	1.93	1.91	1.89	1.87	1.85	1.84	1.82	1.80	1.78	1.76	1.75	1.73	1.71
Men(> 65 years)	1.87	1.86	1.84	1.82	1.81	1.79	1.78	1.76	1.75	1.73	1.71	1.70	1.68	1.67
Ulna length (cm)	32.0	31.5	31.0	30.5	30.0	29.5	29.0	28.5	28.0	27.5	27.0	26.5	26.0	25.5
Women(< 65 years)	1.84	1.83	1.81	1.80	1.79	1.77	1.76	1.75	1.73	1.72	1.70	1.69	1.68	1.66
Women(> 65 years)	1.84	1.83	1.81	1.79	1.78	1.76	1.75	1.73	1.71	1.70	1.68	1.66	1.65	1.63

HEIGHT (m)														
Men(< 65 years)	1.69	1.67	1.66	1.64	1.62	1.60	1.58	1.57	1.55	1.53	1.51	1.49	1.48	1.46
Men(> 65 years)	1.65	1.63	1.62	1.60	1.59	1.57	1.56	1.54	1.52	1.51	1.49	1.48	1.46	1.45
Ulna length (cm)	25.0	24.5	24.0	23.5	23.0	22.5	22.0	21.5	21.0	20.5	20.0	19.5	19.0	18.5
Women(< 65 years)	1.65	1.63	1.62	1.61	1.59	1.58	1.56	1.55	1.54	1.52	1.51	1.50	1.48	1.47
Women(> 65 years)	1.61	1.60	1.58	1.56	1.55	1.53	1.52	1.50	1.48	1.47	1.45	1.44	1.42	1.40

Estimating BMI category from mid upper arm circumference (MUAC)

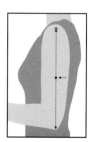

The subject's left arm should be bent at the elbow at a 90 degree angle, with the upper arm held parallel to the side of the body. Measure the distance between the bony protrusion on the shoulder (acromion) and the point of the elbow (olecranon process). Mark the mid-point.

Ask the subject to let arm hang loose and measure around the upper arm at the mid-point, making sure that the tape measure is snug but not tight.

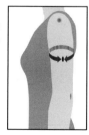

If MUAC is < 23.5 cm, BMI is likely to be < 20 kg/m^2
If MUAC is > 32.0 cm, BMI is likely to be > 30 kg/m^2

Appendix 3
Table of UK and USA dietary reference values for vitamins, minerals and trace elements

Dietary reference values for vitamins, minerals and trace elements, for adults over 18, except where otherwise stated (UK Department of Health 1991[1]; Institute of Medicine of the National Academies 2001[2])

Nutrient	RNI	RDA/AI*	SI	UL
Arsenic	ND	ND	ND	ND
Biotin (µg/d)	ND	30*	10–200	ND
Boron (mg/d)	ND	ND	ND	20
Calcium (mg/d)	700	M&F (19–50 y): 1000	ND	2500
		M&F (50+ yr): 1200		
Chloride (mg/d)	2500		ND	
Choline (mg/d)	ND	M: 550*	ND	3500
		F: 425*		
Chromium (µg/d)	ND	M (19–50 yr): 35*	Above 25	ND
		M (50+ yr): 30*		
		F (19–50 yr): 25*		
		F (50+ yr): 20*		
Copper (µg/d)	1.2 mg/d	900	ND	10 000
Fluoride (mg/d)	ND	M: 4*	0.5 mg/kg	10
		F: 3*		
Folate (µg/d)	200	400	ND	1000
Iodine (µg/d)	140	150	ND	1100
Iron (mg/d)	M: 8.7	M: 8	ND	45
	F (19–50): 14.8	F (19–50 yr): 18		
	F (50+ yr): 8.7	F (50+ yr): 8		
Magnesium (mg/d)	M: 300	M: 420	ND	350
	F: 270	F: 320		
Manganese (mg/d)	Above 1.4	M: 2.3	ND	11
		F: 1.8		
Molybdenum (µg/d)	ND	45	50–400	2000
Niacin (mg/d)	M (19–50 yr): 17	M: 16	ND	35
	M (50+ yr): 16	F: 14		
	F (19–50 yr): 13			
	F (50+ yr): 12			
Nickel (mg/d)	ND	ND	ND	1.0
Pantothenic acid (mg/d)	ND	5*	3–7	ND

Cont.

Nutrient	RNI	RDA/AI*	SI	UL
Phosphorus (mg/d)	550	700	ND	19–70: 4000 70+: 3000
Potassium (mg/d)	3500		ND	
Riboflavin (mg/d)	M: 1.3 F: 1.1	M: 1.3 F: 1.1	ND	ND
Selenium (µg/d)	M: 75 F: 60	55	ND	400
Silicon	ND	ND	ND	ND
Sodium (mg/d)	1600		ND	
Thiamin (mg/d)	M (19–50 yr): 1.0 M (50+ yr): 0.9 F: 0.8	M: 1.2 F: 1.1	ND	ND
Vanadium (mg/d)	ND	ND	ND	1.8
Vitamin A (µg/d)	M: 700 F: 600	M: 900 F: 700	ND	3000
Vitamin B_6 (mg/d)	M: 1.4 F: 1.2	M&F (19–50 yr): 1.3 M (50+ yr): 1.7 F (50+ yr): 1.5	ND	100
Vitamin B_{12} (µg/d)	1.5	2.4	ND	ND
Vitamin C (mg/d)	40	M: 90 F: 75	ND	2000
Vitamin D (µg/d)	M&F (< 65 yr): – M&F (65+ yr): 10	M&F (19–50 yr): 5* M&F (50–70 yr): 10* M&F (70+ yr): 15*	ND	50
Vitamin E (mg/d)	ND	15	M: > 4 F: > 3	1000
Vitamin K (µg/d)	ND	M: 120* F: 90*	1 µg/kg/d	ND
Zinc (mg/d)	M: 9.5 F: 7.0	M: 11 F: 8	ND	40

RNI: reference nutrient intake (UK)
SI: Safe intake (UK)
RDA: Recommended dietary allowance (USA)
AI: Adequate intake (USA)
UL: Tolerable upper intake level (USA)
ND: not defined

1. Department of Health (1991): *Report 41. Dietary reference values for food energy and nutrients for the United Kingdom.* The Stationery Office.
2. Institute of Medicine of the National Academies 2001, *Dietary Reference Intakes* (DRI) reports, accessed through www.nap.edu.

Appendix 4
Elimination diet for rheumatoid arthritis

This is the diet used by Dr Gail Darlington and colleagues in their study published in *The Lancet* {Darlington LG, Ramsey NW, Mansfield JR (1986): Placebo-controlled, blind study of dietary manipulation therapy in rheumatoid arthritis. *The Lancet* 1(8475), 236–38; see section 7.2}. However, Dr Darlington (pers. comm., 2005) comments:

> *'Many patients find it very difficult to comply with the diet at this level of strictness in the elimination phase. For the past five years or so, I have permitted really rare fruits and vegetables such as sweet potatoes, papaya, mango, papaw and kiwi fruit in the elimination phase which aids compliance and at the same time makes it easier for patients to hold their weight. I am not aware of any loss of efficacy as a result of this minor level of leniency although I cannot back up that statement with scientific data.'*

The diet was later retyped into the format below and used by Dr Dorothy Pattison when she was Senior Dietician with St Albans and Hemel Hempstead NHS Trust, 1992–1995, mainly, but not exclusively with RA patients. Undertaking the diet regimen was the patient's decision and agreed by the rheumatologist. Dr Pattison (pers. comm., 2005) reported:

> *'A small number of patients (approximately 6%) identified foods that aggravated symptoms but other positive outcomes were weight loss (when overweight – though surprisingly few patients experienced "unwanted" weight loss), improved eating habits and improved "feeling of wellbeing". Though these are not particularly robust measures, they were important to the patients. There were plenty of people who could not follow the regime, but at least they had given it a try.'*

Dr Darlington (pers. comm., 2005) comments:

> *'The diet sheet you quote for the dietary elimination and reintroduction of foods is at a level of strictness which I used originally, to be a complete purist in our original research studies.'*

The diet

Stage 1

For seven days starting on (date)..........................your diet will be totally restricted to:

Trout, salmon, cod	either grilled, roasted, hot or cold
Pears (fresh)	which can be eaten raw or baked or boiled but with no additions
Carrots (fresh or frozen)	raw or boiled in mineral water
Mineral water	still or sparkling spring water (no additions)
Use only sea salt	

NB Pear juice can be made by removing the skin from pears and liquidising them with spring water.

Optional

On the first day of the diet, in the morning, three teaspoons of Epsom salts in half a pint of warm water may be taken to eliminate previous foods from the bowel. If constipation occurs later in the seven days, a further dose may be given.

It is vital to the whole investigation that there is absolutely no break in this diet. A small sip of coffee, for example, in those seven days could completely change the pattern of response that is crucial for detecting an adverse reaction to a specific food. As well as restricting your diet, it is very important **NOT TO SMOKE**.

It is very possible that initially you will feel worse than usual, especially in the first three days. Keep a comprehensive record of all symptoms you notice on each day of this restricted diet, for example, headaches, tiredness, dizziness, aching muscles, catarrh, joint swelling and other such symptoms.

Medications almost always include food substances. Wheat, corn, potato and yeast are used as base materials or fillers in a wide range of tablets. Try and avoid using medications for symptom relief or keep the use of these to a minimum.

DO NOT ALTER YOUR MEDICATION FOR ARTHRITIS WITHOUT FIRST DISCUSSING THIS WITH YOUR CONSULTANT RHEUMATOLOGIST.

Stage II

The first four foods to be assessed in Stage II are broccoli, runner beans (fresh or frozen), pineapple (fresh) and turkey (fresh). It is worthwhile buying these foods in advance, so that they are ready for use after your seventh day consultation with your dietitian. These foods will be introduced one at a time in the second stage, followed by many others as the week goes on.

The main aim in stage II is to obtain a list of about 20 foods that do not cause you to have an adverse reaction. By the end of Stage II you should have a reasonable range of 'safe' foods to eat while you are testing further foodstuffs. These initial foods have a relatively small risk of producing a reaction – but no food is completely safe.

A suggested order of introduction is given below. It is advisable to keep rigidly to this as the order has been arranged for two specific reasons. Firstly to ensure that the 'safest' foods are introduced first and secondly to ensure that new foods are tested in such a way that members of similar food families are separated by four days. This avoids the possibility of false-negative responses from cross-reaction within the food family.

Stick to the foods that have been suggested for each day **but** these foods can be tested in **any order** on that particular day. Once a food has been tested and found to be 'safe' it can be included in any subsequent meal. It is a cumulative process with each meal usually consisting of the new food to be tested plus any foods already found to be safe.

When testing a food, the most important feature to watch for is the recurrence of symptoms. Symptoms would normally occur within five hours of eating a sensitive food. Therefore, if one food is introduced at breakfast time, e.g. 8am and no adverse response occurs by 1pm, then it is usually safe to introduce another food at approximately 1pm. Similarly, if no response occurs to the lunchtime food by 6pm, it is usually safe to try a further new food then.

Never introduce two new foods at the same time as it will be impossible to tell which food is causing an adverse reaction if one does occur.

Symptoms can vary from person to person, e.g. one person may develop a headache while someone else may have increased joint pain or swelling and others just might feel lethargic or depressed. Reactions may also vary in intensity. There is usually little doubt about strong reactions but mild reactions can be difficult to be certain of. If you are uncertain, a reaction can be confirmed or rejected by re-testing a food at a later stage.

There are two major rules on food testing:

(1) **If in doubt about a food reaction leave the food out of the diet.**
(2) **Never re-test a food in less than five days from the original test.**

Important notes: if an adverse reaction does occur and symptoms return, then **no** further testing should be done until symptoms clear. To assess whether a food reaction has occurred or not you must be quite sure about what symptoms occurred when the new food was tried.

If an adverse reaction does occur then you must restrict yourself to only the foods that have been tested and found to be 'safe' until symptoms clear. This may take between 1 and 3 days.

Remember to keep a strict food and symptom diary to record what you eat and if any reactions occur.

Stage II: list of foods

Day	Date	Food	Comments
7		Broccoli	Fresh or frozen
8		Runner beans	Fresh or frozen
		Pineapple	Fresh
		Turkey	Fresh or frozen, whole or pieces

Day	Date	Food	Comments
9		Tomatoes	Fresh
		Melon	Fresh
		Beef	Fresh or frozen
10		Tap water	
		Rice	Brown, boiled
		Lettuce	
11		Banana	
		Soya beans	This is an important test as soya is present in many processed foods. Soya beans are available in supermarkets and health food shops. Soak the beans first and cook according to instructions on packet
		Grapes	Red or green
12		Cows' milk	Any variety – 2 large glasses
		Cabbage	
		Chicken	Fresh or frozen – whole or pieces
13		Indian tea	With milk if it is 'safe'
		Apple	Fresh
		Yeast	Take two teaspoons of baker's yeast or brewer's yeast powder (raw or dried). This can be quite an unpleasant taste so have some 'safe' food with it. Again this is an important test because of the wide range of products that contain yeast Can be bought from health food shops and supermarkets
14		Butter	Do not do this test if the milk test was positive
		Leeks	Fresh, boiled, baked or cooked in butter if 'safe'
		Pork	Roast pork or pork chops – grilled, roast
15		Lamb	Fresh or frozen
		Plaice	Fresh or frozen (no breadcrumbs)

Stage III

The next stage involves testing the major, staple foods, therefore it is very important that you test them carefully. A maximum of two foods per day is suggested. WHEAT and CORN are absorbed more slowly. They frequently have a delayed or muted response. Therefore, these foods are tested for two full days each.

Stage III: list of foods

Day	Date	Food (morning)	Food (evening)
1		Eggs – not fried in oil	Potatoes – not fried in oil
2 and 3		Wheat as wholemeal bread IF yeast test is negative Use homemade bread or from a bakery in order to reduce the level of additives. Alternatively, use pure wheat flakes or wholewheat macaroni (plain and boiled) You must test wheat at every meal for the next two days	
4		Percolated coffee (coffee beans)	Mushrooms
5		Cane sugar (demerara)	
6		Oranges	Black pepper
7		Beet sugar (white)	Bacon IF pork test negative
8 and 9		Corn test. Using corn on the cob or glucose powder. Use at least two dessertspoons of glucose powder or fresh corn on the cob at every meal for two days	
10		Onion	Natural peanuts (in the shell)
11		Cheddar cheese (if other dairy products test negative)	Spinach

Stage IV

Stage IV: list of foods

Day	Date	Food	Comments
1		White bread	IF yeast and wheat tests negative
		Garlic	
2		Peas	Fresh or frozen (NOT petit pois)
		Grapefruit	Fresh
		Dates	Natural (try health food shop)
3		Cucumber	Fresh
		Celery	Fresh
		Cauliflower	Fresh or frozen
4 and 5		Rye bread – this is a two-day test. IF the yeast test was positive, use yeast-free rye based alternative, e.g. Ryvita. If using bread, try homemade or from a bakery as before	
6		Tuna fish	Fresh tuna steak – in most supermarkets or fishmongers
		*Rhubarb	
		*Honey	Natural, clear
7		*Instant coffee – this is a chemical test. Look for a coffee without corn added. Do not test if you reacted to ordinary coffee.	
		Asparagus	
		Lemon	
8		*Olive oil	

Day	Date	Food	Comments
		Lentils	
		*Tinned carrots – do not test if you reacted to fresh carrots. This is a test for the phenolic resin lining of the tin. Check that the tin says 'no sugar added'	
9 and 10		Oats e.g. porridge oats. Take at every meal for two days	
11		*Monosodium glutamate – this is a flavour enhancer used in many processed foods. Can be obtained from some supermarkets and Chinese supermarkets. To test, sprinkle on top of some meat.	
		*Prawns or shrimps	
		*Brussels sprouts	
12		*Saccharin tablets	
		*Herrings	
		*Almonds	
13		Malt extract – at every meal for 1 day (in supermarket or health food shop)	
14		Avocado pear	
		Green or red peppers	
		Raisins	
15		Chocolate – contains wheat, corn and sugar. Do not test if any of these caused a reaction	
		Spice mixture	

Food items marked with an asterisk* are unrelated to other items and can be interchanged as long as the spacing between other foods is undisturbed. Food dyes, emulsifiers and other additives have not been specifically assessed but when standard foods have been evaluated reactions to such chemicals are usually obvious.

Seasonal fruits such as cherries, plums, apricots, peaches, strawberries, raspberries, gooseberries and blackcurrants have not been included but should be tested during their season.

You have at this point assessed more than 60 different food items, which account for at least 95% of what most people eat.

Glossary

Definitions taken from a number of sources.

Analytic study: A study that is designed to test hypotheses and examine associations, yet does not involve any experimental intervention by the investigator e.g. case control and cohort studies.

A priori: Proceeding from a known or assumed cause to a necessarily related effect; deductive

Acute phase reactants: Used to help diagnose rheumatoid arthritis, which is characterised by high levels of C reactive protein (CRP).

Acute: Afflicted by a disease exhibiting a rapid onset followed by a short, severe course.

Adhesion molecules: Cell Adhesion Molecules (CAMs) are proteins located on the cell surface involved with the binding with other cells or with the extracellular matrix (ECM) in the process called cell adhesion.

Adipocyte: Any of various cells found in adipose tissue that are specialised for the storage of fat.

Aerobic: Living or occurring only in the presence of oxygen.

Aggrecan: Aggrecan is the shortened name of the large aggregating chondroitin sulphate proteoglycan.

α-linolenic acid: An n-3 polyunsaturated fatty acid, $C_{17}H_{29}COOH$, considered essential to the human diet.

Amyloidosis: A disorder marked by the deposition of amyloid in various organs and tissues of the body. It may be associated with a chronic disease such as rheumatoid arthritis, tuberculosis, or multiple myeloma.

Angiogenesis: The formation of new blood vessels.

Angiotensin II: Any of three polypeptide hormones, one of which is a powerful vasoconstrictor, that function in the body in controlling arterial pressure.

Antigenicity: The degree to which a substance induces an immune response.

Antigen: A substance that when introduced into the body stimulates the production of an antibody. Antigens include toxins, bacteria, foreign blood cells, and the cells of transplanted organs.

Antioxidant: A substance, such as vitamin E, vitamin C, or β-carotene, thought to protect body cells from the damaging effects of oxidation.

Apoptosis: Apoptosis consists of a cascade of events leading to the ordered dismantling of critical cell survival components and pathways: sometimes referred to as programmed cell death.

Arachidonic acid: An n-6 polyunsaturated fatty acid, $C_{20}H_{32}O_2$, found in animal fats, that is essential in human nutrition and is a precursor to the biosynthesis of prostaglandins.

Arthritis: Inflammation of a joint, usually accompanied by pain, swelling, and stiffness, and resulting from infection, trauma, degenerative changes, metabolic disturbances, or other causes. It occurs in various forms, such as bacterial arthritis, osteoarthritis, or rheumatoid arthritis.

Arthrodesis: The surgical fixation of a joint, ultimately resulting in bone fusion. Basically, the procedure is artificially induced ankylosis performed to relieve pain or provide support in a diseased or injured joint.

Arthroplasty: The creation of an artificial joint.

Athroscopic debridement: Surgical excision of dead, devitalised, or contaminated tissue and removal of foreign matter from a wound using a type of endoscope that is inserted into the joint through a small incision.

Autoimmune disorder: An immune response by the body against one of its own tissues, cells, or molecules.

β-lactoglobulin: The globulin present in milk, comprising from 50–60% of bovine whey protein.

Bias: Occurs when a sample estimate deviates from the truth due to systematic (i.e. non-random) errors in the collection, analysis, or publication of data. Bias may heighten or attenuate the association that would otherwise have been observed. Unlike confounding, bias occurs as an artefact of study design.

Body mass index (BMI): a mathematical formula [(body weight in kg) ÷ (height in m)^2] to assess relative body weight that correlates highly with body fat.

Bone sclerosis: Thickening or hardening of bone.

Cachexia: Weight loss, wasting of muscle, loss of appetite, and general debility that can occur during a chronic disease.

Capital epiphysis: The end of a long bone that is originally separated from the main bone by a layer of cartilage but later becomes united to the main bone through ossification.

Cartilage: A tough, elastic, fibrous connective tissue found in various parts of the body, such as the joints, outer ear, and larynx.

Cartilage matrix: The intercellular substance of cartilage consisting of fibres and ground substance: composed mainly of proteoglycans, a special type of glycosaminoglycans, the most common of which are chondroitin sulphate and keratan sulphate.

Catabolism: The metabolic breakdown of complex molecules into simpler ones.

Catalase: An iron-containing enzyme found in the blood and in most living cells that catalyses the decomposition of hydrogen peroxide into water and oxygen.

CD4: A glycoprotein predominantly found on the surface of helper T-cells.

Cellular immunity: Immunity resulting from a cell-mediated immune response.

Chemotaxis: The characteristic movement or orientation of an organism or cell along a chemical concentration gradient either toward or away from the chemical stimulus.

Chondrocyte: A connective tissue cell that occupies a lacuna within the cartilage matrix. Also called a *cartilage cell*.

Chondroitin sulphate: One of several classes of sulphated glycosaminoglycans that is a major constituent of various connective tissues, especially in the ground substance of blood vessels, bone, and cartilage.

Chromosome: A threadlike linear strand of DNA and associated proteins in the nucleus of eukaryotic cells that carries the genes and functions in the transmission of hereditary information.

Chronic: A condition that persists for a long time.

Coagulation cascade: The coagulation cascade is a step-by-step process that occurs when a blood vessel is injured. The end result of the coagulation cascade is a blood clot that creates a barrier over the injury site, protecting it until it heals.

Cohort: A group or band of people.

Collagen: The fibrous protein constituent of bone, cartilage, tendon, and other connective tissue.

Collagenase: Any of various enzymes that catalyse the hydrolysis of collagen.

Confounding: Occurs when a variable is associated with *both* the exposure and outcome of interest, yet is not on the causal pathway between the two – and can therefore provide an alternative explanation for the observed relationship between exposure and disease. Unlike bias, confounding is a function of the complex interactions that exist between exposures and outcomes and would exist whether the phenomenon was being studied or not.

Correlation: A measure of the degree of linear association between two variables. Both parametric and non-parametric methods of describing correlation exist. The most common technique is *Pearson's correlation* (a parametric method). The extent of the association is described by the correlation coefficient, r.

Corticosteroids: Any of the steroid hormones produced by the adrenal cortex or their synthetic equivalents, such as cortisol and aldosterone.

Cox-inhibitors: Pharmacological inhibition of cyclo-oxygenase (Cox) can provide relief from the symptoms of inflammation and pain; this is the method of action of well-known drugs such as aspirin and ibuprofen.

Crepitus: Where the cartilage around joints has eroded away and joints grind against one another, producing noise.

CRP: C reactive protein, level related to severity of inflammatory disease and effectiveness of anti-inflammatory treatment.

Cyclo-oxygenase: An enzyme that is responsible for formation of important biological mediators called prostanoids (including prostaglandins, prostacyclin and thromboxane).

Cytokines: A generic term for soluble molecules that mediate interactions between cells.

Cytotoxic: Producing a toxic effect on cells.

Denature: To induce structural alterations that disrupt the biological activity of a molecule. Often refers to breaking hydrogen bonds between base pairs in a double-stranded nucleic acid molecule to produce single-stranded polynucleotides, or altering the secondary and tertiary structure of a protein, destroying its activity.

Dendritic cell: An antigen-presenting immune cell that functions to initiate the immune response by activating lymphocytes and stimulating the secretion of cytokines.

Diarthrodial joint: Any of several types of bone articulation permitting free motion in a joint, as that of the shoulder or hip.

Dioxin: Any of several carcinogenic or teratogenic heterocyclic hydrocarbons that occur as impurities in petroleum-derived herbicides.

Double-blind: Method of allocation concealment designed to reduce bias such that both the investigators and the participants are unaware of the treatment allocated. This involves the use of placebo treatments and properly blinded randomisation procedures.

Effusion: The seeping of serous, purulent, or bloody fluid into a body cavity or tissue.

Eicosanoid: A lipid mediator of inflammation derived from the 20-carbon atom arachidonic acid (20 in Greek is *eicosa*) or a similar fatty acid. The eicosanoids include the prostaglandins, prostacyclin, thromboxane, and leukotrienes.

Endocytosis: A process of cellular ingestion by which the plasma membrane folds inward to bring substances into the cell.

Endothelium: A thin layer of flat epithelial cells that lines serous cavities, lymph vessels, and blood vessels.

Epitope: A unique shape or marker carried on the surface of an antigen that triggers a corresponding antibody response.

Erythropoiesis: The formation or production of red blood cells.

Erythropoietin: A glycoprotein hormone that stimulates the production of red blood cells by stem cells in bone marrow. Produced mainly by the kidneys, it is released in response to decreased levels of oxygen in body tissue.

Extra-articular: Outside the joint – in RA the disease is also systemic in that it often also affects many extra-articular tissues throughout the body including the skin, blood vessels, heart, lungs, and muscles.

Extracellular matrix: Any material part of a tissue that is not part of a cell.

Fatty acid flux: The rate that fat travels through the blood.

Ferritin: An iron-containing protein, found principally in the intestinal mucosa, spleen and liver that functions as the primary form of iron storage in the body.

Fibril: Any threadlike fibre or filament, such as a myofibril or neurofibril, that is a constituent of a cell or larger structure.

Fibrin: An elastic, insoluble, whitish protein produced by the action of thrombin on fibrinogen and forming an interlacing fibrous network in the coagulation of blood.

Fibrinogen: A protein in the blood plasma that is essential for the coagulation of blood and is converted to fibrin by the action of thrombin in the presence of ionised calcium.

Flavonoid: Any of a large group of polyphenolic plant substances.

Free radical: An atom or group of atoms that has at least one unpaired electron and is generally unstable, highly reactive and can cause damage.

Genotype: The entire genetic identity of an individual, including alleles, or gene forms, that do not show as outward characteristics.

Gliadin: Any of several simple proteins derived from rye or wheat gluten. It is capable of inducing a toxic response among individuals who lack the enzyme necessary for its digestion.

Glucocorticoids: Any of a group of steroid hormones, such as cortisone, that are produced by the adrenal cortex, are involved in carbohydrate, protein, and fat metabolism, and have anti-inflammatory properties.

Glycosaminoglycan: Any of a group of polysaccharides with high molecular weight that contain amino sugars and often form complexes with proteins.

Glycosylation: The addition of glycosyl groups to a protein to form a glycoprotein.

Herberden's nodes: A common complication of OA, especially in women. The nodes tend to run in families and usually appear first in one finger, then may develop in others. Herberden's nodes often cause redness, swelling, tenderness and aching.

HLA-DR: Gene locus in the human HLA complex region encoding an MHC class II molecule strongly associated with rheumatoid arthritis.

Homocysteine: An amino acid used normally by the body in cellular metabolism and the manufacture of proteins. High levels of homocysteine are a risk factor for coronary artery disease.

Homozygosity: The condition of having identical genes at one or more loci in homologous chromosome segments.

Human leucocyte antigen: A gene product of the major histocompatibility complex.

Humoral immunity: The component of the immune system involving antibodies that are secreted by B cells and circulate as soluble proteins in blood plasma and lymph.

Hyperplasia: An abnormal increase in the number of cells in an organ or a tissue with consequent enlargement.

Hypertrophy: A non-tumorous enlargement of an organ or a tissue as a result of an increase in the size rather than the number of constituent cells.

Hypochromic: An anaemic condition in which the percentage of haemoglobin in red blood cells is abnormally low.

Immunoglobulin: Any of a group of large glycoproteins that are secreted by plasma cells and that function as antibodies in the immune response by binding with specific antigens. There are five classes of immunoglobulins: IgA, IgD, IgE, IgG, and IgM.

Incidence: The proportion of individuals who develop new instances of a disease or event in a given population over a specified time interval.

Incidence rate: A measure of incidence that expresses the number of individuals who develop a new disease or condition over a specified time interval as a proportion of the total population at risk *throughout* that interval. Incidence rate is calculated using person-time as the denominator.

Inflammation: A localised protective reaction of tissue to irritation, injury, or infection, characterised by pain, redness, swelling, and sometimes loss of function.

Joint capsule: A sac enclosing a joint, formed by an outer fibrous membrane and an inner synovial membrane.

Lectin: Any of several plant proteins that bind to specific carbohydrate groups on proteins or on cell membranes and are used in the laboratory to isolate glycoproteins, to stimulate proliferation of lymphocytes, and to agglutinate red blood cells.

Leptin: A neurotransmitter produced by fat cells and involved in the regulation of appetite.

Lequesne Index: An index of arthritis severity that includes the measurement of pain (5 questions), walking distance (1 question), and activities of daily living (4 questions), with versions available for the hip and knee.

Leucocyte: White blood cell. Any of various blood cells that have a nucleus and cytoplasm, separate into a thin white layer when whole blood is centrifuged, and help protect the body from infection and disease. White blood cells include neutrophils, eosinophils, basophils, lymphocytes, and monocytes.

Leukotriene: Any of several lipid compounds that contain 20 carbon atoms, are related to prostaglandins, and mediate the inflammatory response.

Ligament: A sheet or band of tough, fibrous tissue connecting bones or cartilages at a joint or supporting an organ.

Lipoxygenase: An enzyme that plays a pivotal role in the synthesis of inflammatory mediators known as leukotrienes.

Lysosome: A membrane-bound organelle in the cytoplasm of most cells containing various hydrolytic enzymes that function in intracellular digestion.

Macromolecule: A very large molecule, such as a polymer or protein, consisting of many smaller structural units linked together.

Macrophage: Any of the large phagocytic cells of the reticuloendothelial system.

Major histocompatability complex: A group of genes that codes for cell surface histocompatibility antigens and are the principal determinants of tissue type and transplant compatibility.

Meniscectomy: Excision of a meniscus, usually from the knee joint.

Metalloproteinases: A family of enzymes from the group of proteinases. They play an important role in tumour metastasis, embryonic development, wound healing – generally in processes including matrix degradation.

Microcyte: An abnormally small red blood cell that is less than five microns in diameter and may occur in certain forms of anaemia.

Mitogen: An agent that induces mitosis.

Molybdenum: An essential trace element.

Monozygotic: Derived from a single fertilised ovum or embryonic cell mass.

Neutrophil: A neutrophil cell, especially an abundant type of granular white blood cell that is highly destructive of micro-organisms.

Nucleotide: Any of various compounds consisting of a nucleoside combined with a phosphate group and forming the basic constituent of DNA and RNA.

Odds: A method of representing probability. The odds is the ratio of the probability of an event occurring to that of it not occurring. For example, if in a group of 10 individuals 6 die and 4 do not, the odds of death is 6/4, or 1.5. Odds have several statistical properties that are useful in the analysis of case control studies; however, they are not a particularly intuitive measure.

Osteoblast: A cell from which bone develops.

Osteoclast: A large multinucleate cell found in growing bone that resorbs bony tissue, as in the formation of canals and cavities.

Osteopenia: A condition of bone in which decreased calcification, decreased density, or reduced mass occurs.

Osteophyte: A small, abnormal bony outgrowth, typically associated with OA.

Osteoporosis: A disease in which the bones become extremely porous, are subject to fracture, and heal slowly, occurring especially in women following menopause and often leading to curvature of the spine from vertebral collapse.

Oxidative stress: A condition of increased oxidant production in animal cells characterised by the release of free radicals/reactive oxygen and nitrogen species and resulting in cellular degeneration.

Pannus: A membrane of granulation tissue covering the normal surface of the articular cartilages in rheumatoid arthritis.

Pathogenesis: The development of a diseased or morbid condition.

Peptidoglycan: A polymer found in the cell walls of prokaryotes that consists of polysaccharide and peptide chains in a strong molecular network.

Peripheral neuropathy: A problem with the functioning of the nerves outside the spinal cord.

Peroxidation: The oxidative degradation of lipids. This process proceeds by a free radical chain reaction mechanism.

Phagocytosis: The engulfing and ingestion of bacteria or other foreign bodies by phagocytes.

Placebo: An inert medication or treatment designed to be identical to the active intervention in all but its effect. Use of placebos helps to reduce bias in randomised controlled trials.

Plasminogen: The inactive precursor to plasmin that is found in body fluids and blood plasma.

Polymorphism: The occurrence together in the same population of more than one allele or genetic marker at the same locus with the least frequent allele or marker occurring more frequently than can be accounted for by mutation alone i.e. conventionally in 1% or more individuals in the population.

Polyphenols: A group of vegetable chemical substances, characterised by the presence of more than one phenolic group. Their phenolic reactions produce gelatines, alkaloids and other proteins. The polyphenols are responsible for the colouring of some plants. Polyphenols have been shown to be strong antioxidants with potential health benefits.

Polysaccharide: Any of a class of carbohydrates, such as starch and cellulose, consisting of a number of monosaccharides joined by glycosidic bonds.

Prevalence: The proportion of individuals in a population at risk who have the outcome of interest at a specified time.

Prostaglandin: Any of a group of potent hormone-like substances that are produced in various mammalian tissues, are derived from arachidonic acid, and mediate a wide range of physiological functions, such as control of blood pressure, contraction of smooth muscle, and modulation of inflammation.

Protease: Any of various enzymes, including the endopeptidases and exopeptidases, that catalyse the hydrolytic breakdown of proteins into peptides or amino acids.

Proteoglycan: Any of various mucopolysaccharides that are bound to protein chains in covalent complexes and occur in the extracellular matrix of connective tissue.

Randomisation: A probabilistic method of assigning individuals to categories, such that each individual has a known chance of receiving any of the treatments, independent of what categories the other individuals are assigned to. In a large enough sample, randomisation effectively removes allocation bias, and balances all known and unknown covariates evenly across the allocated categories.

Rate: A measure of the frequency with which an event occurs in a population at risk over a specified time period.

Refractory disease: Resistant to treatment.

Synovium: The connective tissue membrane that lines the cavity of a synovial joint and produces the synovial fluid.

T-cells: Any of the lymphocytes that mature in the thymus and have the ability to recognise specific peptide antigens through the receptors on their cell surface.

Teratogenic: Causing malformations of an embryo or fetus.

Thromboxane: Any of several compounds originally derived from prostaglandin precursors in platelets that stimulate aggregation of platelets and constriction of blood vessels.

Tidemark: Line between the articular and calcified cartilage zones.

Transferrin: A β-globulin in blood serum that combines with and transports iron.

Triacylglycerol: A naturally occurring ester of three fatty acids and glycerol that is the chief constituent of fats and oils.

Tumour necrosis factor: A protein produced by macrophages in the presence of an endotoxin and shown experimentally to be capable of attacking and destroying cancerous tumours.

Vascularisation: The process of vascularising; the formation of vessels, especially blood vessels.

Vasodilation: Dilation of a blood vessel, as by the action of a nerve or drug.

Index

Items highlighted in bold indicate main entries.